The Public Shaping of Medical Research

Patient organizations and social health movements offer one of the most important and illuminating examples of civil society engagement and participation in scientific research and research politics. Influencing the research agenda and initiating, funding and accelerating the development of diagnostic tools, effective therapies and appropriate healthcare for their area of interest, they may champion alternative, sometimes controversial, programs or critique-dominant medical paradigms. Some movements and organizations advocate for medical recognition of contested illnesses, as with fibromyalgia or ADHD, while some attempt to "de-medicalize" others, such as obesity or autism.

Bringing together an international selection of leading scholars and representatives from patients' organizations, this comprehensive collection explores the interaction between civil society groups and biomedical science, technology development and research politics. It takes stock of the key findings of the research conducted in the field over the past two decades and addresses emerging problems and future challenges concerning the interrelations between health movements and patient organizations on the one hand, and biomedical research and research policies on the other. Combining empirical case studies with conceptual discussion, the book discusses how public participation can contribute to, as well as restrict, the democratization of scientific knowledge production.

This volume is an important reference for academics and researchers with an interest in the sociology of health and illness, the sociology of knowledge, science and technology studies, medical ethics or healthcare management and research, as well as medical researchers and those involved with health-related civil society organizations.

Peter Wehling is currently Senior Researcher at the Institute of Sociology at Goethe-University, Frankfurt/Main, Germany. Until the end of 2013 he directed the research project "Participatory Governance of Science" at the University of Augsburg, Germany. His research interests include science and technology studies, sociology of knowledge and ignorance, sociology of health and illness, and sociological theory and critical sociology.

Willy Viehöver is a Senior Researcher at the University of Augsburg, Germany, and is currently Visiting Professor at the Department of Sociology. His main research interests include discourse and narrative analysis, qualitative social research, sociology of health and illness, policy analysis, science and technology studies, sociology of knowledge and sociological theory.

Sophia Koenen is currently working at the Department of Medical Sociology at the University of Regensburg, Germany, as a researcher and teacher of undergraduate studies. She is involved in an interdisciplinary project on the public communication of genetic risk factors of widespread diseases, specifically Age Related Macular Degeneration (AMD). Until the end of 2013, Sophia Koenen was part of the research project "Participatory Governance of Science" at the Institute of Sociology at Augsburg University Germany. She successfully earned her Master of Arts at the University of Augsburg, Germany, in March 2014. Her scientific interest focuses on qualitative research in the sociology of health and illness.

Routledge Studies in the Sociology of Health and Illness

Available titles include:

Dimensions of Pain
Humanities and social science perspectives
Edited by Lisa Folkmarson Käll

Caring and Well-being
A lifeworld approach
Kathleen Galvin and Les Todres

Aging Men, Masculinities and Modern Medicine
Edited by Antje Kampf, Barbara L. Marshall and Alan Petersen

Disclosure in Health and Illness
Edited by Mark Davis and Lenore Manderson

The Public Shaping of Medical Research
Patient associations, health movements and biomedicine
Edited by Peter Wehling, Willy Viehöver and Sophia Koenen

Forthcoming titles:

Abuse, Mental Illness and Recovery in Everyday Lives
Beyond trauma
Nicole Moulding

Systems Theory and the Sociology of Health and Illness
Observing healthcare
Edited by Morten Knudsen and Werner Vogd

The Public Shaping of Medical Research

Patient associations, health movements and biomedicine

Edited by Peter Wehling, Willy Viehöver and Sophia Koenen

Routledge
Taylor & Francis Group
LONDON AND NEW YORK

First published 2015 by Routledge

2 Park Square, Milton Park, Abingdon, Oxfordshire OX14 4RN
52 Vanderbilt Avenue, New York, NY 10017

Routledge is an imprint of the Taylor & Francis Group, an informa business

First issued in paperback 2019

British Library Cataloguing in Publication Data
A catalogue record for this book is available from the British Library

Library of Congress Cataloging-in-Publication Data
The public shaping of medical research : patient associations, health movements and biomedicine / edited by Peter Wehling, Willy Viehöver, and Sophia Koenen.
p. ; cm. – (Routledge studies in the sociology of health and illness)
Includes bibliographical references.
I. Wehling, Peter, 1954– editor. II. Viehöver, Willy, editor. III. Koenen, Sophia, editor. IV. Series: Routledge studies in the sociology of health and illness.
[DNLM: 1. Biomedical Research. 2. Public Opinion. 3. Patient Advocacy. 4. Patient Participation. W 20.5]
R852
610.72'4–dc23
2014021196

ISBN: 978-0-415-85823-6 (hbk)
ISBN: 978-0-367-34141-1 (pbk)

Typeset in Baskerville
by Cenveo Publisher Services

Contents

Notes on contributors

Madeleine Akrich

Madeleine Akrich is Research Director at the *Centre de sociologie de l'innovation* (Mines ParisTech). She compared obstetrical practices in France and in the Netherlands in the 1990s. Recently, she has studied internet discussion groups on health issues, and conducted research projects on the role of patient organizations in the production and circulation of knowledge. Recently, she has published notable works including "Policing exchanges as self description in internet groups" (in Brousseau et al., *Governance, Regulations and Powers on the Internet*, 2012) and "From Communities of Practice to Epistemic Communities: Health Mobilizations on the Internet" (*Sociological Research Online* 15(2), 2010).

Lori Baralt

Lori Baralt is an Assistant Professor of Women's, Gender & Sexuality Studies at California State University, Long Beach, USA. Her research focuses on the intersection of reproductive and environmental health, primarily with regard to environmental links to breast cancer. Her recent publications appear in the journals *Women's Health Issues* and *Environmental Health Perspectives.*

Sharon Batt

Sharon Batt lives in Halifax, Canada, where she teaches social determinants of health and ethics to medical students at Dalhousie University. Her prize-winning doctoral research examines changes in Canada's breast cancer movement as neoliberal governments withdrew funds and groups turned to the pharmaceutical industry for support. She began writing about cancer patients' issues as a journalist following her own diagnosis of breast cancer in 1988. Her book *Patient No More: The Politics of Breast Cancer* documents the early breast cancer movement in Canada. A book based on her doctoral research is under contract with the University of British Columbia Press.

Massimiano Bucchi

Massimiano Bucchi is Professor of Science and Technology in Society at the University of Trento, Italy, and has been visiting professor in several academic and research institutions in Asia, Europe and North America. He has received several recognitions for his work, including the Mullins Prize awarded by the Society for Social Studies of Science (1997) and the Merck Serono special jury award for science books (2007). He has served as advisor and evaluator for several research and policy bodies, including the US National Science Foundation, the Royal Society, and the European Commission, and has chaired (with B. Trench) the program of the XII world conference of Public Communication of Science and Technology (2012). His publications include *Science in Society* (2004), *Handbook of Public Communication of Science and Technology* (with B. Trench, 2008), *Beyond Technocracy: Citizens, Politics, Technoscience* (2009, published also in Chinese) and essays in journals such as *Nature* and *Science.* His website is www.massimianobucchi.it.

Peter Conrad

Peter Conrad is Harry Coplan Professor of Social Sciences and Professor of Sociology at Brandeis University, Massachusetts, USA. He is the author of over a hundred articles and chapters and has published nine books including *Deviance and Medicalization: From Badness to Sickness* (with Joseph W. Schneider, 1980) and *The Medicalization of Society: On the Transformation of Human Conditions into Treatable Disorders* (2008). In addition to his continuing work on medicalization, Professor Conrad is engaged in research on the expansion of Attention Defi cit Hyperactivity Disorder (ADHD) and the impact of the Internet on the experience of illness.

Monica Ensini

Monica Ensini holds a PhD in Neurobiology obtained from the University of Pisa and Scuola Normale Superiore of Pisa, Italy. During her postdoctoral training at Columbia University, New York, USA, she focused her research studies on the development of the vertebrate motor system. Subsequently, her research interests extended to the development of the vertebrate forebrain while working at University College and King's College in London, UK, and at the École Normale Supérieure in Paris, France. Her engagement in the rare disease field started with the Italian Telethon Foundation as grant review and Personal Award Program manager. Currently she is Scientific Director at EURORDIS.

David J. Hess

David J. Hess is a professor of sociology at Vanderbilt University, Tennessee, where he is also the Director of the Program in Environmental and

Sustainability Studies. He has written extensively on mobilized publics, science and technology, with ongoing support from the Science, Technology, and Society Program of the National Science Foundation. He has published several books and articles on the movement in support of complementary and alternative approaches to cancer therapy, and he has also published on social movements and environmental health issues. His website is www.davidjhess.net.

Sophia Koenen

Sophia Koenen is currently working at the Department of Medical Sociology at the University of Regensburg, Germany, as a researcher and teacher of undergraduate studies. She is involved in an interdisciplinary project on the public communication of genetic risk factors of widespread diseases, specifically Age-related Macular Degeneration (AMD). Until the end of 2013, Sophia Koenen was part of the research project "Participatory Governance of Science" at the Institute of Sociology at Augsburg University, Germany. She gained her Master of Arts at the University of Augsburg in March 2014. Her scientific interest focuses on qualitative research in sociology of health and illness.

Henriette Langstrup

Henriette Langstrup is associate professor at Centre for Medical Science and Technology Studies at University of Copenhagen, Denmark. She is organizing to undertake a PhD and has studied various consequences of the increased involvement of patients and citizens in and through medical technological innovation. Apart from her work on patient associations, she has written extensively on issues related to chronic care and telemedicine and is presently studying how welfare technologies travel globally. A recent publication is "Chronic Care Infrastructures and the Home" (*Sociology of Health and Illness*, 35(7), 2010).

Thomas Lemke

Thomas Lemke is Professor of Sociology with focus on Biotechnologies, Nature and Society at the Faculty of Social Sciences of the Goethe-University Frankfurt/Main in Germany. His research interests include social and political theory, biopolitics, and social studies of genetic and reproductive technologies. Recent publications include: *Governmentality: Current Issues and Future Challenges* (co-edited with Ulrich Bröckling and Susanne Krasmann, 2010); *Biopolitics: An Advanced Introduction* (2011); *Foucault, Governmentality and Critique* (2011); *Perspectives on Genetic Discrimination* (2013); and *Die Natur in der Soziologie: Gesellschaftliche Voraussetzungen und Folgen biotechnologischen Wissens* (2013).

Mercedes C. Lyson

Mercedes C. Lyson earned her PhD in Sociology from Brown University, Rhode Island, USA, in 2013. Her dissertation was a qualitative study on the class politics of the alternative food movement, based on two years of participant observation and 83 in-depth interviews in Rhode Island. Her primary research interests include agri-food studies, governance/governmentality studies, the politics of obesity and bodies, class distinction and urban sociology. Currently, Mercedes C. Lyson is a Research Fellow at a higher education consulting firm outside of Boston.

Maria Mavris

Maria Mavris has a PhD in Molecular Microbiology from the University of Adelaide, Australia. Her two post-doctoral positions were in the field of infectious diseases, at the Institut Pasteur, Paris, and the École Vétérinaire d'Alfort. She joined EURORDIS in 2008 where she is responsible for the implication of patients in regulatory activities at the European Medicines Agency and is also an observer on the Committee for Orphan Medicinal Products. In addition she is responsible for organizing training for these activities for patients via the EURORDIS Summer School in clinical trials and drug development, a capacity-building project for patients' advocates in Europe.

Christel Nourissier

Christel Nourissier was one of the founders of the association Prader-Willi France, then of the French National Alliance for Rare Diseases (2000). Christel's daughter, now 37 years old, was born with a rare disease and experienced diffi culties in accessing diagnosis, medical and social care. Living with her daughter's diagnosis sparked Christel's long career in rare disease advocacy. She advocated for the Commission Communication "Rare Diseases, Europe's challenge" and for the Council Recommendations for Rare Diseases. She was a member of the European Committee of Experts on Rare Diseases, and of the Board of Directors of EURORDIS for 13 years. She is extensively involved in National Plans for Rare Diseases in France as well in a regional Committee for Rights and Autonomy of people with disabilities. She is a EUROPLAN advisor.

Órla O'Donovan

Órla O'Donovan is based in the School of Applied Social Studies in University College Cork, Ireland, where much of her research and teaching has been focused on questions about democracy, expertise and social movements. In recent times, co-editing a supplement to the *Community Development*

Journal, "Common Senses: New Thinking about an Old Idea" has nourished her interest in commoning and has led to work on the idea of the body as a commons. Recent publications include: "Tracking Transformations in Health Movement Organisations: Alzheimer's Disease Organisations and their Changing 'Cause Regimes'" (with T. Moreira and E. Howlett, *Social Movement Studies*, 12(3), 2013); and *Mobilising Classics: Reading Radical Writing in Ireland* (edited with F. Dukelow, 2010).

Vololona Rabeharisoa

Vololona Rabeharisoa is Professor of Sociology at Mines ParisTech and Senior Researcher at Centre de Sociologie de l'Innovation, France. Her main research interests are in science and technology studies, notably sociology of biomedicine, in disability studies and patients' activism. Recent publications include "From 'Politics of Numbers' to 'Politics of Singularisation': Patients' Activism and Engagement in Research on Rare Diseases in France and Portugal" (with M. Callon, A.M. Filipe, J.A. Nunes, F. Paterson and F. Vergnaud, *BioSocieties*, 9(2), 2014); and, "Staging and Weighting Evidence in Biomedicine: Comparing Clinical Practices in Cancer Genetics and Psychiatric Genetics" (with P. Bourret, *Social Studies of Science*, 39(5), 2009).

Andreas L. G. Reimann

Following pharmacy studies and registration as Pharmacist, Andreas Reimann earned his PhD in pharmacology from the University of Frankfurt, Germany, and an executive MBA from the University of Bradford, UK. He has a total of 22 years of experience in science, the pharmaceutical industry and in patient organizations. Currently he serves as the Managing Director of Mukoviszidose Institute gGmbH, a not-for-profit limited company wholly owned by the German patient organization Mukoviszidose e.V. Andreas is also Vice-President of the Germany Alliance for Rare Diseases (ACHSE e.V.). His main interest is in patient-centered health care including the development of new therapeutic options in particular for patients living with rare diseases. Amongst other publications, he co-authored a landmark study investigating the needs of patients with rare diseases in the German Health Care System.

Matthias Roche

Matthias Roche is researcher and teacher of undergraduate studies at the Department of Sociology and member of the Institute for Canadian Studies at the University of Augsburg, Germany. He specializes in memory studies, science and technology studies, discourse research and sociological theory. Past involvement in research projects includes "Participatory Governance of Science", funded by the German Ministry of Science and Research (BMBF) until the end of 2013.

Silke Schicktanz

Silke Schicktanz is Professor of Cultural and Ethical Studies of Biomedicine at the Institute of Medical Ethics and History of Medicine at the University Medical Center Göttingen, Germany. Her research focuses on empirical studies of and ethical reflection on public and patient involvement in bioethics, currently in fields such as aging medicine and genetics. Additionally, she examines the theoretical relationship between empirical, sociological, ethical-normative methods. Recent publications include *Genetics as Social Practice* (with Barbara Prainsack and Gabriele Werner-Felmayer, 2014), and "The Ethics of 'Public Understanding of Ethics'" (in *Medicine, Healthcare and Philosophy*, 15 (2), with Mark Schweda and Brian Wynne, 2012).

Catherine Tan

Catherine Tan is currently a doctoral student in sociology at Brandeis University. She received her MA in sociology from Columbia University and her BA in sociology from the University of California, San Diego. Catherine's interests include medical sociology, social stratification, and science, knowledge and technology. Her previous work examined how therapy providers maintain a sense of efficacy despite medical uncertainty.

Willy Viehöver

Willy Viehöver is a Senior Researcher at the University of Augsburg (Germany) and currently visiting professor at the Department of Sociology. His main research interests include discourse and narrative analysis, qualitative social research, sociology of health and illness, policy analysis, science and technology studies, sociology of knowledge and sociological theory. His recent publications include "Governing the Planetary Greenhouse in Spite of Scientific Uncertainty" (*Science, Technology & Innovation Studies*, 6(2), 2010); and "Zivilgesellschaft und Wissenschaft: Ein Spannungsfeld zwischen Konfl ikt und Kooperation" (with Peter Wehling, *Sozialwissenschaften und Berufspraxis* (SuB), 35(2), 2010).

Peter Wehling

Peter Wehling is currently Senior Researcher at the Institute of Sociology at Goethe-University, Frankfurt/Main (Germany); until the end of 2013 he directed the research project "Participatory Governance of Science" at the University of Augsburg, Germany. His research interests include science and technology studies, sociology of knowledge and ignorance, sociology of health and illness, sociological theory and critical sociology. His recent publications include *Entgrenzung der Medizin* (co-edited with Willy Viehöver, 2011); "Fighting a Losing Battle? The Right Not to Know and the Dynamics of Biomedical Knowledge Production" (in M. Gross and L. McGoey (eds) *Routledge International Handbook of Ignorance Studies*, London/New York, forthcoming).

Stephen Zavestoski

Stephen Zavestoski, Associate Professor of Sociology and Environmental Studies at the University of San Francisco, USA, is the co-editor, with Phil Brown, of *Social Movements in Health* (2005), and with Phil Brown and Rachel Morello-Frosch, of *Contested Illnesses: Citizens, Science and Health Social Movements* (2012). His research areas include environmental sociology, social movements and sociology of health and illness. Dr. Zavestoski's previous research has also covered topics such as ecological identity, consumerism and, with David Schlosberg and Stuart Shulman, the effects of the Internet on public participation in environmental regulatory rulemaking processes.

Acknowledgements

This book would not have come to fruition without the generous support of many people and institutions. First of all, we would like to express our gratitude to all contributors to this volume for their inspiring ideas, interest, and commitment as well as their patience during the editorial process. The present book was only made possible thanks to the financial support by the German Federal Ministry of Education and Research (BMBF), which is very much appreciated. The BMBF not only funded our research project "Participatory Governance of Science" (funding code: 01UZ0907) from 2009 to 2013, but also the international conference on "Patient organizations, health movements and medical research: varieties, effects and future of civil society engagement in science, technology development and research policies" that we organized at the University of Augsburg, Germany, on May 10–12, 2012. This conference was the inspiration and starting point for this volume; we would therefore like to thank all participants, and in particular Kristin Barker, Nadja Kanellopoulou, Sabrina McCormick, Shobita Parthasarathy, Frank Stehr and Uta Wagenmann for their inspiring presentations. We are very grateful as well to Monika Wächter from the German Aerospace Center (DLR), the project management agency of the BMBF, for coordinating the research programme on "New Governance in Science" as well as to the members of the programme's Scientific Board, notably Edgar Grande, Dorothea Jansen, Otfried Jarren, Arie Rip, Uwe Schimank and Peter Weingart for their commitment and support of our research. In addition, we very much appreciated the fact that a number of German patient associations, mainly from the field of rare diseases, as well as their umbrella organization ACHSE constructively cooperated in our research project notwithstanding their limited financial, organizational, and personal resources. Ever reliable and meticulous in his critique, we would like to thank Gerard Holden for his help in translating and proofreading whenever we needed assistance. Our editors at Routledge, James Watson and Louisa Vahtrick, gave us excellent guidance along the way: we are grateful for their support.

Many colleagues and friends accompanied and supported our research project, critically commented on early drafts of our contributions to this volume, or gave helpful advice during the editorial process. For their valued time and effort, we would like to thank Silke Beck, Alex Bogner, Peter Conrad, Heiner Fangerau, David J. Hess, Karen Kastenhofer, Thomas Lemke, and Silke Schicktanz, as well as our colleagues or former colleagues at the Institute of Sociology at Augsburg University, Stefan Böschen, Sasa Bosancic, Oliver Dimbath, Eva Holzinger, Fabian Karsch, Reiner Keller, Matthias Klaes and, most notably, Christoph Lau. Last but not least, we would like to express tremendous gratitude to all those colleagues and student assistants who have worked with us during the past five years in the research project, helped us to organize the conference in 2012 and engaged in the production of the present volume: Lea Baumeister, Michael Ernst-Heidenreich, Debora Frommeld, Nikolas Güttler, Andreas Hechtel, Harald Hofer, Benedikt Laubert, Tobias Lehmann, Miriam Molter, Simon Oschwald and Brigitte Ploner. Finally, we are indebted to Matthias Roche for his co-authorship and his invaluable support in editing and proofreading our book chapters.

Sophia Koenen, Willy Viehöver and Peter Wehling, in May 2014

Patient associations, health social movements and the public shaping of biomedical research

An introduction

Peter Wehling, Willy Viehöver and Sophia Koenen

The emergence of the public shaping of medical research

In their study *No safe place: Toxic waste, Leukemia, and Community Action*, first published in 1990, Phil Brown and Edwin Mikkelsen describe how the residents of Woburn, a town in Massachusetts near Boston, came to realize in the mid-1970s "that their children were contracting leukemia at exceedingly high rates. By their own efforts affected families discovered a leukemia cluster, which they attributed to carcinogens leached into their drinking water supply from industrial waste" (Brown and Mikkelsen 1997: 1). The authors termed this engagement in knowledge production of the concerned people of Woburn "popular epidemiology" (ibid.: 2), thereby accounting for emerging new constellations of "lay and professional ways of knowing" (Brown 1992; see also Brown 1997). In retrospect, Brown recently pointed to both the novelty of the phenomenon and the lack of an adequate conceptual approach to it in the early 1990s: "I needed a framework to understand this phenomenon of laypeople engaging in science, and found nothing in the literature to explain it in enough detail" (Brown 2013: 148).

In the mid-1990s, Steven Epstein (1996) impressively told the story of how in the previous decade AIDS activists in the United States had become "lay experts" with regard to scientific knowledge production on "their" disease. He gave an account of how these activist groups influenced or even transformed ways of doing biomedical research (especially of doing clinical trials), challenged the hierarchical relations of experts and laypeople, and insisted "on the rights of those affected by biomedical science to participate in its production" (Epstein 1995: 428).[1] In the field of "rare" or "orphan" diseases, Vololona Rabeharisoa and Michel Callon some years later investigated the activities of the Association Français contre les Myopathies (AFM), the French Muscular Dystrophy Association, which were aimed at initiating, funding and even conducting medical research into these previously largely neglected conditions. As they argue, these efforts have given rise to a new model of both patient associations and their relations to medical experts: the "partner association" or "partnership model". In this model, the patient organization acts on a par with scientists and doctors; by pooling and comparing the experience of its members, it "builds up a collective expertise just as objective and authentic as that of the specialists, even if it is different" (Rabeharisoa and Callon 2002: 62).

These three cases are rather prominent and successful examples of what we understand in this volume as the "public shaping" of medical research and research politics, using a term introduced by David J. Hess (2004) to both medical sociology and science and technology studies (STS). By the term "public shaping" we mean the growing involvement and participation of civil society groups and organizations, such as local communities (as in the Woburn case), patient associations, advocacy groups, and health social movements in knowledge production on medical issues or even in advanced biomedical research.[2] We are in agreement with many social-scientific studies which have found that since 1990, when Brown and Mikkelsen first published their study, the phenomenon of the public shaping of medical research has become ever more important. It has attracted growing attention from different social-scientific fi elds such as medical sociology, medical anthropology, and STS, and also from public health research, governance theory, democratic theory, political philosophy and medical ethics.[3] In our view, the term "public shaping" of medical research (and research policies) is analytically useful and appealing since it covers a wide range of science-related activities of patient associations and health social movements. These activities include, in particular, the great variety of forms of "uninvited participation" (Wynne 2007) or "spontaneous participation" (Bucchi and Neresini 2008), that have developed both in addition and in contrast to "invited" and "sponsored" participatory exercises such as consensus conferences or "stakeholder" dialogues (see also Wehling 2012).

In detail, the public shaping of medical research by patient and advocacy groups, activists and health social movements comprises a number of partly overlapping activities. These include:

- lobbying for (or against) certain research fields and methodological approaches such as neuropharmacological interventions or stem cell research (Ganchoff 2008);
- initiating and/or funding (or co-funding) research projects, research grants, or even entire institutes, as can be observed in the field of rare diseases, for instance;
- networking with researchers and building collaborative networks among scientists, not least among researchers from different medical or scientific fields, countries and/or epistemic approaches;
- recruiting patients for clinical trials as well as issuing guidelines for such trials;

- influencing and shaping the research agendas and priorities of medical fields (Abma and Broerse 2010; Elberse et al. 2011), in particular identifying areas of "undone science" that have been neglected by mainstream research (Frickel et al. 2010);
- challenging mainstream medical science, in particular what Brown and his colleagues have termed the "dominant epidemiological paradigm" (Brown et al. 2006; Brown 2007) and its assumptions about the etiology, prevention and therapy of diseases;
- contesting medical definitions of health, normal behavior, illness, and disease (Moss and Teghtsoonian 2008; Brown et al. 2012), including efforts to medicalize or demedicalize certain conditions (Conrad 2007);[4]
- contributing in various ways to medical knowledge production (Caron-Flinterman et al. 2005, 2007), or even directly and personally participating in biomedical research (Terry et al. 2007; Kanellopoulou 2009);
- participating in or conducting specific, independent or cooperative forms of research and knowledge production, such as "research in the wild" (Callon and Rabeharisoa 2003), "popular epidemiology" or "community based participatory research" (Minkler and Wallerstein 2008).

In the last two or three decades these facets of the public shaping of medical research have become increasingly relevant in a wide range of medical fields. Among the most important are research on AIDS (Epstein 1996; Barbot and Dodier 2002; Barbot 2006), cancer research (Hess 1999), in particular breast cancer research (Brown 2007; Klawiter 2008; Ley 2009; McCormick 2009a, 2009b), rare diseases (Rabeharisoa and Callon 1999; Panofsky 2011; Huyard 2012), mental illnesses (Crossley 2006; Tomes 2011), Alzheimer's disease (Innes et al. 2004; O'Donovan et al. 2013) as well as various contested illnesses and spheres of medicalization or demedicalization such as Gulf War syndrome (Zavestoski et al. 2002), attention deficit/hyperactivity disorder (ADHD) (Conrad and Potter 2000), fibromyalgia (Barker 2005), or deafness (Blume 2010). The public shaping of science is of course not unique to the medical field, and has occurred in a number of other areas such as environmental or sustainability research (Hess 2007; Ottinger 2010), nanotechnology (Hess 2009, 2010), and gender and "queer" studies. The engagement of patient groups and social movements in medical research has, however, attracted particular attention from social scientists, not least due to the diversity of cases, of forms of participation and knowledge production, social actors involved, medical fields and scientific or political outcomes. Thus there have been a number of attempts to develop classifications and typologies of health movements and patient associations with regard to their interactions with healthcare and medical research.[5] Among the most prominent typologies are the distinctions drawn by Rabeharisoa and Callon (2002: 60) between the auxiliary, the partner and the opposing patient association, as well as the three types of health social movements identified by Brown and his co-authors: first, health access movements which seek equitable access to health care; second, embodied health movements, which challenge established science on etiology, diagnosis, treatment, and prevention; third, constituency-based health movements addressing health inequality and inequity based on categories such as race, ethnicity, gender, class or sexuality differences (Brown et al. 2008: 522–523). While these classifications are of course still valuable, the chapters in this volume will demonstrate that there is now a much greater variety of groups and movements such as "virtual", internet-based patient and advocacy groups (see Conrad and Tan in Chapter 6 of this volume), advocacy groups and movements who act on behalf of other groups of (putative) patients (Lyson and Zavestoski in Chapter 5 of this volume), and various "hybrid" groups which combine seemingly contradictory orientations towards medical research and/or economic actors (see, for instance, Hess in Chapter 8 of this volume).

Recurrent topics, open questions and new developments

Given the heterogeneity of cases, activities and medical fields presented in the previous section, it is unsurprising that in recent years a wide range of different conceptual and methodological approaches have developed within the social sciences that are designed to explore the shaping of biomedical research by patient groups and health social movements, as well as its preconditions and results.[6] Social-scientific work includes detailed individual case studies as well as more generalizing and occasionally also comparative analyses. While both types of studies offer numerous illuminating insights into the varieties and dynamics of the public shaping of medical research, there are nevertheless a number of open questions and recurrent issues that are addressed, albeit quite differently or even controversially, by almost all conceptual approaches in the field. These questions are therefore dealt with throughout this volume.

One of the most fundamental and prominent of these issues is the question of how to conceptualize the knowledge which patients, their relatives or carers, and activists are able to mobilize and of how this knowledge relates to scientific knowledge and contributes to medical research. Should we understand patients' knowledge as "lay knowledge", which seems to imply that it is not merely distinct from but also deficient and ultimately inferior to scientific knowledge (see, for instance, Prior 2003)? Or should we rather understand it as "experiential knowledge", that is to say independent knowledge in its own right – patients' "intimate, firsthand knowledge" of their bodies and illnesses, as Brown et al. (2012: 19) have put it – which might be considered equal or in certain respects even superior to scientific knowledge (see e.g. Whelan 2007)? This basic distinction is mirrored in the one that is drawn between "lay" and "experiential experts" or "experts of experience" (Akrich et al. 2008: 19ff.) While these terms are of course not always used in an unambiguous manner (Prior 2003: 45), a lay expert is usually held to be a lay person who has acquired scientific knowledge to a certain degree, whereas an "experiential expert" is understood as someone who has become an expert on her or his own experience of living with an illness or caring for a person with an illness.

Contrary to both these concepts stressing the distinctiveness of patients' and experts' knowledge, Jeanette Pols (2014) has recently suggested that we should understand "patient knowledge" as a hybrid and "messy" form of knowledge, which is indeed influenced and shaped by scientific knowledge, but is nevertheless distinct from it in that it results from transforming and adapting medical knowledge to the daily lives of patients. Popular epidemiology (Brown 1992, 1997) and "research in the wild" (Callon and Rabeharisoa 2003) may also be seen as activities that productively combine patients' knowledge and certain forms of scientific research and inquiry, and potentially transform the ways in which medical research is conducted (see also Akrich et al. in Chapter 4 of this volume). However, this does not preclude the possibility that patients' knowledge (and perhaps even their bodily experiences) may be more or less dominated by biomedicine, thus fostering the emergence not only of "professionalized" lay experts (Thompson et al. 2012), but also of biomedicalized "technoscientific illness identities" (Sulik 2009; Clarke et al. 2010). In a less rigorous manner, patient groups and health movements may be "interpellated" as potential users of future biomedical technologies (Langstrup in Chapter 9 of this volume) or constructed as "biosocialities", that is social communities which are held to constitute themselves and their identities on the basis of a seemingly objective and scientifically attested biological or genetic condition (Lemke in Chapter 10 of this volume). Or, by contrast, do (putative) patients form their identities in explicit opposition to medical science, thereby often demanding demedicalization of their conditions, as has been the case with many mental or sexual "disorders"? Similar questions and tensions arise in relation to the interactions of patient and scientific knowledge: to what extent and under what circumstances is patients' knowledge complementary to and instrumental for scientific knowledge production, and how far is it opposed to it, contesting its background assumptions and conceptual approaches or even transforming the latter? As the contributions to this volume will demonstrate, the answers to all these questions vary considerably and largely depend on the specific cases examined. However, while there is of course no "one best solution" to these conceptual problems, we need ongoing debates aiming at an adequate and comprehensive understanding of patients' expertise and its productive interactions as well as potential conflicts with scientific medical knowledge.

A second important issue concerns the "problem of representation" (Epstein 2011) mentioned above. On the one hand, this includes the question of who legitimately speaks for patients, in particular in those cases where they are unable to speak for themselves because they are too young or too severely impaired by their illness. The problem of how to authentically and accurately represent the interests and experiences of the directly affected persons (and more basically of how to know and understand these interests) has always been far from trivial, even in those cases where parents speak for their children. Recently, however, this problem has become even more complicated due to a number of developments. One of these developments lies in the fact that in many cases different, often competing patient associations or advocacy groups have emerged which nevertheless claim to speak for all patients having the same condition; see Batt on breast cancer (Chapter 7); Conrad and Tan on autism (Chapter 6); Lyson and Zavestoski on obesity (Chapter 5). Which of these groups and their contradictory views, then, authentically represent the experiences and needs of the patients? On the other hand, not least due to the increasingly important role of the media in contemporary societies and politics, the "problem of representation" also includes the question of which patient and advocacy groups are taken notice of in the public sphere and in political or scientific debates – and which are not (see Blume 2010; Grob 2011; Wehling and Viehöver in Chapter 12 of this volume; Schicktanz in Chapter 13). What are the criteria and mechanisms that draw attention to some diseases and/or patient associations while marginalizing others? What role do financial resources, access to the media, and compliance (or, by contrast, explicit non-compliance) with biomedical definitions of illness and disease play for the public "visibility" and acceptance of patient associations and health movements? How would it be possible to strengthen and support those patient groups who, for whatever reasons, lack financial resources and easy access to the media, politics or medical science? This question of the authentic and unbiased representation of patients, their experiences and needs is also linked to what Epstein (2011: 267f.) has termed the "problem of incorporation and co-optation" (see Batt in Chapter 7 of this volume; Hess in Chapter 8). To what extent and in what ways are the science-related activities and statements of patient groups influenced or biased as a consequence of their dependence on funding from the pharmaceutical industry (or state agencies), or of their struggle for access to medication and for recognition from biomedical science?

All these aspects – the specificity and role of patients' knowledge, the representativeness of patient associations and their spokespersons, and the authenticity of their demands – are crucial for the legitimacy, and the recognition of the legitimacy, of their participation in medical knowledge production and research policies. However, there are different and, at first sight, contrasting conceptions or models of what constitutes that legitimacy. Very generally speaking, one can distinguish two main rationales for patient participation: one of these is based on the more representational idea that all those who are affected by a certain condition should be involved and participate in knowledge production and decision-making concerning this condition, and the other is more "technical" in that it emphasizes the useful contributions of patient knowledge or expertise to scientific research.[7]

According to this second view, lay people such as patients or social movement activists should indeed participate in research, but only insofar as they are able to make substantive contributions to scientific knowledge production (Collins and Evans 2002; Prior 2003).

However, both of these rationales actually raise a number of questions. Regarding the democratic, representational approach one might ask whether the primary aim should be to actually involve all affected people (which often might be impossible) or at least the majority of them. Yet going beyond a merely statistical, quantitative concept of representation, it might be equally or even more important to consider and include all the different experiences, interests and needs that patients have and express. With respect to the "technocratic" rationale, the question arises of who is authorized and legitimized to decide which forms of patient expertise are useful for scientific knowledge production and which are not. If only scientists decide on this, the result is likely to be biased.[8] Indeed, patients' experience frequently does not contribute to biomedical knowledge in a narrow "technical" sense (and therefore might appear to be of little scientific interest), but it may nevertheless further a better understanding of the social contexts of living with a disease as well as of the normative values which are at stake. In addition, patients can make reasoned contributions to research agenda-setting even if they are unable to contribute to the research itself. Moreover, even radical challenges to firmly established "dominant epidemiological paradigms" may in the long run turn out to be beneficial to medical research, as might be the case with activists' insistence on environmental causes of breast cancer (see Baralt in Chapter 1 of this volume). Thus, on closer inspection the two justifications for patient involvement are not so distinct or even incompatible as might appear at first sight: the representative model tends to go beyond statistical representation of patients to the representation of the variety of experiences and interests they voice in public debates and decision-making, and the expertise-based model tends to shift (or *should* tend to shift) attention from a "technocratic" understanding of expertise to recognizing a variety of patients' views, even opposing ones, as (potentially) valuable and instrumental for medical research and healthcare. There is, therefore, a kind of convergence of both rationales towards including a (more or less) wide range of affected people, forms of knowledge, interests and demands. Nevertheless, it continues to be an open and contested question how the two requirements for legitimate patient participation, democratic representation and/or valuable expertise, are to be fulfilled in general, and to what extent they are actually found in specific situations. It remains highly debatable how an adequate representation of persons or groups as well as of views and interests might be achieved, and what should be understood as useful, reliable and authentic lay or experiential expertise; on these issues see Bucchi (Chapter 11), Schicktanz (Chapter 13), Wehling and Viehöver (Chapter 12).

Many of these questions coalesce into the issue of the *success* or *failure* of the public shaping of biomedical research, including the difficult problem of how to assess or even "measure" such success (Epstein 2011). As Epstein (ibid.: 258) rightly emphasizes, there are two reasons why we should not link success too narrowly to the achievement of a group's stated goals. First, it might be the case that, while a patient group or health social movement is not or only partly successful in realizing their own objectives, the outcomes of their activities may benefit a larger social group or even society as a whole. Second, in some cases patients may actually achieve their goals, but this success may at the same time be questioned and overshadowed by indirect outcomes and unintended consequences. In addition, even if a desired goal (such as more medical research on a certain disease) has been realized, it may be difficult to determine to what extent this has been the result of patient engagement or of other developments in science or politics. Epstein (ibid.: 260) therefore reasonably warns against exaggerating the effects of patient advocacy; however, social-scientific research should not underestimate these effects either, be they direct or indirect. In any event, it is an important aim of that research (and of this volume as well) to identify and compare conditions that are likely to result in the success (or failure) of patient group and movement participation in medical research and research politics (see, for instance, Brown 2007; Akrich et al. 2008; Parthasarathy 2010; Panofsky 2011).

Up until now, empirical research has drawn a complex and ambiguous picture of the success and failure of patient activism – and so do the contributions to this volume. Prominent cases of success can be seen in the impact of AIDS activists on medical research (Epstein 1996), and in the efforts of various rare disease patient organizations who not only successfully drew the attention of medical science, politics and the general public to this group of "orphaned" diseases but also initiated and funded numerous research projects on their respective diseases (see Terry 2007; Callon and Rabeharisoa 2008; Nourissier et al. in Chapter 3 of this volume; Reimann in Chapter 2 of this volume). Patient activism in the field of rare diseases led to the constitution of communities formed by sufferers, their families, peers and concerned groups, and also forged new, sometimes powerful forms of cooperation between scientists and patient organizations, politics and market actors, thereby bringing together different kinds of "epistemic communities" (Akrich 2010; Panofsky 2011). In addition, not least due to the activities of patient associations and umbrella organizations such as EURORDIS (European Organisation for Rare Diseases), all European Union (EU) member states have been obliged to prepare national action plans for rare diseases up to the year 2013. Among other things, these plans embrace coordinated and intensified efforts in the field of medical research on rare diseases, including increased participation of patients and patient organizations.[9] More generally, in some countries such as the United Kingdom, patient and public involvement (PPI) in decision-making on healthcare and medical research has become part of governmental politics – though with seemingly mixed results (Thompson et al. 2012) and a serious recent backlash (Tritter and Koivusalo 2013).[10] In other countries, for instance in the Netherlands, individual patients and/or patient associations have frequently and successfully been engaged in coordinated and collaborative processes of research agenda-setting in various medical fields such as asthma, diabetes, burns and dementia (Abma and Broerse 2010).

A more ambivalent picture emerges from the activities of the Environmental Breast Cancer Movement (EBCM) in the USA, Canada, and some other countries (see Ley 2009; McCormick 2009a; Baralt in Chapter 1 of this volume; Batt in Chapter 7 of this volume). On the one hand, this movement of patients, activists and sympathetic scientists in the United States succeeded in initiating publicly funded research programs and research centers and even in establishing an independent research institute. On the other hand, the EBCM had only limited success in changing the research priorities of mainstream biomedical research or in achieving political regulation of environmental toxins. Moreover, in some countries such as Germany, this movement is rather weak and has seen little by way of response from either medical research or breast cancer patient organizations. In some other cases, however, patient groups and health social movements failed even more dramatically to achieve their goals, for instance in the campaign to gain medical and scientific recognition for contested conditions such as multiple chemical sensitivity (MCS) or so-called "electrosensitivity". One of the most significant examples of failure has been the struggle of parts of the Deaf Community against the development and spread of cochlear implants in order to maintain the community's social and cultural identity based on the use of sign language. As Stuart Blume (2010: 197) argues, this community's failure "points to the limits imposed on empowerment and suggests that patient groups can gain acknowledgement and influence only insofar as their demands are compatible with certain fundamental assumptions of medical science, medical authority, and the consumption of medical goods and services". Blume self-critically adds that social scientists should bear in mind such failures instead of focusing mainly on presumed "success stories", and he demands that they reflect on the extent to which they themselves might be influenced by or even complicit with the dominant ways of framing scientific and medical issues.

Aims of the volume and overview of the chapters

Given the background of ongoing debates on the aforementioned issues, the aim of the present volume is threefold. First, after more than two decades of social science and STS research on patient associations and health social movements, it attempts to summarize some of the most significant empirical findings and theoretical developments in the field.[11] The second aim is to explore what new developments and challenges health movements and patient organizations are going to face in the near future. Among these are the growing importance of internet-based patient groups, the emergence of competing advocacy groups for the same condition, the rise of adverse political contexts such as neoliberalism, and the increasing "technoscientization" of biomedicine (Clarke et al. 2010; Sulik 2009), including a seemingly persistent tendency to favor basic research over health care research. Third, the volume seeks to improve our understanding of the conditions of legitimacy of patients' engagement with medical knowledge production and to explore the opportunities (and possible difficulties) for the democratization of medical science and research politics resulting from this engagement.

With these aims in view, the book is structured in three parts. The first part, "Empirical cases and theoretical perspectives", presents, inevitably selectively, both significant examples of patients' engagement with medical research in fields such as breast cancer, rare diseases, obesity, ADHD and Alzheimer's, and some of the conceptual perspectives (such as "contested illnesses", "evidence-based activism", and "health social movements") developed in social science research in order to theoretically account for such engagement. In the first chapter of this part, "A seat at the table, 'a lab of our own' and working with what we know now: how the US Environmental Breast Cancer Movement shapes research", *Lori Baralt* describes in detail the development of the EBCM in the USA. This is doubtless one of the most prominent cases of patient involvement in medical knowledge production, in particular of patients and activists challenging the "dominant epidemiological paradigm" of mainstream biomedical research. Baralt analyzes three different ways in which the EBCM has engaged with cancer research: activists have, first, collaborated in partnerships with non-mainstream scientists; second, founded their own, independent research institute, the Silent Spring Institute; and, third, advocated for policy change based on the existing state of the evidence on environmental links to breast cancer. Although the movement has faced a number of serious challenges it can, Baralt argues, serve as an example for other environmental health movements in terms of developing multidimensional strategies for engaging with scientific research to further movement goals.

In his chapter "Initiating and funding medical research on a rare disease: the approach of the German Cystic Fibrosis Association", *Andreas Reimann*, managing director of Mukoviszidose e.V., gives an insight into the quite sophisticated practices of a patient organization with regard to funding and assessing research on cystic fibrosis (CF), or mucoviscidosis. He shows how Mukoviszidose e.V. found a way to ensure that funded projects are of high scientific quality on the one hand and of significant relevance to the patients on the other. Reimann explains in detail how a multi-step peer-review evaluation process and a procedure to assess the patient impact of the associations' funding programs were designed, and also examines their limitations. Moreover, he summarizes the lessons learned from 15 years of participation in CF research and argues for a social entrepreneurship approach which combines the strengths of an idealistic non-profit organization with those of an entrepreneurial context. Among these lessons is the need to communicate expectations about research outcomes as transparently and honestly as possible, because otherwise the patients' and donors' trust in science might be threatened. Shifting the focus to the European level, *Christel Nourissier*, *Monica Ensini* and *Maria Mavris* describe the various roles and tasks of the transnational umbrella organization EURORDIS in the field of medical research and research policies. In their chapter "EURORDIS: empowering patients living with rare diseases to participate in biomedical knowledge production", the authors present important data and findings regarding the broad range of science-related and political activities undertaken by both EURORDIS itself and its nearly 600 member organizations throughout Europe. The authors, who themselves work or have worked with EURORDIS, place particular emphasis on the need to encourage targeted medical research and research policies in the field of rare diseases. Empowerment and capacity-building of the member organizations, in order to improve their abilities to both participate in medical knowledge production and get access to medical and social care, is another important issue for EURORDIS.

In the fourth chapter, "The entanglement of scientific and political claims: towards a new form of patients' activism", *Madeleine Akrich*, *Órla O'Donovan* and *Vololona Rabeharisoa* examine what they term the "evidence-based activism" of patient organizations in four specific condition areas: rare diseases, childbirth, attention deficit hyperactivity disorder (ADHD) and Alzheimer's disease, in different European countries, mainly France and Ireland. The authors use the term "evidence-based activism" to suggest a new view of knowledge for these groups and for the social scientists who study them: instead of contemplating knowledge as a mere resource "out there" which patients' organizations and activists rely on to defend their causes, knowledge should be considered as "something" to be produced and discussed. By working on and with both academic and experiential knowledge, patients and activists contribute to creating epistemic networks and developing new understandings of their conditions and the problems these give rise to for themselves and for medical experts. While Akrich, O'Donovan and Rabeharisoa emphasize that we should avoid romanticizing patients' evidence-based activism, they nevertheless argue that it introduces a form of collective reflexivity in the shaping of research and research policies. *Mercedes C. Lyson* and *Stephen Zavestoski* seek to advance the theoretical concept of health social movements by analyzing how the "alternative food" movement and the "complete streets" movement (demanding, for example, walkable neighborhoods and greater investment in public spaces and transit) strive to address the ostensible "obesity epidemic" in the USA. In their chapter "Obesity, the alternative food movement, and complete streets: new forms of 'patient' activism and the evolution of health social movements", they examine how dynamics of race, class and power are implicated when advocacy is driven by one group of individuals acting on behalf of a "target population" such as those diagnosed as obese, many of whom fiercely reject being addressed as "patients". Through an analysis of the complex field of social movement actors who seek to define and redefine obesity, the authors explore whether activism around obesity can be considered a novel – and in some respects dubious – form of "patient" activism, and how this example helps us advance our understanding of the emergence and performance of health social movements.

The second part of the book, "Shifting contexts and new challenges" addresses new political, cultural, scientific, and technological developments and their ambivalent implications for the field of patient activism and advocacy. It is introduced by *Peter Conrad* and *Catherine Tan's* examination of "Autism, the internet, and medicalization", which focuses on the emergence of quite disparate and partly competing patient advocacy groups as facilitated by the internet. Starting from the recent strong increase in autism diagnoses, the authors examine how the three main perspectives that are representative of the "autism world on the internet" relate to the medicalization or demedicalization of this condition. In the first view, autism is understood as a medical disease and therefore needs more biomedical research. In the second perspective autism is also seen as a medical condition, but is held to be caused by environmental toxins (particularly vaccines), which means that its prevention requires reducing exposure to toxins. According to the third perspective autism is not a disease at all, but rather part of a normal range of human "neurodiversity" which must be demedicalized and protected from social discrimination. Although there is obviously only very little overlap between the opinions and goals of these three groups, all see themselves as actors that advocate for autism and adequate scientific research related to autism.

Sharon Batt's research focus is on the influence of shifting political contexts on patient activism and, specifically, on the impact of emerging neoliberal government policies on the Canadian women's health and breast cancer movement during the last two to three decades. In her chapter "A community fractured: Canada's breast cancer movement, pharmaceutical company funding, and science-related advocacy", she examines the breast cancer movement through the double lens of pre- and post-neoliberal politics. While in the 1990s the movement was able to act rather independently and had significant influence on the breast cancer research agenda, the subsequent neoliberal reduction of government funding for advocacy groups led to a struggle within the Canadian breast cancer activists' community which ultimately split the movement. Many groups turned to the pharmaceutical industry for support and adopted research advocacy goals which are consistent with a corporatized health research agenda, while only a minority resisted this problematic alliance. *David J. Hess'* chapter, "Beyond scientific controversies: scientific counterpublics, countervailing industries, and undone science", also deals with the relations of cancer patients and activists with industry, albeit from a different angle. Hess argues that health advocacy organizations can be conceptualized on a continuum from an interest group pole, which generally does not challenge mainstream assumptions about etiology and treatment, to a social movement pole, which often challenges the dominant epidemiological paradigm and calls attention to "undone science" such as research on the value of nutritional and nutraceutical cancer therapies. Looking at the case of complementary and alternative medicine (CAM) in the field of cancer research and therapy, he observes the emergence of a genuine scientific counterpublic consisting of researchers, clinicians, patient advocacy leaders, nutritional companies, political officials, and health freedom organizations and opposing the mainstream of cancer research. Given the fact that without the constant surveillance of the nutraceutical industry this counterpublic would have achieved only limited political success, Hess argues that the case of CAM cancer therapies disturbs the idea of industrial cooptation of social movements by drawing attention to coalitions of civil society organizations, scientists and countervailing industries.

How do patients and patient associations come to regard themselves as users of future medical technologies such as stem cell therapies, the success of which currently remains rather uncertain? Why do some groups refrain from doing so? These are the questions on which *Henriette Langstrup* focuses in her chapter "Interpellating patients as future users of biomedical technologies: the case of patient associations and stem cell research". Drawing on the notion of "interpellation" as developed by the French philosopher Louis Althusser, she analyzes the engagement of various Danish patient associations with stem cell research in the early 2000s and their relations to what she terms (following John Law) the "projectness" of technoscience, that is to say its enactment as a series of targeted, entrepreneurial projects of technology development. However, as Langstrup's study shows, this does not mean that patient associations are subject to a deterministic logic of being obliged to support the development of stem cell therapies for their respective diseases. To the contrary, while some groups responded to the interpellation affirmatively others remained reluctant to do so, and still others "counter-interpellated" biomedical researchers by striving to place their condition "on the list" of diseases to be possibly cured by future stem cell therapies.

Thomas Lemke's chapter, entitled "Patient organizations as biosocial communities? Conceptual clarifications and critical remarks", also deals with the complex interrelations of patient activism with biomedical and, in particular, genetic research. It starts from an analytical stance on the powerful concept of "biosociality" developed by the anthropologist Paul Rabinow in the early 1990s in the context of the Human Genome Project. This concept, Lemke argues, points to two closely related developments: first, an emerging new arrangement of the relation between nature and culture that is no longer characterized by a clear borderline, and second, new forms of identities and alliances between patients, scientists, politicians, medical doctors, and biotech companies that give rise to new kinds of socialities formed around particular biological conditions. In the following years, however, the focus of the literature on biosociality has been selectively and enthusiastically on self-help groups and patients' associations. Lemke points out that this led to some empirical shortcomings and analytical deficits, such as a remarkable narrowing of the issue of biosociality, the questionable idea of a stable and univocal biology, and a failure to adequately examine power relations.

The third part of the volume, entitled "Democratizing biomedicine? The role of patient associations and health social movements", focuses on the political and epistemic legitimacy of patients' engagement in medical research. These chapters examine how patient activism might contribute to the democratization of science and science-society interactions, and develop a reflective understanding of what such democratization should look like. *Massimiano Bucchi*'s chapter "Changing contexts for science and society interaction: from deficit to dialogue, from dialogue to participation – and beyond?" introduces this part by focusing on the development of different models of science-society interactions which form the political and discursive context of patient activism. However, despite a general historical trend towards more participatory forms of science-society interactions, the change of keywords observable in funding schemes or policy documents, for instance from "public awareness of science" to "citizen engagement", does not necessarily reflect a corresponding change in the actual practice and understanding of science-society interactions. In any case, as Bucchi emphasizes, we should resist the temptation to understand such changes of keywords or practices as a linear and normative sequence of stages in which the emerging forms ("participation") necessarily obliterate the previous ones ("dialogue"). Instead of asking "which model accounts best" for expert-public interactions, we should acknowledge both the open-endedness of participation and the simultaneous coexistence of different patterns of interaction that emerge depending on specific conditions and on the issues at stake.

In their chapter entitled "The virtues (and some perils) of activist participation: the political and epistemic legitimacy of patient activism", *Peter Wehling* and *Willy Viehöver* argue from both a democratic theory and a sociology of science perspective. Drawing on what might be termed "post-deliberative" political theory, they suggest that activist participation in science and technology is likely to be more effective than deliberative participatory exercises such as consensus conferences. In addition, it can claim at least as much democratic legitimacy as it brings in the interests of particular and often marginalized groups. Moreover, the sociology of science has repeatedly shown that civil society actors such as patient associations perform important tasks for knowledge production, including acting as an epistemic "corrective" of mainstream research, thus urging science to operate more adequately and in a more socially responsible way. However, there are also some challenges to the legitimacy of activist participation. Using examples from advocacy for newborn screening and preconception genetic testing, the authors point to the problem of legitimate representation not only *within* patient associations but also *among* them, a problem which becomes more salient the more these associations enter the public and political sphere with their market-like mechanisms of drawing attention to some issues while denying it to others. In the last chapter of this part, "The ethical legitimacy of patient organizations' involvement in politics and knowledge production: epistemic justice as a conceptual basis", *Silke Schicktanz* develops an ethical approach to the issue of legitimacy by asking how we can do justice (or avoid being unjust) to patients' contributions to knowledge production and ethical discourse. Drawing on the concept of "epistemic (in) justice" introduced by the philosopher Miranda Fricker, as well as on Donna Haraway's notion of "situated knowledge", Schicktanz points to existing epistemic injustices in public debates on medical issues. Epistemic injustice occurs, according to Fricker, when statements made by members of particular groups (such as patients) are routinely (though often inadvertently) discredited or neglected, for instance because of negative social stereotypes (lack of objectivity, idiosyncrasy, etc.) which are associated with those groups. This theoretical perspective helps to identify unfair exclusion, on the one hand, and unjustified advantages given to particular discourse participants, such as experts, on the other. Schicktanz argues that the inclusion of patients' perspectives is justified by the two criteria of "being affected" and of sharing particular situated knowledge.

In the concluding chapter, *Willy Viehöver*, *Peter Wehling* and *Matthias Roche* seek to summarize some of the findings presented in the contributions to this volume and point to open questions as well as promising areas of future research. As they emphasize, the public shaping of medical research by patient and advocacy groups and health social movements will doubtless continue to be an important (and contested) topic of social science research, ethical reflection and political debate.

Notes

1 Epstein was quick to point out, however, a potential tension within health social movements and patient groups (and a complication of the project of democratizing expertise) which still appears to be relevant: the risk of replicating the expert/lay division within the movements and groups themselves by producing a divide between "lay expert" activists and "lay lay" activists (Epstein 1995: 429; see also Thompson et al. 2012). In a recent insightful paper, Epstein (2011: 264) refers to this as both "the problem of representation", drawing attention to the "symbolic practices of representation by which spokespersons come to stand in for a group", and the "problem of expertise" possibly resulting from the "scientization" of a patient group or movement (ibid.: 265–267).

2 According to Hess (2004: 695), the public shaping of science includes "both greater agency of social movement/lay advocacy organisations and greater recognition of the legitimacy of that agency." While we agree with the statement that the involvement of civil society organizations (CSOs) in research and technology development has increased in recent decades, we are less sure whether this

applies equally to recognition of the legitimacy of this involvement which, by contrast, still seems to be contested in a number of cases. Therefore, the third part of this volume is dedicated to exploring the democratic and epistemic legitimacy of the public shaping of research by patient groups and health social movements.

3 For recent overviews, see Akrich et al. 2008; Epstein 2008; Banaszak-Holl et al. 2010; Hoffman et al. 2011; Löfgren et al. 2011; Brown et al. 2012.

4 The term *medicalization* refers to the framing of (social) phenomena and conditions in medical terms whereas *demedicalization* points to cases in which the phenomenon in question is no longer understood in terms of disease, illness or disorder.

5 However, most patient associations continue to act as self-help groups whose members share their experiences of living with the disease, organize support and mutual aid, demand access to healthcare and medications, circulate information among their members and frequently strive to empower each other to enter into the political sphere (see Banaszak-Holl et al. 2010; Hoffman et al. 2011). Nevertheless, particularly during the last two or three decades, many patient associations and health movements have increasingly engaged in medical research. While many of these groups have successfully funded, initiated and evaluated medical research projects, they are also facing the problem of how to balance these new objectives with the more "traditional" tasks of a self-help group (see, for instance, Reimann in Chapter 2 of this volume).

6 A still-illuminating synopsis of the rapidly growing body of social-scientific work on patient associations and health movements is given by Epstein (2008).

7 Martin (2008: 36) terms these the "democratic" and the "technocratic" rationales for public involvement. While the first one is primarily linked to the problem of representation, the second is more closely related to the issue of patients' expertise.

8 Thus, for patients and activists the problem arises of how to break the "expertise barrier" (Parthasarathy 2010) which often denies them full recognition by scientists and policy-makers. Among the four activist strategies which Shobita Parthasarathy identifies, she includes "deploying established expertise" as well as "introducing new kinds of facts".

9 However, even the case of rare diseases is not an unambiguous example of success, since the hopes for therapeutic breakthroughs initially pinned on genetic research were only partly realized. However, this research did develop more and more tools for prenatal or preconceptional genetic testing for rare diseases, thus raising the issue of prevention which at least for some patient associations is difficult to deal with (see Wailoo and Pemberton 2006).

10 For recent challenges to patient participation on the European Union level, see Koivusalo and Tritter 2011.

11 There is, however, a regrettable limitation, as the book focuses primarily on patient group and health movement activism in Europe and North America while largely neglecting the apparently quite different challenges and difficulties which patients, activists and advocates are facing in poor and developing countries. Since this bias more or less mirrors the mainstream of social science research, we should understand it as an urgent appeal to broaden the scope of research and to draw attention to patient activism outside the industrialized world as well as to the interrelations and possible conflicts between the views and interests of patients and movement activists in the "North" and "South" (see Sunder Rajan 2008).

References

Abma, Tineke A. and Broerse, Jacqueline (2010) Patient Participation as Dialogue: Setting Research Agendas, *Health Expectations*, 13(2), 160–173.

Akrich, Madeleine (2010) From Communities of Practice to Epistemic Communities: Health Mobilizations on the Internet, *Sociological Research Online*, 15(2). Available online at <www.socresonline.org.uk/15/2/10.html> (accessed 8 June 2013).

Akrich, Madeleine; Nunes, João; Paterson, Florence and Rabeharisoa, Vololona (2008) *The Dynamics of Patient Organizations in Europe*, Paris: Presses de l'École des Mines.

Banaszak-Holl, Jane C.; Levitsky, Sandra R. and Zald, Mayer N. (eds) (2010) *Social Movements and the Transformation of American Health Care*, Oxford: Oxford University Press.

Barbot, Janine (2006) How to Build an "Active" Patient? The Work of AIDS Associations in France, *Social Science and Medicine*, 62(3), 538–551.

Barbot, Janine and Dodier, Nicolas (2002) Multiplicity in Scientific Medicine: The Experience of HIV-Positive Patients, *Science, Technology & Human Values*, 27(3), 404–440.

Barker, Kristin (2005) *The Fibromyalgia Story: Medical Authority and Women's Worlds of Pain*, Philadelphia, PA: Temple University Press.

Blume, Stuart (2010) *The Artificial Ear. Cochlear Implants and the Culture of Deafness*, New Brunswick, NJ: Rutgers University Press.

Brown, Phil (1992) Popular Epidemiology and Toxic Waste Contamination: Lay and Professional Ways of Knowing, *Journal of Health and Social Behavior*, 33(3), 267–281.

Brown, Phil (1997) Popular Epidemiology Revisited, *Current Sociology*, 45(3), 137–156.

Brown, Phil (2007) *Toxic Exposures: Contested Illnesses and the Environmental Health Movement*, New York: Columbia University Press.

Brown, Phil (2013) Integrating Medical and Environmental Sociology with Environmental Health: Crossing Boundaries and Building Connections through Advocacy, *Journal of Health and Social Behavior*, 54(2), 145–164.

Brown, Phil and Mikkelsen, Edwin (1997) *No Safe Place: Toxic Waste, Leukemia, and Community Action*, 2nd edition, Berkeley, CA: University of California Press.

Brown, Phil; McCormick, Sabrina; Mayer, Brian; Zavestoski, Stephen; Morello-Frosch, Rachel; Gasior Altman, Rebecca and Senier, Laura (2006) "A Lab of Our Own": Environmental Causation of Breast Cancer and Challenges to the Dominant Epidemiological Paradigm, *Science, Technology & Human Values*, 31(5), 499–536.

Brown, Phil; Zavestoski, Stephen; McCormick, Sabrina; Mayer, Brian; Morello-Frosch, Rachel and Gasior Altman, Rebecca (2008) Embodied Health Movements: New Approaches to Social Movements in Health, in P. Brown (ed.) *Perspectives in Medical Sociology*, 4th edition, Long Grove, IL: Waveland Press, 521–538.

Brown, Phil; Morello-Frosch, Rachel; Zavestoski, Stephen and the Contested Illnesses Research Group (eds) (2012) *Contested Illnesses: Citizens, Science and Health Social Movements*, Berkeley, CA: University of California Press.

Bucchi, Massimiano and Neresini, Federico (2008) Science and Public Participation, in E.J. Hackett; O. Amsterdamska; M. Lynch and J. Wajcman (eds) *The Handbook of Science and Technology Studies*, 3rd edition, Cambridge, MA: MIT Press, 449–473.

Callon, Michel and Rabeharisoa, Vololona (2003) Research "In the Wild" and the Shaping of New Social Identities, *Technology in Society*, 25(2), 193–204.

Callon, Michel and Rabeharisoa, Vololona (2008) The Growing Engagement of Emergent Concerned Groups in Political and Economic Life: Lessons from the French Association of Neuromuscular Disease Patients, *Science, Technology & Human Values*, 33(2), 230–261.

Caron-Flinterman, Francisca; Broerse, Jacqueline and Bunders, Joske F.G. (2005) The Experiential Knowledge of Patients: A New Resource for Biomedical Research, *Social Science and Medicine*, 60(11), 2575–2584.

Caron-Flinterman, Francisca; Broerse, Jacqueline and Bunders, Joske F.G. (2007) Patient Participation in Decision Making on Biomedical Research: Changing the Network, *Science, Technology & Human Values*, 32(3), 339–368.

Clarke, Adele E.; Mamo, Laura; Fosket, Jennifer Ruth; Fishman, Jennifer R. and Shim, Janet K. (eds) (2010) *Biomedicalization. Technoscience, Health and Illness in the U.S.*, Durham, NC: Duke University Press.

Collins, Harry M. and Evans, Robert (2002) The Third Wave of Science Studies: Studies of Expertise and Experience, *Social Studies of Science*, 32(2), 235–296.

Conrad, Peter (2007) *The Medicalization of Society: On The Transformation of Human Conditions into Treatable Disorders*, Baltimore, MD: Johns Hopkins University Press.

Conrad, Peter and Potter, Deborah (2000) From Hyperactive Children to ADHD Adults: Observations on the Expansion of Medical Categories, *Social Problems*, 47(4), 559–582.

Crossley, Nick (2006) *Contesting Psychiatry. Social Movements in Mental Health*, Abingdon: Routledge.

Elberse, Janneke E.; Caron-Flinterman, Francisca and Broerse, Jacqueline (2011) Patient-Expert Partnerships in Research: How to Stimulate Inclusion of Patient Perspectives, *Health Expectations*, 14(3), 225–239.

Epstein, Steven (1995) The Construction of Lay Expertise: AIDS Activism and the Forging of Credibility in the Reform of Clinical Trials, *Science, Technology & Human Values*, 20(4), 408–437.

Epstein, Steven (1996) Impure Science: AIDS, Activism, and the Politics of Knowledge, Berkeley, CA: University of California Press.

Epstein, Steven (2008) Patient Groups and Health Movements, in E.J. Hackett, O. Amsterdamska, M.E. Lynch and J. Wajcman (eds) *The Handbook of Science and Technology Studies*, 3rd edition, Cambridge, MA: MIT Press, 499–539.

Epstein, Steven (2011) Measuring Success: Scientifi ç Institutional, and Cultural Effects of Patient Advocacy, in B. Hoffman, N. Tomes, R. Grob and M. Schlesinger (eds) *Patients as Policy Actors*, New Brunswick, NJ and London: Rutgers University Press, 257–277.

Frickel, Scott; Gibbon, Sahra; Howard, Jeff; Kempner, Joanna; Ottinger, Gwen and Hess, David J. (2010) Undone Science: Charting Social Movement and Civil Society Challenges to Research Agenda, *Science Technology & Human Values*, 35(4), 444–473.

Ganchoff, Chris (2008) Speaking for stem cells. Biomedical Activism and Emerging Forms of Patienthood, in S. Chambré and M. Goldner (eds) *Patients, Consumers, and Civil Society*, Bingley: Emerald, 225–245.

Grob, Rachel (2011) A House on Fire: Newborn Screening, Parents' Advocacy, and the Discourse of Urgency, in B. Hoffman, N. Tomes, M. Schlesinger and R. Grob (eds) *Patients as Policy Actors*, New Brunswick, NJ and London: Rutgers University Press, 231–256.

Hess, David J. (1999) *Evaluating Alternative Cancer Therapies*, New Brunswick, NJ: Rutgers University Press.

Hess, David J. (2004) Medical Modernisation, Scientifi c Research Fields, and the Epistemic Politics of Health Social Movements, *Sociology of Health and Illness*, 26(6), 695–709.

Hess, David J. (2007) *Alternative Pathways in Science and Industry: Activism, Innovation, and the Environment in an Era of Globalization*, Cambridge, MA: MIT Press.

Hess, David J. (2009) The Potentials and Limitations of Civil Society Research: Getting Undone Science Done, *Sociological Inquiry*, 79(3), 306–327.

Hess, David J. (2010) Environmental Reform Organizations and Undone Science in the United States: Exploring the Environmental, Health, and Safety Implications of Nanotechnology, *Science as Culture*, 19(2), 181–214.

Hoffman, Beatrix; Tomes, Nancy; Grob, Rachel and Schlesinger, Mark (2011) *Patients as Policy Actors*, New Brunswick, NJ and London: Rutgers University Press.

Huyard, Caroline (2012) *Rare: Sur la Cause Politique des Maladies Peu Fréquentes*, Paris: Editions de l'Ecole des Hautes Etudes en Sciences Sociales.

Innes, Anthea; Archibald, Carole and Murphy, Charlie (eds) (2004) *Dementia and Social Inclusion: Marginalised Groups and Marginalised Areas of Dementia Research, Care and Practice*, London and Philadelphia, PA: Jessica Kingsley Publishers.

Kanellopoulou, Nadja (2009) Advocacy Groups as Research Organizations: Novel Approaches in Research Governance, in C. Lyall, T. Papaioannou and J. Smith (eds) *The Limits to Governance: The Challenge of Policy-making for the New Life Sciences*, Farnham and Burlington, VT: Ashgate, 193–216.

Klawiter, Maren (2008) *The Biopolitics of Breast Cancer: Changing Cultures of Disease and Activism*, Minneapolis, MN: Univ. of Minnesota Press.

Koivusalo, Meri and Tritter, Jonathan (2011) Citizens, Consumers and Stakeholders in European Health Policy, in H. Löfgren, E. de Leeuw and M. Leahy (eds) *Democratizing Health: Consumer Groups in the Policy Process*, Cheltenham and Northampton, MA: Edward Elgar, 47–60.

Ley, Barbara (2009) *From Pink to Green: Disease Prevention and the Environmental Breast Cancer Movement*, New Brunswick, NJ: Rutgers University Press.

Löfgren, Hans; de Leeuw, Evelyne and Leahy, Michael (eds) (2011) *Democratizing Health: Consumer Groups in the Policy Process*, Cheltenham and Northampton, MA: Edward Elgar.

Martin, Graham (2008) "Ordinary People Only": Knowledge, Representativeness, and the Publics of Public Participation in Healthcare, *Sociology of Health and Illness*, 30(1), 35–54.

McCormick, Sabrina (2009a) *No Family History: The Environmental Links to Breast Cancer*, Lanham, MD: Rowman & Littlefield.

McCormick, Sabrina (2009b) *Mobilizing Science: Movements, Participation, and the Remaking of Knowledge*, Philadelphia, PA: Temple University Press.

Minkler, Meredith and Wallerstein, Nina (eds) (2008) *Community-Based Participatory Research for Health: From Process to Outcomes*, 2nd edition, San Francisco, CA: Jossey-Bass.

Moss, Pamela and Teghtsoonian, Katherine (eds) (2008) *Contesting Illness: Process and Practices*, Toronto, Buffalo, NY and London: University of Toronto Press.

O'Donovan, Órla; Moreira, Tiago and Howlett, Etaoine (2013) Tracking Transformations in Health Movement Organisations: Alzheimer's Disease Organisations and their Changing "Cause Regimes", *Social Movement Studies: Journal of Social, Cultural and Political Protest*, 12(3), 316–334.

Ottinger, Gwen (2010) Buckets of Resistance: Standards and the Effectiveness of Citizen Science, *Science, Technology & Human Values*, 35(2), 244–270.

Panofsky, Aaron (2011) Generating Sociability to Drive Science: Patient Advocacy Organizations and Genetics Research, *Social Studies of Science*, 41(1), 31–57.

Parthasarathy, Shobita (2010) Breaking the Expertise Barrier: Understanding Activist Strategies in Science and Technology Policy Domains, *Science and Public Policy*, 37(5), 355–367.

Pols, Jeanette (2014) Knowing Patients: Turning Patient Knowledge into Science, *Science, Technology & Human Values*, 39(1), 73–97.

Prior, Lindsay (2003) Belief, Knowledge and Expertise: the Emergence of the Lay Expert in Medical Sociology, *Sociology of Health and Illness*, 25(3), 41–57.

Rabeharisoa, Vololona and Callon, Michel (1999) *Le Pouvoir des Malades: L'association Française Contre les Myopathies et la Recherche*, Paris: Presses de l'École des Mines.

Rabeharisoa, Vololona and Callon, Michel (2002) The Involvement of Patients' Associations in Research, *International Social Science Journal*, 54(171), 57–65.

Sulik, Gayle A. (2009) Managing Biomedical Uncertainty: the Technoscientific Illness Identity, *Sociology of Health and Illness*, 31(7), 1059–1076.

Sunder Rajan, Kaushik (2008) Biocapital as an Emergent Form of Life: Speculations on the Figure of the Experimental Subject, in S. Gibbon and C. Novas (eds) *Biosocialities, Genetics and the Social Sciences: Making Biologies and Identities*, London and New York: Routledge, 157–187.

Terry, Sharon F.; Terry, Patrick F.; Rauen, Katherine A.; Uitto, Jouni and Bercovitch, Lionel G. (2007) Advocacy Groups as Research Organizations: The PXE International Example, *Nature Reviews Genetics*, 8(2), 157–164.

Thompson, Jill; Bissell, Paul; Cooper, Cindy; Armitage, Chris J. and Barber, Rosemary (2012) Credibility and the "Professionalized" Lay Expert: Reflections on the Dilemmas and Opportunities of Public Involvement in Health Research, *Health*, 16(6), 602–618.

Tomes, Nancy (2011) From Outsiders to Insiders: The Consumer-Survivor Movement and Its Impact on U.S. Mental Health Policy, in B. Hoffman, N. Tomes, R. Grob and M. Schlesinger (eds) *Patients as Policy Actors*, New Brunswick, NJ and London: Rutgers University Press, 113–131.

Tritter, Jonathan and Koivusalo, Meri (2013) Undermining Patient and Public Engagement and Limiting its Impact: The Consequences of the Health and Social Care Act 2012 on Collective Patient and Public Involvement, *Health Expectations*, 16(2), 115–118.

Wailoo, Keith and Pemberton, Stephen (2006) *The Troubled Dream of Genetic Medicine: Ethnicity and innovation in Tay-Sachs, Cystic Fibrosis, and Sickle Cell Disease*, Baltimore: Johns Hopkins University Press.

Wehling, Peter (2012) From Invited to Uninvited Participation (and Back?): Rethinking Civil Society Engagement in Technology Assessment and Development, *Poiesis & Praxis. International Journal of Technology Assessment and Ethics of Science*, 9(1–2), 43–60.

Whelan, Emma (2007) "No One Agrees Except for Those of Us Who Have It": Endometriosis Patients as an Epistemological Community, *Sociology of Health and Illness*, 29(7), 957–982.

Wynne, Brian (2007) Public Participation in Science and Technology: Performing and Obscuring a Political–Conceptual Category Mistake, *East Asian Science, Technology and Society: an International Journal*, 1(1), 99–110.

Zavestoski, Stephen; Brown, Phil; Linder, Meadow; Mayer, Bryan and McCormick, Sabrina (2002) Science, Policy, Activism, and War: Defining the Health of Gulf War Veterans, *Science, Technology & Human Values*, 27(2), 171–205.

Part I

Empirical cases and theoretical perspectives

1 A seat at the table, "a lab of our own" and working with what we know now

How the US environmental breast cancer movement shapes research

Lori Baralt

Introduction

Breast cancer is the most common cancer in women in the United States and the second leading cause of cancer death in US women after lung cancer (American Cancer Society 2013). Given the prevalence of breast cancer, particularly in the US, where one in eight women will develop breast cancer in her lifetime, it is not surprising that many women became concerned and began to advocate for more research on this disease. While early breast cancer advocacy in the 1970s and 1980s focused on providing support for women with breast cancer, reducing the social stigma surrounding breast cancer, increasing funding for medical research on the disease, and promoting breast cancer screening, the trajectory of breast cancer advocacy over the past 40 years in the US has been and continues to be complex and multifaceted.

In this chapter, I discuss the breast cancer advocacy landscape in the US, focusing on the challenges that environmental breast cancer advocates have posed, both to mainstream biomedical breast cancer advocacy and to the current limited biomedical approach to breast cancer research. I propose that the environmental breast cancer movement in the US is successfully challenging the deeply entrenched individual and genetic focused biomedical approach to breast cancer by advocating for and engaging in federally-funded environmental breast cancer research projects, developing "a lab of their own" and conducting their own research into environmental causes of breast cancer, and critiquing the call for "proof of harm" itself and advocating for the precautionary principle. Nevertheless, the environmental breast cancer movement faces challenges in demonstrating and remedying the environmental links to breast cancer, which will be discussed throughout this chapter.

The landscape of US breast cancer advocacy

Biomedical screening and early detection advocacy is the most prominent form of breast cancer advocacy in the US. Biomedical breast cancer advocates focus on the problem of lack of awareness and access to screening for breast cancer. They promote early detection and often fundraise to contribute to medical research on breast cancer in the name of finding a cure. Komen for the Cure, founded in 1982 by the younger sister of Susan G. Komen, who had died from breast cancer two years before, and today the largest and most financially successful breast cancer organization in the US, is largely associated with this approach to breast cancer advocacy. Given the biomedical focus of this type of advocacy, these advocates generally have a positive view of the medical establishment overall, seeing them as allies in the quest to conquer breast cancer. Many of the organizations associated with this approach to breast cancer advocacy have elite and often professional origins, often having been initiated by corporations (e.g. Avon, Estée Lauder) and celebrity or wealthy families who formed organizations after losing a member of their family to breast cancer (e.g. Komen for the Cure). Drawing on the rhetoric of the 1970s women's health movement, these organizations in practice often function more as philanthropic charities, but have self-identified as social movements (King 2006; Klawiter 2008). They do not challenge the biomedical model of addressing breast cancer, but rather engage with medical research by raising money that can be funneled into breast cancer research, which typically focuses on genes, individual risk factors (e.g., body fat, diet, exercise, alcohol consumption), and pharmacological treatments. Representatives from these organizations often have a seat at the table on government panels for cancer research, but they do not usually challenge the status quo with regard to research priorities. Rather, they seek to increase the funding for biomedical breast cancer research.

In stark contrast to biomedical breast cancer advocacy, environmental and cancer prevention activist organizations (e.g. Breast Cancer Action, Massachusetts Breast Cancer Coalition, Breast Cancer Fund, Zero Breast Cancer), which first emerged in the early 1990s have grassroots origins, often developing in communities where cancer clusters appear to exist, predominantly in Cape Cod, Massachusetts, Long Island, New York, and the San Francisco Bay Area in California. Rather than working toward gaining greater access to biomedical screening and treatment in its current state, they advocate a new inclusive scientific paradigm. The environmental breast cancer movement can be understood as an "embodied health movement," in which activists address "disease, disability or illness experience by challenging science on etiology, diagnosis, treatment and/or prevention" (Brown and Zavestoski 2005: 7). Environmental breast cancer activists take a critical stance toward science and medical professionals. They have sought to strategically partner with scientists to investigate the increased cancer incidence rates in their communities. These activists and the organizations that they have developed draw on the feminist tradition of health activism and AIDS activism, and also have strong connections to environmental health and justice movements (Klawiter 2008).

The development of environmental and prevention-oriented breast cancer activism is largely due to the fact that many women who were affected by breast cancer, particularly in communities where they noticed many other women being diagnosed with breast cancer, began to question the causes of the disease more deeply and began to see breast cancer as a "contested illness." Contested illnesses are conditions that are "either unexplained by current medical knowledge or have purported environmental explanations that are often disputed by medical professionals and scientists" (Brown and Zavestoski 2005: 7). People concerned with these illnesses may collectively organize to achieve medical recognition, treatment, and/or increased medical research (Brown and Zavestoski 2005). In some cases where environmental factors are suspected, advocacy groups may strive to shift attention away from strictly medical explanations of the disease and call for research into environmental causes and prevention of the illness (Brody and Rudel 2003; Brody et al. 2005; Brown et al. 2006; Eisenstein 2001; Krimsky 2000; McCormick et al. 2004; Steingraber 2000).

Breast cancer is a contested illness due to the lack of a definitive explanation of its etiology. Because much medical research is focused on individual bodies at the cellular, hormonal and genetic levels, the context beyond this bodily level of understanding is often absent. Additionally, in the current "human genome era" the emphasis of biomedical research is primarily focused on genetic understandings of diseases (Rooser 2000). Despite the much celebrated discovery of the BRCA-1 and BRCA-2 gene mutations in the 1990s, genetic predispositions to breast cancer account for only about five to ten percent of all breast cancer cases (Klawiter 2002). These genetic mutations are not particularly prevalent in the population and cannot explain the majority of women who are diagnosed with breast cancer and do not have genetic mutations. "Medical researchers supplement this account of breast cancer causation, which fails to explain 90–95% of breast cancer cases, with a focus on 'lifestyle factors' (e.g., diet, exercise) to explain the rest of the occurrences" (Baralt 2010: 288). In particular, medical professionals tend to explain the increasing rates of breast cancer, particularly among women in industrialized countries, by citing changing reproductive behaviors (Aronowitz 2007). Delayed childbearing or lack of childbearing, birthing fewer children, not breastfeeding (or breastfeeding for only a short period of time), and using hormone replacement therapy all increase a woman's lifetime exposure to estrogen, which is associated with increased breast cancer risk (Aronowitz 2007). Additionally, the increasing rate of breast cancer, particularly in (but not limited to) more developed countries, is often explained within the medical field as an artifact of improved medical detection and increased screening (Aronowitz 2007). This explanation alone, however, only accounts for between 25 and 40 percent of the increase. The rest of the increase remains unexplained (Brody 2010; McCormick 2010). Thus, in contrast to a disease like lung cancer, where a clear link has been drawn between smoking and lung cancer risk and only a limited number of cases remain unexplained, breast cancer remains an elusive disease despite much medical research.

To date, the large majority of breast cancer research has been on detection and treatment, even though a growing number of women with breast cancer and environmental breast cancer activists are concerned with causes of the disease and prevention. While research on breast cancer risk factors such as genetic mutations, childbearing history, body fat, alcohol consumption and sedentary lifestyle has been well-documented and publicized in an effort to reduce women's risk of developing the disease, environmental breast cancer activists have been calling for more research into environmental factors that may be contributing to breast cancer risk. These activists focus on particular environmental links to breast cancer (Brown et al. 2006; Eisenstein 2001; Potts 2004; Steingraber 2000). This push for research into breast cancer and the environment has led to a fruitful area of research that is demonstrating the complexity of breast cancer causation and the role that various environmental factors play in contributing to breast cancer risk (Gray 2010).

Since the early 1990s, environmental breast cancer activists have engaged with medical researchers to shape the breast cancer research agenda. Their methods of engaging with scientifi c research have been varied. One approach has involved advocating for research into environmental links to breast cancer that would include some form of participatory research, meaning that the breast cancer activists themselves would be involved in the research process (see 26ff.). Based on the potential as well as the challenges of this approach, which will be discussed later, environmental breast cancer activists decided to take environmental breast cancer research into their own hands by creating "a lab of their own", the Silent Spring Institute (Silent Spring Institute 2013a) (see 31ff.). Finally, also fueled by the frustration that environmental breast cancer activists have experienced regarding the standard of proof in traditional medical and epidemiological research, many environmental breast cancer activists are shaping medical research from the outside by 1) publicly challenging the biomedical narrative of medical progress toward fi nding a cure, 2) pushing medical researchers as well as other breast cancer advocacy organizations to demand research into environmental causes of breast cancer, and 3) calling for corporate accountability and governmental regulation based on the existing scientific knowledge on environmental links to breast cancer (see 34ff.).

A seat at the table: advocating for and collaborating on federally-funded breast cancer research projects

As stated previously, environmental breast cancer activism emerged in areas of the US where women who had breast cancer noticed that women around them were increasingly being diagnosed with the same disease. In the wake of environmental disasters such as Love Canal and the publication of Rachel Carson's groundbreaking *Silent Spring*, many of these women began questioning whether there was something in their environment that was contributing to the seemingly high levels of breast cancer cases. Early engagement with research often involved breast cancer mapping projects that activists conducted themselves by going door-to-door to find out where women who were being diagnosed with breast cancer were living. They were looking for patterns in the geography of breast cancer diagnoses to begin to better understand what was happening in their communities. Environmental breast cancer activists began these mapping projects in the San Francisco Bay Area in California, which was reported in the early 1990s to have the highest incidence rate of breast cancer in the world (Zero Breast Cancer 2013) as well as Long Island, New York, and Cape Cod, Massachusetts. All of these regions had breast cancer incidence rates that were higher than the national average (McCormick et al. 2003; McCormick et al. 2004).

The Long Island breast cancer research study project

In all three of these geographic locations of what are now commonly referred to as "cancer clusters", environmental breast cancer activists began working to shape and engage in research into environmental causes of breast cancer. Breast cancer activists sought public funding for environmental breast cancer research. In Long Island, local breast cancer organizations joined together to form the Long Island Breast Cancer Network (Kabat 2008; National Cancer Institute 2002). The organization consisted of women who were politically savvy and well-educated about breast cancer. They worked to form the National Breast Cancer Coalition to advocate for increased funding for breast cancer research in Congress. These environmental breast cancer activists lobbied Congressional Representatives in the early 1990s and in 1993 Congress passed Public Law 103–43 (Kabat 2008). The law, entitled "Study of Elevated Breast Cancer Rates in Long Island", would become the first federally funded study of potential environmental causes of breast cancer (National Cancer Institute 2013). The law called on the head of the National Cancer Institute (NCI) in collaboration with the head of the National Institute of Environmental Health Sciences (NIEHS) to conduct research in two of the counties in Long Island that were of particular concern to activists. The law specified the location of the study, the methodology of the study, and certain elements of the study, such as the use of a geographic information system to evaluate current and past exposures of individuals to certain contaminants (National Cancer Institute 2013). Although the law was generated by activist support, the research grants themselves were awarded to academic scientists, who had some discretion regarding the specific chemicals that would be investigated. Some activists felt left out of this part of the process and many were dissatisfied with the researchers' choice to focus on organochlorine compounds (e.g., DDT, DDE, chlordane) (Brody et al. 2005; McCormick et al. 2003). There were many chemicals of concern that activists wanted to have included in the study, which were not included. Furthermore, activists wanted a study that could potentially produce actionable results, meaning recommendations regarding chemical regulation and exposure reduction. The organochlorine compounds chosen by the researchers were already banned from use, so the findings would not be directly actionable (Brody et al. 2005).

Although environmental breast cancer activists succeeded politically in demonstrating the importance of environmental breast cancer research, which led to the development of this $31 million federally funded research project, the end results were mixed for activists. Before the long-awaited results of the study were published in 2002, activists already felt discontented with the study. Their participation was not clearly outlined in the research mandate and many felt that the researchers pursued their own agendas and did not take their priorities or concerns into consideration (McCormick et al. 2003). The study found no association between blood serum levels of DDE, chlordane, or dieldrin measured near the time of diagnosis with breast cancer (Gammond et al. 2002). Environmental breast cancer activists felt disillusioned by the results and by the process that led to them (Brody et al. 2005; McCormick et al. 2003).

This early collaboration between environmental breast cancer activists and medical researchers highlighted some of the challenges that these activists continue to face in their attempts to shape an environmental breast cancer research agenda. One of the main challenges is deciding who sets the research agenda. By calling for research into environmental links to breast cancer and actually getting funding for this research, Long Island breast cancer activists made significant progress in shaping the medical research agenda by actually getting environmental breast cancer research funded. That said, activists were frustrated that chemicals of concern went unstudied. The researchers themselves set this part of the agenda, leaving the activists feeling left out of a significant part of the research process. Additionally, medical research itself is limited in its ability to address environmental causes of diseases. Methodologically, this study in particular was based on serum measures close to the time of diagnosis (Brody et al. 2005). What environmental breast cancer researchers and activists are increasingly understanding about environmental links to breast cancer is that the timing of exposures is likely significant and that there are windows of susceptibility in breast development where exposures to certain toxins may increase the risk of breast cancer many years later (Brody et al. 2005; Brody 2010). Finally, the medical research paradigm is based on a standard of proof in which a study must demonstrate that A causes B (Brody et al. 2005). In other words, mainstream scientific approaches tend "to err on the side of uncertainty" (McCormick et al. 2004). The accumulation of strong evidence of correlation is not enough to meet this standard of proof. This poses a great challenge to environmental breast cancer activists, who want to act on the current evidence regarding environmental causes of breast cancer in creating individual and policy recommendations, while continuing to conduct more research and develop more appropriate methodologies to study the effects of various chemicals on humans.

Breast cancer and the environment research program

Even before the Long Island Breast Cancer Study Project (LIBCSP) was completed, officials at the NIEHS as well as environmental breast cancer activists anticipated the need for further study. In 2002, the NIEHS convened a brainstorming workshop, which included breast cancer activists, researchers and clinicians to "identify data gaps, bottlenecks and research needs" (BCERP 2010). The workshop participants reached a general decision to "promote research that would characterize environmental exposures over the lifetime that could alter the risk of breast cancer development" (BCERP 2010). Based on this decision, the NCI and the NIEHS released a Request for Applications (RFA). The RFA stated that the primary goal was to establish a

> network of research centers in which multidisciplinary teams of scientists, clinicians, and breast cancer advocates work collaboratively on a unique set of scientific questions that focus on how chemical, physical, biological and social factors in the environment work together with genetic factors to cause breast cancer.
>
> (National Institute of Health 2002)

In 2003, they established the Breast Cancer and Environment Research Centers (BCERCs) Network, which consisted of four BCERCs throughout the US, specifi ally in San Francisco, California; Cincinnati, Ohio; Philadelphia, Pennsylvania; and East Lansing, Michigan (Baralt and McCormick 2010). The BCERCs were created to study the "impact of prepubertal exposures that may affect pubertal development and predispose a woman to breast cancer" (BCERP 2010). Pubertal development is considered to be one of the "windows of susceptibility," "where the developing breast may be more vulnerable to environmental exposures" (BCERP 2010). The BCERC program spanned from 2003–2010, with the NCI and NIEHS committing $35 million over the seven years.

Knowing the frustrations that many environmental breast cancer activists experienced coming out of the LIBCSP, the NCI and NIEHS structured the BCERCs differently. For one thing, as mentioned previously, activists were included in the brainstorming workshop that would frame the focus of the research. Additionally, the NCI and NIEHS designed a "more formalized structure for advocate participation in the centers, particularly with regard to translation and dissemination of research findings" (Baralt and McCormick 2010: 1669). Breast cancer activists were included in the centers through the RFA-mandated Community Outreach and Translation Cores (COTC) that would develop and implement strategies to translate the scientific findings of the centers into information for the public and policy makers (National Institute of Health 2002).

Despite activists being included in the initial brainstorming workshop for the centers and being included in the COTCs of each center, there were still gaps in activist participation. Once the RFA was released, researchers from across the country could apply for the funding. They had to at least name breast cancer advocacy organizations that they could collaborate with in their application, but the advocacy organizations were not necessarily involved in the application process or in deciding the research emphasis of the proposal (Baralt and McCormick 2010). Additionally, based on our research on the BCERCs from 2005 to 2007, McCormick and I found that there were two main challenges to the advocate/researcher collaboration: first, a lack of understanding and training in community based participatory research as an alternative inquiry paradigm and, second, divergent prior assumptions as well as desired and expected outcomes regarding environmental causes of breast cancer (Baralt and McCormick 2010).

Although the BCERCs used elements of community based participatory research (CBPR) philosophy by developing research centers based on researchers collaborating with community activists, there were still challenges to implementing this research model. CBPR is based on contextualizing scientific research within particular communities and legitimizing knowledge, understandings, and priorities of advocates that represent the affected groups (Israel et al. 1998; Minkler 2005; Minkler and Wallerstein 2008). CBPR has been particularly relevant for researching health issues such as breast cancer, where traditional biomedical approaches have proven insufficient (Brody et al. 2005, 2007; Brody and Rudel 2003; Brown et al. 2006; McCormick et al. 2004; O'Fallon and Dearry 2002). Based on an alternative inquiry paradigm, in which those affected by the issue at hand participate in the research process, the role of advocates is crucial in this research model. This is in direct contrast to the positivist paradigm that remains the dominant model of scientific inquiry, in which an emphasis is placed on objectivity and the researcher is thought to be neutral and free of bias (Baralt and McCormick 2010). Many of the researchers and some of the activists were new to this type of research model, leading to some confusion about the appropriate role of the activists in the research process.

Additionally, a crucial aspect to conducting research on environmental causes of breast cancer involves defining what is meant by "environment." This is a recurring issue of contention for environmental breast cancer activists with medical research on breast cancer. The RFA for the BCERCs defined the environment very broadly, so that it could include things like diet, stress, smoking, alcohol consumption, as well as pesticide exposure and other chemical exposures. Environmental breast cancer activists are particularly concerned with research on environmental toxicants as they relate to breast cancer. They argue that research on things like diet, stress, smoking and other individual risk factors have been extensively researched and the focus needs to shift to studying environmental toxins (Baralt and McCormick 2010). Similar to the LIBCSP, activists engaged with the BCERCs were also interested in actionable results. They desired findings that could lead to public health policy and chemical regulation changes that can work toward breast cancer prevention. Researchers, on the other hand, tend to emphasize the small scale of projects like this, and based on a medical model standard of proof, the unlikelihood of having certain results from just this project.

Despite the challenges faced by environmental breast cancer activists working with the LIBCSP and the BCERCs, this type of collaborative research has much potential and many activists and researchers are committed to continuing these types of projects. In 2009, the NIEHS and the NCI extended the funding for the BCERCs, now Breast Cancer and Environment Research Program (BCERP), to "complete the initial population studies, expand upon recent findings, and continue efforts to include and inform the engaged breast cancer community" (BCERP 2010). These projects are helping to develop innovative forms of alternative inquiry paradigms, not based on "objective" of "bias-free" science, but based on the concerns of those impacted by the disease being studied. In particular, these alternative inquiry paradigms base research on activists' concerns and often early-stage research by activists in affected communities. By engaging in these collaborative research projects with medical researchers, environmental breast cancer activists are shifting the research paradigm from a strictly medical model to a more environmental health and public health model. The environmental breast cancer movement is using these research projects to support public health prevention efforts and chemical regulation, which will be further discussed later in the chapter.

"A lab of our own": an activist-led research agenda

As discussed above, strong scientific evidence of links between particular environmental toxins and breast cancer have been difficult to find, largely due to the standard of proof used in traditional scientific research. This has led to skepticism on the part of some researchers and much frustration for breast cancer activists who are seeking answers that can be translated into actionable precautionary measures and policies. A group of breast cancer activists from the Massachusetts Breast Cancer Coalition in conjunction with scientists founded Silent Spring Institute in 1994 in response to the above-average rates of breast cancer in 11 of the 15 towns on Cape Cod (Silent Spring Institute 2007a) and to define their own research priorities and engage in research collaborations on their own terms. Similar to the activists in Long Island, these activists sought public funding for research into breast cancer and the environment. In 1994, they succeeded when they won passage of a bill in Massachusetts that would provide $1 million a year for research on breast cancer and the environment. This was another significant political achievement for the environmental breast cancer movement. The passage of the bill was facilitated both by the active political engagement of environmental breast cancer activists and the existing research that demonstrated that Cape Cod, Massachusetts had "a history of elevated breast cancer incidence – 20 percent above the state average"

(McCormick et al. 2004: 632). With this funding, they founded "a laboratory of their own" and "named it Silent Spring Institute in tribute to Rachel Carson, whose landmark book, *Silent Spring*, launched the modern environmental movement" (Silent Spring Institute 2007a). The activists and scientists who founded Silent Spring Institute felt that too much money for breast cancer research was going toward treatment and detection and not enough toward finding preventable causes of the disease (Brody and Rudel, personal communication). The Institute states that its research agenda is defined by the following priorities.

- Focus on the environment, an under-studied area that can lead to the discovery of preventable causes of cancer, particularly in communities with higher risk.
- Make women's health, especially breast cancer, a central rather than peripheral research priority.
- Support innovation, including new research methods and pilot studies to test new hypotheses.
- Foster multidisciplinary teams of researchers to integrate their strengths.
- Foster true collaboration among scientists, physicians, and community members (Silent Spring Institute 2007a).

These priorities are driven by breast cancer activists themselves and demonstrate an important shift in the understanding of medical research itself. By defining their own priorities and approaches to research, the collaborating activists and scientists at Silent Spring Institute are able to avoid some of the challenges faced by advocate/scientist collaborations in the LIBCSP and the BCERC/BCERPs. For one, environmental breast cancer activists prioritize research focusing on the environment, as they define it, which as discussed above is often different from how it is defined by medical researchers and in federal health agencies. The activists at Silent Spring Institute state that despite decades of the "War on Cancer" in the US, breast cancer incidence continues to increase. They argue that this may be due to increased exposure to environmental toxins that have greatly increased in our environment since World War II, "when industry began pumping out pesticides, plastics, solvents, and other chemicals, leaving residues in our air, water, and soil" (Silent Spring Institute 2007b). Despite growing evidence that environmental factors may contribute to breast cancer risk, "few studies have investigated the effects of modern chemicals on women's breast health" (Silent Spring Institute 2007b). Research focusing on such effects may find ways to prevent breast cancer from developing or, at least, to reduce the risk of breast cancer. This is the main priority of environmental breast cancer activist-initiated research.

Silent Spring Institute represents a community-based participatory research model with an activist-led agenda. The Institute is run and staffed by researchers who are dedicated to "science that serves the public interest"

(Silent Spring Institute 2007c). The Institute "partners with physicians, public health and community advocates and other scientists to identify and break the links between environmental chemicals and women's health, especially breast cancer" (Ruthann Rudel, personal communication). Whereas projects like the LIBCSP and the BCERP are based on federally-funded grants that are given directly to scientists, who then collaborate with community activists, Silent Spring Institute was not only initiated by environmental breast cancer activists, but remains under their direction. According to Julia Brody, executive director, and Ruthann Rudel, director of research, the Institute's "pioneering community-based approach to research has transformed the traditional dynamic between 'scientist' and 'subject' so both are working side-by-side to uncover findings that can help save lives and stop people from getting sick in the first place" (personal communication). Because environmental breast cancer activists set the research agenda, in its 15 years of existence the Institute has been able to focus on health risks associated with toxins "where we live and work – areas that have been ignored in cancer research" (Brody and Rudel, personal communication).

The work of Silent Spring Institute has fundamentally challenged the medical research paradigm's ability to address environmental causes of breast cancer. Medical research paradigms rely on human clinical trials and epidemiologic studies of exposures. As discussed previously, they are based on a standard of proof of definitive causation. This approach is very limited when it comes to studying environmental links to breast cancer, as it is not possible to conduct human clinical trials with a control group when investigating the potential relationship between environmental toxins and breast cancer. This is because there is no control group. We are all exposed to varying extents to a variety of chemicals over the course of a lifetime. Additionally, breast cancer is not a disease that develops immediately after an exposure, making understanding the potential significance of the timing of exposures difficult. It is also difficult to separate out the effects of individual toxins, since we are exposed to a variety of toxins at once, and there is potential that they interact with each other in unknown ways as well. Additionally, whereas toxicology relies on a dose-response model to understand the effects of chemicals on the body, this is not a useful model when examining long term exposures and exposures to multiple chemicals at once.

The researchers at Silent Spring Institute, on the other hand, are developing a different way of understanding environmental links to breast cancer. They argue that we should rely on "animal and cell studies of biological mechanisms coupled with human exposure studies, using these types of evidence as a basis for public health intervention to reduce exposure" (Brody 2010: 2). Their goal is to develop information on the role that various toxic chemicals play with regard to breast cancer so it can be used to reduce exposures to suspect chemicals (Brody and Rudel, personal communication). The Institute is developing an "environmental health paradigm" (Brody 2010: 2). This research paradigm is fundamentally distinct from medical research paradigms, in that it does not rely on definitive proof for action. Rather, it utilizes a different standard of proof in which the Institute recommends acting in the interest of public health based on "early warnings from studies that show a chemical affects cancer mechanisms in animals or cells, and that people are substantially exposed to" (Brody 2010: 2). Rather than waiting for definitive proof that certain chemicals cause human harm before acting, the activists and researchers at Silent Spring Institute are calling for a new emphasis on cancer prevention that is focused on reducing and eliminating people's exposures to toxic chemicals. According to Brody and Rudel, "this change is exemplified in recent authoritative reports from the Institute of Medicine and the President's Cancer Panel, which have adopted our perspective that we should reduce exposure to chemicals shown in laboratory studies to potentially affect breast cancer, because evidence in humans is so difficult to get that waiting for it is tantamount to doing nothing" (Brody and Rudel, personal communication). The fact that that these large scale reports are echoing the call for research into environmental links to breast cancer demonstrates the wide-reaching effects that Silent Spring Institute and other activist-initiated research into environmental causes of breast cancer have had on the medical research agenda.

Working with existing evidence and demanding systemic change

In addition to engaging in collaborative and activist-led research initiatives, the environmental breast cancer movement also plays an important role in shaping medical research from outside. Environmental breast cancer organizations do this by critically responding to medical research agendas, inspiring public awareness and concern about the role of the environment in breast cancer risk, and calling for a public health approach to breast cancer risk by advocating for implementation of the precautionary principle to create systemic change to reduce everyone's risk of breast cancer. However, despite the tireless efforts of environmental breast cancer activists in initiating and engaging in research on environmental links to breast cancer, most physicians, breast cancer researchers, advocates, and the public remain predominantly focused on individual risk factors (e.g., diet, alcohol consumption, reproductive behavior) rather than systemic change focused on preventing chemical exposures that might be contributing to increasing rates of breast cancer. The environmental breast cancer movement nevertheless plays an important role in shifting the dominant discourse around breast cancer from an individual risk focus to a public health and prevention focus. By drawing attention to potential environmental links to breast cancer, the environmental breast cancer movement shapes medical research by shifting the public's focus and concern.

Even environmental breast cancer activists who are not engaged in the actual research process influence breast cancer research and the public's perception of this research through providing critical assessment of research agendas and reports. Breast Cancer Action, an environment and prevention-focused breast cancer organization in San Francisco and the self-proclaimed watchdog of the breast cancer movement, regularly provides critical comments on widely-publicized medical reports. In 2011, for example, the Institute of Medicine (IOM) released a report based on their review of the current state of the evidence on breast cancer and the environment, gene-environment interactions, and challenges in investigating environmental links to breast cancer. Although the report was viewed by some as being supportive of more research into environmental links to breast cancer, Breast Cancer Action issued a press release critical of the report. In the press release, Karuna Jaggar, Executive Director of Breast Cancer Action, stated that "The IOM Report fails to turn the tide on this epidemic because it misses some important opportunities to implement real changes" (Breast Cancer Action 2011). As Jaggar states, the IOM researchers "too broadly define the environment as all factors not directly inherited through DNA which includes anything from genetic changes to tissue, to stress, to lifestyle choices and changes in abdominal fat rather than the chemicals we are all exposed to in our everyday lives" (Breast Cancer Action 2011). Once again, breast cancer activists lamented the fact that mainstream medical research continues to define the environment so broadly that it leads to research on the same individual and lifestyle factors that have been studied for years, while, as Jaggar states, missing "an opportunity to focus on relatively unknown areas of the environment" (Breast Cancer Action 2011). Breast Cancer Action, as well as other environmental breast cancer organizations, regularly follow and provide feedback on such medical reports, which often set the agenda for medical research. In doing so, they push medical science further, particularly with regard to their conceptualization of the environment.

Additionally, the environmental breast cancer movement has also worked to shift the culture of breast cancer advocacy in the US. While many breast cancer advocacy organizations still focus on the same messages of early detection as the answer to the breast cancer epidemic, environmental breast cancer activists challenge this narrative, shifting public understanding of the disease, which may lead to a broader push for research on environmental causes of breast cancer. For example, since 2002, Breast Cancer Action has engaged in a Think Before You Pink Campaign during the month of October, which is National Breast Cancer Awareness Month. For years, the campaign focused on challenging corporations that were selling pink ribbon products while at the same time contributing to breast cancer risk due to chemicals in their products. The organization coined the term "pinkwashing" to refer to this practice. In recent years, the campaigns have taken on a broader focus. In 2012, the campaign urged people to call on their elected officials to sign on to Breast Cancer Action's Mandate for Government Action, which urged governmental officials to make a commitment to support research on causes of breast cancer and regulate harmful chemicals that are linked to breast cancer (Think Before You Pink 2013). In 2013, the Toxic Time Is Up campaign encouraged people to sign a petition demanding that elected officials "enact meaningful chemical safety reform to reduce the risk of a range of devastating diseases and disorders, including breast cancer" (Breast Cancer Action 2013). The organization gathered over 30,000 signatures on the petition, which called on the Senate Committee on Environment and Public Works to "overhaul and update the Toxic Substance Control Act (TSCA) of 1976." These types of campaigns put the burden of proof of chemical safety on the government, rather than on individual consumers or even on breast cancer or other health activists. They are based on the precautionary principle, which environmental breast cancer activists broadly support, which argues that the burden of proof should be on the government or corporations to determine that a chemical is safe for public health, rather than on individuals to prove that it is not.

By promoting the precautionary principle, environmental breast cancer activists shift the medical research paradigm that many mainstream breast cancer organizations promote. Commitment to the precautionary principle is part of a public health and prevention-oriented paradigm. In a way, it sidesteps the issue of medical research by calling for the government to take responsibility for regulation of toxic chemicals based on the current state of knowledge, rather than waiting for certainty from medical research studies. In this way, the environmental breast cancer movement is changing the public understanding of and conversation around breast cancer, including shifting the focus away from detection, treatment, and cure to causes and prevention, which impacts the medical research agenda.

Conclusion

While the general trend of breast cancer activism in the US has focused on medical research on detection and treatment as well as lifestyle risk factors, over the past 30 years the environmental breast cancer movement has played an important role in challenging this culture of health activism. Breast cancer activists have organized in communities with particularly high rates of breast cancer and have successfully lobbied the national and state governments for more funding on potential environmental links to breast cancer. Many of these activists have become fluent in scientific language and have engaged in collaboration with scientists and, in the case of Silent Spring Institute, have created their own activist-led research agenda. In doing so, they have challenged the definition of "environment" often used in medical research and the standard of proof often called for in scientific research. Additionally, they have noted the limits of current scientific methodologies in addressing the complexities of multiple environmental exposures over the life course. They posit that we must rely on the research that currently exists that suggests that certain chemicals are linked to increased breast cancer risk.

Based on current knowledge, environmental breast cancer activists have been at the forefront of advocating for the precautionary principle. They have worked to educate the public about environmental links to breast cancer in addition to insisting on corporate transparency and accountability and governmental chemical regulation.

Largely due to well-educated and politically savvy breast cancer activists who have organized and lobbied for environmental breast cancer research and have educated themselves in science to engage in collaborative research projects, the environmental breast cancer movement in the US has been successful in shaping medical research on breast cancer. That said, they are still swimming against the stream of medical research, where the vast majority of funding remains geared toward detection and treatment. Even when research is touted as environmental, it is often still focused on individual risk factors, not on the environmental concerns of activists. By engaging in collaborative research through federally-funded programs and through Silent Spring Institute, researchers are working to develop new methodologies to address the complexities of environmental exposures and gene–environment interactions. This might be one of the most fruitful aspects of the environmental breast cancer movement's engagement with research. Their engagement, through bringing to light new priorities for research, is actually challenging medical researchers, epidemiologists, and toxicologists to develop new methodologies and potentially new standards of proof to address areas of research that they may not otherwise have explored.

Given the frustration of many environmental breast cancer activists with the slow pace of medical research and the divide between the existing evidence that many chemical exposures do in fact contribute to breast cancer risk and the medical certainty of this, activists have also focused on creating awareness among the public about the evidence on environmental links to breast cancer. In this way, the environmental breast cancer movement simultaneously engages with medical research, while trying to sidestep it by encouraging the public and policymakers to act on existing evidence, rather than waiting for defi nitve proof. This two-pronged strategy has allowed the movement more flexibility in that, while medical research is an important aspect of environmental breast cancer advocacy, they are not beholden to the medical establishment. That said, environmental breast cancer activists have much work ahead of them in terms of increasing the funding for environmental breast cancer research. Governmental research budgets, and even the budget of Komen for the Cure, focus much more heavily on biomedical research questions. While environmental breast cancer research has increased, the process is slow-going and much more funding is needed. Given that only 200 of the over 100,000 chemicals currently used and produced in the US have been tested for safety, there is a lot of work to be done in the area of environmental health in general. Environmental breast cancer activists are continuing to push for research funding to understand the effects of these chemicals on mammary glands at different stages of development and on gene-environment interactions. Despite the challenges that they face, as the relationship between environmental breast cancer activists and medical researchers continues to be refined over years of collaboration, there seems to be much promise in the work that they can achieve together.

Acknowledgements

I would like to thank Karuna Jaggar, Executive Director of Breast Cancer Action, Julia Brody, Executive Director of Silent Spring Institute, and Ruthann Rudel, Director of Research at Silent Spring Institute for taking the time to share their thoughts with me.

References

American Cancer Society (2013) What are the Key Statistics about Breast Cancer? 24 October. Available online at: <www.cancer.org/cancer/breastcancer.detailed-guide/breast-cancer-key-statistics> (accessed 1 December 2013).

Aronowitz, Robert. A. (2007) *Unnatural History: Breast Cancer and American Society*, Cambridge: Cambridge University Press.

Baralt, Lori B. (2010) Breast cancer and the environment, in R. Friis (ed.) *Praeger Handbook of Environmental Health*, Volume Four, *Current Issues and Emerging Debates*, Westport, CT: Praeger Publishers, 287–310.

Baralt, Lori B. and McCormick, Sabrina (2010) A review of advocate-scientist collaboration in federally funded environmental breast cancer research centers, *Environmental Health Perspectives*, 118(12), 1668–1675.

BCERP (Breast Cancer and the Environment Research Program) (2010) *Background Information*. Available online at: <www.bcerp.org/about.htm> (accessed 1 December 2013).

Breast Cancer Action (2011) Breast Cancer Action says IOM Report Misses Important Opportunities to turn the tide on the epidemic. Available online at: <http://bcaction.org/2011/12/07/breast-cancer-action-says-iom-report-misses-important-opportunities-to-turn-the-tide-on-the-epidemic> (accessed 1 December 2013).

Breast Cancer Action (2013) Think Before You Pink: Toxic Time is Up! Available online at: <http://org2.salsalabs.com/o/6098/p/dia/action3/common/public/?action_KEY=15464> (accessed 1 December 2013).

Breast Cancer Action (2013) Chemical Safety Improvement Act Doesn't Go Nearly Far Enough Available online at: <http://bcaction.org/2013/05/31/chemical-reform-update-chemical-safety-improvement-act> (accessed 6 January 2014).

Brody, Julia G. (2010) Everyday exposures and breast cancer, *Reviews on Environmental Health*, 25(1), 1–7.

Brody, Julia G. and Rudel, Ruthann A. (2003) Environmental pollutants and breast cancer, *Environmental Health Perspectives*, 111(8), 1007–1019.

Brody, Julia G.; Tickner, Joel and Rudel, Ruthann A. (2005) Community-initiated breast cancer and environment studies and the precautionary principle, *Environmental Health Perspectives*, 113, 920–925.

Brody, Julia G.; Morello-Frosch, Rachel; Brown, Phil; Rudel, Ruthann A.; Altman, Rebecca G.; Frye, Margaret; Osimo, Cheryl C.; Perez, Carla and Seryak, Liesel M. (2007) Improving disclosures and consent: "is it safe?" New ethics for reporting personal exposures to environmental chemicals, *American Journal of Public Health*, 97(9), 1547–1554.

Brown, Phil and Zavestoski, Stephen (2005) Social movements in health: an introduction, in P. Brown and S. Zavestoski (eds) *Social Movements in Health*, Malden, MA: Blackwell Publishing, 1–16.

Brown, Phil; McCormick, Sabrina; Mayer, Brian; Zavestoski, Stephen; Morello-Frosch, Rachel; Altman, Rebecca G. and Senier, Laura (2006) "A lab of our own": Environmental causation of breast cancer and challenges to the dominant epidemiological paradigm, *Science, Technology, & Human Values*, 31(5), 499–536.

Eisenstein, Zillah R. (2001) *Manmade Breast Cancers*, Ithaca, NY: Cornell University Press.

Gammon, Marilie, D.; Wolff, Mary S.; Neugut, Alfred I.; Eng, Sybil M.; Teitelbaum, Susan L.; Britton, Julie A.; Terry, Mary Beth; Levin, Bruce et al. (2002) Environmental toxins and breast cancer on Long Island. II. Organochlorine compound levels in blood, *Cancer Epidemilogy Biomarkers & Prevention*, 11, 686–697.

Gray, Janet (2010) *State of the Evidence: The Connection between Breast Cancer and the Environment*, 6th edition, San Francisco: Breast Cancer Fund.

Israel, Barbara A.; Schultz, Amy J.; Parker, Edith A. and Becker, Adam B. (1998) Review of community-based participatory research: assessing partnership approaches to improve public health, *Annual Review of Public Health*, 19, 173–202.

Kabat, Geoffrey C. (2008) *Hyping Health Risks: Environmental Hazards in Daily Life and the Science of Epidemiology*, New York: Columbia University Press.

King, Samantha (2006) *Pink Ribbons, Inc.: Breast Cancer and the Politics of Philanthropy*, Minneapolis: University of Minnesota Press.

Klawiter, Maren (2002) Risk, prevention and the breast cancer continuum: the NCI, the FDA, health activism and the pharmaceutical industry, *History and Technology*, 18(4), 309–353.

Klawiter, Maren (2008) *The Biopolitics of Breast Cancer: Changing Cultures of Disease and Activism*, Minneapolis, MN: University of Minnesota Press.

Krimsky, Sheldon (2000) Environmental endocrine hypothesis and public policy, in P. Brown, S. Kroll-Smith and V.J. Gunter (eds) *Illness and the Environment: A Reader in Contested Medicine*, New York: New York University Press, 95–107.

McCormick, Sabrina; Brown Phil and Zavestoski, Stephen (2003) The personal is scientifi c, the scientifi c is political: The public paradigm of the environmental breast cancer movement, *Sociological Forum*, 18(4), 545–576.

McCormick, Sabrina; Brody, Julia G.; Brown, Phil and Polk, Ruth (2004) Public involvement in breast cancer research: An analysis and model for future research, *International Journal of Health Services*, 34(4), 625–646.

McCormick, Sabrina (2010) *No Family History: The Environmental Links to Breast Cancer*, Plymouth and Lanham, ML: Rowman and Littlefield.

Minkler, Meredith (2005) Community-based research partnerships: Challenges and opportunities, *Journal of Urban Health*, 82(S2), ii3–ii12.

Minkler, Meredith and Wallerstein, Nina (eds) (2008) *Community-Based Participatory Research for Health: From Process to Outcomes*, San Francisco: Jossey-Bass.

National Cancer Institute (2002) Long Island Breast Cancer Study Project (LIBCSP). Available online at: <www.cancer.gov/newscenter/qa/2002/long-island-environmentqa> (accessed 22 July 2014).

National Cancer Institute (1993) Study of elevated breast cancer rates in Long Island (past initiative), *Public Law* 103–43, 10 June. Available online at: <http://epi.grants.cancer.gov/past-initiatives/LIBCSP/PublicLaw.html> (accessed 1 December 2013).

National Institute of Health (2002) *Breast Cancer and the Environment Research Centers.* Available online at: <http://grants.nih.gov/grants/guide/rfa-files/RFA-ES-03-001.html> (accessed 1 December 2013).

O'Fallon, Liam R. and Dearry, Allen (2002) Community-based participatory research as a tool to advance environmental health sciences, *Environmental Health Perspectives,* 110(S2), 155–159.

Potts, Laura K. (2004) An epidemiology of women's lives: The environmental risk of breast cancer, *Critical Public Health,* 14(2), 133–147.

Rooser, Sue V. (2000) Controversies in breast cancer research, in A. S. Kasper and S. J. Ferguson (eds) *Breast Cancer: Society Shapes an Epidemic,* New York: St. Martin's Press, 245–271.

Silent Spring Institute (2007a) *The History of Silent Spring Institute.* Available online at: <www.silentspring.org/history-silent-spring-institute> (accessed 1 December 2013).

Silent Spring Institute (2007b) *Breast Cancer and the Environment.* Available online at: <www.silentspring.org/breast-cancer-and-environment> (accessed 1 December 2013).

Silent Spring Institute (2007c) *About Us.* Available online at: <www.silentspring.org/about-us> (accessed 1 December 2013).

Steingraber, Sandra (2000) The environmental link to breast cancer, in A. S. Kasper and S. J. Ferguson (eds) *Breast Cancer: Society Shapes an Epidemic,* New York: St. Martin's Press, 271–302.

Think Before You Pink (2013) *It's an Epidemic, Stupid!* Available online at: <www.thinkbeforeyoupink.org/?page_id=2089> (accessed 1 December 2013).

Zero Breast Cancer (2013) *Breast Cancer in Marin.* Available online at: <www.zerobreastcancer.org/breast-cancer-in-marin> (accessed 1 December 2013).

2 Initiating and funding medical research on a rare disease

The approach of the German Cystic Fibrosis Association

Andreas L. G. Reimann

Introduction

The German Cystic Fibrosis (CF) association, Mukoviszidose e.V., is an untypical patient organization comprising not only patients and relatives but also clinicians, scientists and allied health professionals as integrated yet self-organized groups within the association. This unique setting facilitates a structured research funding process that is both rigorous and participative. A multi-step peer review evaluation process aims at ensuring that funds are allocated to projects of high scientific quality and significant relevance to patients. The association has spent approximately 11.5 million euros directly on research funding during the past decade. Ongoing projects are more leveraged with third parties, e.g. the European Union, contributing major amounts. These projects are worth another 9 million euros. To organize research administration and the organization of clinical trials professionally and to keep liability issues away from the association, Mukoviszidose Institute (MI), a limited liability non-profit affiliate wholly owned by the association, was established in 2006. Applying a social entrepreneurship approach, MI has been or is currently the sponsor of several non-commercial clinical trials that would not otherwise have been undertaken. An evaluation of the research effort using the input-output-outcome-impact typology revealed that approximately 360,000 euros had to be spent per project with a high-rated patient impact. This paper discusses the limitations of that analysis and further reveals critical issues that need to be addressed in the future. Amongst these issues is the need for open and transparent communication between scientists, research administrators and patients' representatives as a pre-requisite for efficient patient-centered research promotion. This paper will first describe the background of the disease followed by a discussion of the research funding efforts of Mukoviszidose e.V. and their evaluation, a summary of the attempts to assess the impact on patients and some details on new approaches towards patient-centered research. It will be concluded by a section discussing and summarizing the content.

Why patient involvement matters: the background of the disease

Cystic Fibrosis (CF) is a monogenetic disease caused by mutations in the cystic fibrosis transmembrane conductance regulator (CFTR). This results in dysfunction of the CFTR protein, a chloride channel involved in the regulation of the ion and water balance in secretory epithelial cells. Consequently, CFTR dysfunction has an impact on the fluidity, salt concentration and pH of the mucus layer on secretory epithelial cells. Clinically essential organ systems, in particular the lungs, the exocrine pancreas, the liver, and the small intestine are impaired in their functions by a high viscous mucus (hence the synonym "Mucoviscidosis") (Kerem et al. 2005). Today, more than 1800 mutations[1] have been identified. They are usually grouped into six different mutation classes with different disease-causing potential. Generally speaking, the complete lack of protein synthesis in class-I (stop mutations, approx. 5–10 per cent of patients) or the lack of functioning protein in class II (folding defect, 50–80 per cent of patients) and the synthesis of a low-conductance protein in class III mutations (gating defect, approx. 5 per cent of patients) are the most important classes causing serious disease.

Life expectancy was as low as 5–10 years back in the 1950s and 60s. With the introduction of symptomatic treatments, e. g. pancreatic enzyme therapy in the 1970s and advanced physiotherapy in the 80s, life expectancy improved quite considerably. Later on, anti-infective therapy was revolutionized by inhalative antibiotics with which acute and chronic infections of the lung could be treated effectively. Today, median survival is approximately 41 years in Germany and most of the western countries. 50 per cent of all patients are 18 years or older (Sens and Stern 2012). However, no causal treatment is available. CF is still a life-limiting disease, with progressive loss of lung function being the most common cause of death. The detection of the gene in 1989 (Riordan et al. 1989) made it possible to target directly the underlying gene defect. Gene therapy seemed to be the most logical approach. At this time, the hopes of patients and relatives were raised by so-called experts voicing over-optimistic expectations, even suggesting that a cure would be found within a 5–10 year period. However, while the use of viral vectors helped to express the healthy gene quickly, the effect was only transient because of immune defense (Parsons 2005). Early in the new millennium, therefore, the CF Trust in the UK launched a new research program aiming at the development of gene therapy based on non-viral vectors (Griesenbach et al. 2006). More than 30 million pounds were raised, and the gene therapy consortium was able to develop a liposomal, i.e. non-viral, vector that successfully passed first trials in humans. This so-called "Wave-1" product is now being studied in a phase II trial. However, it seems clear that even that product may not be the final cure for CF for various reasons (e.g. lack of tissue specificity, transient effect). Further research, and most likely the development of a "Wave-2" product, will be required. 24 years after the gene was discovered, gene therapy is still not much more than a potential light at the end of the tunnel. A true breakthrough, however, was achieved by a drug development program in the United States mainly financed by a $70 million grant from the US Cystic Fibrosis Foundation (CFF). Using high-throughput drug screening, small molecules were identified targeting specific mutation classes. In 2012, the first mutation-specific therapy coming out of this program, Ivacaftor (Kalydeco®), was approved in both the US and Europe. It is what is known as a CFTR potentiator, which improves the chloride conductance of the CFTR channel in patients with at least one G551D mutation (McPhail and Clancy 2013). In Germany, only approximately 200 out of the 8000–9000 CF patients are eligible for this pharmacotherapy. While it is too early to assess the long-term benefits of this product, the results of clinical trials and first reports from patients on this drug are quite encouraging. However, this success comes with two major limitations. The treatment cost per patient are as high as 250,000 € each year for the entire life-span of the individual. While in Germany and a couple of other western countries the product is mostly reimbursed, the price is unaffordable for many other systems and for patients without proper insurance (such as many in the US). True access to that innovation is therefore limited for many potentially eligible patients. The second limitation is the mutation-specific nature of this therapy. Patients with other mutations, in particular those with the most important 508del mutation that affects approximately two-thirds of the German patients, cannot benefit from the product. However, clinical research investigating the safety and efficacy of Ivacaftor in combination with several so-called CFTR correctors, aiming to overcome the folding defect in this most common mutation, is underway. The initial results have been promising, but it may still be years before new products are ready for approval. Of course, the health-economic impact of those presumably very expensive treatments is already being discussed in view of the much higher number of patients potentially eligible for these products. Given this background, three major lessons can be learned (Schlangen and Reimann 2011a, 2011b):

1. Managing expectations of patients is crucial, in order to avoid frustration and jeopardizing trust in science and medicine.
2. Symptomatic treatment may have a big impact on patients' life expectancy and quality.
3. Without massive support from patient organizations, no progress would have been made. However, taking inventions from the bench to the bedside requires co-operation between patient organizations and industry, particular small and medium-sized companies.

Research funding of Mukoviszidose e.V. in Germany

Ten years after the Cystic Fibrosis Foundation (CFF) in the United States was established, the German CF association, Mukoviszidose e.V., was founded in 1965 under the name of "German society for fighting mucoviscidosis". The founders of the German association were physicians who wanted to join forces, sharing knowledge and best practice and seeking to improve the situation of their CF patients. Shortly thereafter, parents of children suffering from CF joined the association. Today, Mukoviszidose e.V. has a membership of 5,500 including approximately 800 professionals (physicians, researchers, and allied health professionals), 3000 parents, and 1200 adult CF patients. While there was always a wish to foster research on a disease that was poorly understood in the 1960s, no systematic approaches are reported from that period. This changed when the corresponding organizations in the United States and the United Kingdom started attempts in the 1980s to organize and foster more systematic research into the background and symptomatic treatment of the disease. In particular, the CFF acted as a role model in making research funding a major topic of interest in the activities of Mukoviszidose e.V. The first research grants, amounting at that time to no more than 3000 or 5000 euros per year, were issued in 1995. However, the organization benefited from its celebrity patron, Christiane Herzog, wife of the German federal president, who attracted a lot of attention to the disease in general and the organization in particular. Fighting fierce opposition from parents who wished to use the newly available funds directly for research funding, the association's board of directors made a strategic decision: they decided to invest in the establishment of systematic and professional fundraising rather than spending the funds immediately on research. While this led to a shortage of funding for research at the beginning, it made the effort sustainable when Mr Herzog's term as president ended and his wife died shortly thereafter in 2000. In addition to social support and counseling, research funding became the major activity of the association with annual funds for research amounting to approximately 1–1.2 million euros in the past three years, i.e. 22% of the association's total budget. Since 2002, the association has spent about 11.5 million euros from its funds. Combined with third party funds, the total volume of ongoing research projects is as high as 9 million euros (Figure 2.1).

In the late 1990s, when research funding was becoming an increasingly prominent activity of the association, it became clear that a proper evaluation process was needed to ensure that funds were allocated to those projects with the greatest scientific merit. An evaluation process was therefore set up analogous to that of the German Research Foundation (DFG), including external peer review. The association's board delegated scientific evaluation to its scientific arm, which was called the CF Research Community (Forschungsgemeinschaft Mukoviszidose, FGM). Members of the FGM are clinicians and scientists from amongst the association's membership. They elect a board which is responsible for the scientific evaluation of research proposals, and the final decision on funding is made by the association's board. In 2000, a scientific secretariat was established

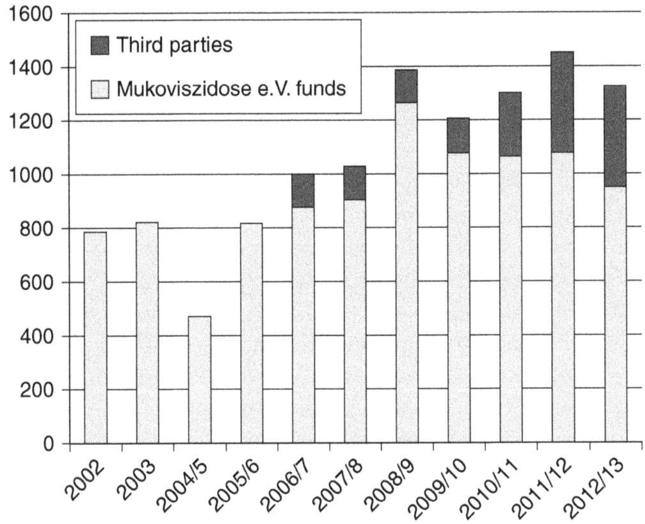

Figure 2.1 Total spending on research from Mukoviszidose e.V. (light grey columns) or third-party funds (dark grey columns). (The financial year changed on 1 July 2004 to a mid-year period. Hence, the period 1 January 2004 until 30 June 2004 is not included).

at the association's office in Bonn. While the secretariat was staffed at the beginning only by one part-time biologist and a part-time secretary, its tasks developed from only administrating the evaluation process to actively steering the acquisition of new projects and fostering networking among scientists. In 2004, the law governing clinical trials in Germany implemented the new EU clinical trial directive. Undertaking clinical trials became much more organizationally burdensome. This included the necessity to define a "sponsor", i.e. the organization held responsible for the entire conduct of a clinical trial. It became apparent that an association was not well placed to do this job. As indicated above, the Mukoviszidose Institute (MI) was therefore established in 2006 as a separate legal entity, a non-profit limited company (gGmbH) wholly owned by Mukoviszidose e.V. Subsequently, all scientific activities were shifted to MI. Using a social entrepreneurship approach, the MI acts as a center of competence for all activities in the area of research funding, organizing non-profit clinical trials, quality-management for CF care, and scientific and medical information. In the beginning, almost all of MI's funds were provided by the association. Today, more than 60 per cent of the income is generated by other parties, mainly the European Union and the Germany Ministry of Health. Increasingly, however, major donors wishing to support specific projects are also donating directly to MI.

Evaluating research proposals submitted to the Mukoviszidose Institute (MI)

Patients, relatives and donors rely on a scientific evaluation process that does not guarantee ideal results but is set up so that funds can be allocated to those projects that are scientifically sound and most likely to have an impact on patients.

The evaluation process at MI as it stands today is the result of 17 years' experience in research funding. It aims at avoiding bias as far as possible and at coming up with a fair and balanced statement on the priority a project should enjoy in Mukoviszidose e.V.'s research funding program.

It is the goal of the Mukoviszidose e.V. to foster CF-relevant research aiming at extending the lifespan and improving the quality of life of patients with cystic fibrosis. Therefore, Mukoviszidose e.V. provides funding exclusively for CF-relevant research projects and clinical studies likely to contribute significantly to patient-relevant therapeutic outcomes.

The funding scheme comprises four different programs. There are three different project funding programs: "Non-clinical research projects to generate new knowledge relevant for CF diagnosis and therapy", "Clinical research projects", "Small projects", and an additional career funding program for young scientists – "Young investigator grants". All programs have dedicated deadlines and a competitive evaluation process including international peer review. The project funding program is not restricted to Germany, and the call for proposals is distributed throughout Europe.

In addition, support for scientific meetings and travel grants for young scientists actively participating is available if CF-relevance can be demonstrated. A structural improvement program (SIP) may also be offered on a case-by-case basis. This type of funding is dedicated to supporting the implementation of certain advanced methodologies in CF centers in Germany, such as CFTR function diagnostics for clarification of the CF diagnosis in questionable cases or new and more informative outcome parameters (e.g. Lung Clearance Index measurements) for German CF sites. To avoid bias, external assessment is conducted in these cases by an international advisory board.

Funding of "Non-clinical research projects" is dedicated to projects providing important knowledge within the field of CF and with the potential to initiate new therapeutic options. This funding is provided for CF-relevant research projects, with the expectation of a clinical application in CF care and/or the generation of new CF-relevant knowledge. However, funding of basic science without any application perspective is not within the scope of MI's funding scheme, as other sources of funding, in particular from the DFG, are available and better suited to meet the needs of these researchers.

"Clinical research projects" cover clinical research in the field of CF with the intention to develop new therapies or diagnostic tools for clinical application in CF patient-centered care. This comprises all clinical studies where patients will be recruited actively for examination within the study. Apart from interventional trials, it may also include observational studies.

While these two types of project are basically limited only by the available budget, they are subject to annual calls with set submission deadlines. At the specific deadline, either a non-clinical or a clinical project can be applied for depending on the subject of the call. In contrast, "small projects" are limited to maximum funding up to 20,000 euros. These can cover either clinical or non-clinical subjects, and can be applied for at any time. Applicants for these three types of project funding do not need to be based in Germany, but co-operation with a German scientific team is strongly encouraged.

"Young investigator grants" provide funding for up to 3 years. They are only available for applicants from German CF working groups and are specifically dedicated to PhD students, young clinicians and medical post-doctoral researchers. They can apply for their own salary during their academic training in a CF-specific research field, e.g. CF therapy, diagnostic or preclinical research. This funding will therefore enable young scientists to deepen their knowledge in CF research and to establish themselves within the network of CF scientists. In the long term, this should enable such scientists to establish their own CF research group.

All proposals have to be submitted in English and electronically, using the appropriate form for a "short application", "full application" or "small-project application". These forms are downloadable from the internet (see www.cf-germany.org for more details).

The evaluation process for all applications except "small projects" is at least a two-step procedure. In steps I and II, the evaluation of the application involves considering the qualifications of the applicant/working group, the scientific quality of the proposal including quality management procedures, and the relevance to CF in terms of the improvement of diagnosis and/or therapy.

In step I, a 10-page "short application" form must be submitted first. In addition to administrative information, it is basically structured along the lines of a full application: background, the applicant's own preliminary work, the objectives of the project, the working program, anticipated CF relevance, and a section dealing with the financial plan. In addition, the Curricula Vitae of the scientists involved and the most relevant publications supporting the hypothesis should be provided. Particular emphasis should be placed on applicants' publications which demonstrate their ability to carry out the working program, and the expertise of the scientific group. The application is completed by a statement on third party funding. This is possible if the situation is made transparent. Applicants must waive their rights of confidentiality with regard to public funding agencies, so that MI can request information on potential parallel applications. As there is no second evaluation step for "small projects", in this case the specific form sheet requests more detailed information and is longer.

After the form has been submitted electronically, the MI scientific officer will check the application for completeness and any obvious problems. If the deadline has not already been passed, applicants may have the chance to revise their application to rectify any flaws. All final applications are then presented in step I of the evaluation process to the board of FGM, acting as the scientific advisory board and consisting of seven experts covering different research areas. The main criteria during the evaluation are CF relevance, i.e. the therapeutic or diagnostic application which should be indicated in the proposal, and scientific quality. At that stage, approximately 50 per cent of the applications fail on the grounds that they do not meet one or both of these criteria.

If successful at this stage, applicants move to step II. They are now asked to submit a "full application" providing in sufficient detail background, methodology, working program and potential benefit for patients. In addition, a comprehensive bibliography and a detailed financial plan must be presented.

The "full application" will be subject to external peer review by three independent, internationally recognized experts in the relevant field. These experts are chosen jointly by the FGM board and the scientific officer of the MI. Applicants can request the exclusion of certain reviewers on the grounds of competitive bias, but they will not be told the names of the peer reviewers. The reviewers are asked to provide their statements on a structured form. Rarely do they recommend funding without any revision. More likely, they will either ask for minor or major revisions or recommend declining the application. Unlike in many public and other private funding programs, the applicant may have the option to revise his/her application or to provide explanations and comments based on the expert opinions that will be sent to him/her for consideration in anonymized version.

In the light of these expert opinions and the comments or revisions of the applicant, the FGM board will discuss the application. In the cases of "young investigator grants" and "non-clinical research" applications the board may decline, ask for a major revision and re-review, or recommend funding. "Clinical projects" that are scientifically recommended for funding will be subject to a third step. Applicants will now be asked to provide a full-scale clinical trial protocol according to good clinical practices. That protocol will again be externally reviewed for feasibility and completeness. A final funding recommendation based on that methodological review will then be made by the FGM board.

All projects recommended for funding within either the "non-clinical" or "clinical" programs will be ranked according to priority. That ranked list of projects is then submitted to the administrative board of Mukoviszidose e.V., which will decide on the basis of the ranking and the availability of funds whether or not a project can be funded. In the latter case, MI drafts a contract with the investigator and his/her institution and will then also be responsible for following up on the project. The entire evaluation process is designed to be completed normally within 11 months, although the step III evaluation of "clinical projects" will require additional time. An intention to fund the project can be stated on the step II evaluation, but the submission and evaluation of a clinical trial protocol is mandatory before project funding can start. If no funds from the association are available, MI may still contract with successful applicants if funding can be obtained from other sources.

Once the contract is signed and the project has officially commenced, progress and interim reports are required to be submitted regularly. For all projects, an implementation report has to be provided three months after the project has started. For clinical projects, a status report on recruitment and any particular problems has to be submitted every three months. For all other projects, reports are due every six months. After an initial installment, usually 10 per cent of the total sum, further payments will be made according to project progress, but 5 per cent is withheld until a final report has been submitted and another 5 per cent is subject to the submission of a manuscript and/or patent filing.

In the final report, the investigator is requested to demonstrate whether and to what extent the original objectives have been achieved. Detailed information about the results and a scientific discussion must be provided. Particular emphasis must be put on any potential follow-up research. In addition to an internal assessment at the end of the project, the final report was for a time also subject to an end-of-project external peer review. This practice was discontinued following the findings of the analysis described in detail below.

Assessing patient impact of research programs

After more than a decade of intensive research funding, a comprehensive analysis of the research effort was undertaken. Most importantly, an attempt was made to assess the impact on patients' health. That analysis comprised all projects that were approved and completed from the beginning in 2000 until 30 September 2011. Two further studies of particular importance that were commenced in the late 90s but completed after 1 January 2000 were included as well.

The assessment was based on a modified Input-Output-Outcome-Impact analysis used by the European Commission for development of projects. In short, input indicators measure the resources that are put into a project. For the sake of this analysis we used only the monetary value of project funds, leaving out researchers' time and effort as well as institutional infrastructure used since detailed information on external resource use was not available to us. Output indicators quantify the technical result, in our case the project reports. Outcome indicators appraise the direct benefit, i.e. publications, postgraduate qualifications (e.g. PhD theses) or patents based on the project. Of utmost importance is eventually, however, the impact on patients' mortality, morbidity or quality of life.

While input was known from our accounting system and the output could easily be retrieved from our report database, researchers' views on both outcome and impact were assessed by a questionnaire sent to the project leaders. This was complemented by a literature search for relevant publications generated out of the funded projects and external peer reviews of the project reports whenever these were available. The latter, however, turned out to be of limited if any value, as peer reviewers appeared to have paid little attention to the actual reports. This may have been caused by lack of time devoted to the report and the fact that at the time of evaluation, i.e. immediately following the completion of the report, the outcome was not always retrievable. In addition, reviewers who also did the pre-project evaluation may have been biased towards the project in a kind of self-affirmative thinking.

When assessing publications, only original articles in peer-reviewed journals were taken into account. As the impact factors of the journals were changing over the period of the analysis, they were not figured in the quantitative analysis.

The final impact evaluation was done independently by three scientific staff members of MI using a seven-score rating system.

- A+: patient-relevant clinical development with proven significance for either routine diagnosis or therapy.
- A: Patient-relevant clinical development with potential significance for routine diagnosis or therapy.
- B+: Patient-relevant clinical development with the option to be further developed into routine diagnosis or therapy, or alternatively an important gain of knowledge with paramount scientific value.
- B: Gain of knowledge with high scientific value.
- C: Gain of knowledge with scientific value.
- D: Gain of knowledge with limited scientific value.
- E: Scientific significance either lacking or not assessable.

Of 81 projects analyzed, 75 were completed with a final report. 49 of these were published, and 26 were not. Of the six projects without a final report, three were nevertheless published. Three projects have been neither reported nor published.

Of the projects, 36 were part of a post-graduate qualification of the young scientists involved, three resulted in a patent filing, and 35 led to further research mostly funded by third parties. The input/output ratio was 64,000 euros per project with a final report that, for the sake of these analyses, is defined as output. The input/outcome ratio amounted to 93,000 euros per project published, and the input/impact ratio was 359,000 euros per project with an A+/A/B+ rating. The results of the impact rating are shown in Table 2.1.

The total funds used for projects covered in this analysis amounted to 4.8 million euros. 52 per cent of those funds were used for projects eventually rated A+/A/B+/B. 22 per cent of the funds were invested in projects

Table 2.1 Results of project assessment and invested funds

Rating	*No. of projects*	*Funds provided*	*%*
A	6 (7%)	336,801.68 €	7%
A+	1 (1%)	113,240.06 €	2%
B	11 (14%)	911,092.05 €	19%
B+	7 (9%)	1,152,817.06 €	24%
C	21 (26%)	616,968.59 €	13%
D	8 (10%)	462,883.83 €	10%
E	24 (30%)	1,077,629.74 €	22%
ND	1 (1%)	49,938.15 €	1%
NA	2 (2%)	113,026.00 €	2%
Total	81 (100%)	4,834,397.16 €	100%

Key
ND: Not determinable as project completed only in 2011.
NA: Not applicable, i.e. projects still running or never commenced.

ending up with an E rating. While this figure may be perceived high by an audience unfamiliar with biomedical research, it is actually not surprising for those involved regularly in funding biomedical projects. Not only can projects fail due to poor management and conduct, they may also fail to produce a meaningful result just because the methodology used was inappropriate and this was not elucidated during the peer-review process. To avoid any misunderstanding, negative results, i.e. falsifications of the hypothesis, are of course very valuable and are augmenting scientific knowledge. An "E-rating" signifies in this context rather a work that is not leading to any conclusion because the reporting is either completely lacking or too poor to obtain a meaningful message.

As shown in Figure 2.2, the funds actually paid tend to be higher in projects with a high rating as opposed to those projects with a less favorable rating.

In 2004 the structure of research funding was amended (for details, see page 000), and from then on projects with a greater likelihood of direct patient impact within a defined focus area stood a better chance of being funded. The idea behind this was to have more patient value per euro spent.

When analyzing projects before and after implementation of that new policy, it becomes apparent that the basic idea worked: 52 per cent of the projects in the period from 2004 onwards received an A/B+/B rating, while only 21 per cent of the earlier projects could achieve those scores. Inversely, fewer projects received the unfavorable E rating (26 per cent) under the new policy as opposed to the earlier period (34 per cent, Table 2.2).

The analysis has several methodological weaknesses that must be taken into account when interpreting the results. More recent projects may still be in the publication process (as claimed by several researchers), so the outcome may have been underestimated. It therefore makes sense to repeat this kind of analysis on a regular basis. In addition, not all information provided by the project leaders could be verified by means of a literature search. Again, this should be the case in future evaluations.

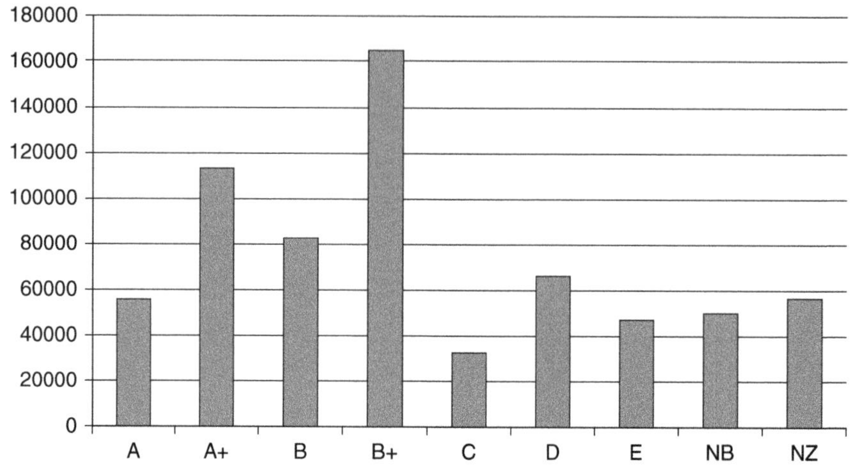

Figure 2.2 Average funds provided in projects rated.

Two major projects could not be included in the analysis because they were officially not yet completed at the set deadline:

The *IGOR/GSH-4* trial investigated the safety and effi cacy of inhaled glutathione in a randomized, placebo-controlled, double-blind clinical trial in 153 CF patients (Griese et al. 2013). While safety was proven, no significant efficacy when compared to placebo could be demonstrated. Although this "negative" result was disappointing for patients hoping for a new treatment option, it was still an important step forward in the association's research funding program in several respects. (1) It was the first noncommercial clinical trial successfully carried out and completed under the sponsorship and direction of MI. (2) It was made possible only by a consortium of scientists, clinical trial sites, small and middle-sized industry partners (providing drug substance and inhalers), loan manufacturers (producing the drug product), and non-profi t organizations funding and organizing the

Table 2.2 Rating of research projects 2000–2003 and, after a new focus area model of research funding was implemented, 2004–2011

Rating	*2000–2003*	*2004–2011*
A+	0 (0%)	0 (0%)
A	3 (6%)	3 (13%)
B+	3 (6%)	4 (17%)
B	5 (9%)	5 (22%)
C	17 (32%)	4 (17%)
D	7 (13%)	1 (4%)
E	18 (34%)	6 (26%)
Total	53 (100%)	23 (100%)

effort. (3) Approximately 40 per cent of the project funds were provided by the US partner organization Cystic Fibrosis Foundation, which meant that the project was also a working example of global co-operation. (4) Mukoviszidose e.V. had successfully applied together with the Committee for Orphan Medicinal Products (COMP) to the European Medicines Agency in London for an orphan drug designation for inhaled Glutathione. That status was granted in 2006 (EU/3/06/361) and potentially provided free access to several incentives in development and marketing.[2] (5) Patients who have participated in clinical trials frequently demand publication of all results even if they are negative. MI supports this policy of full transparency and has signed the ALL-TRIALS[3] initiative. We take pride in having ensured that our first "negative" trial was appropriately communicated. The cost per patient was approximately 6860 euros, and therefore significantly below the industry standard for phase II trials. Mukoviszidose e.V. had contributed approximately 600,000 euros of the 1,050,000 euros budget for this study. Retrospectively applying the rating typology, a B rating could be justified as an important clinical question has been answered.

The CF Diabetes trial investigated the comparative safety and efficacy of insulin and repaglinide, a sulfonyl-urea oral anti-diabetic drug, in the treatment of CF-associated diabetes mellitus. In this case, the trial established that repaglinide was not inferior to insulin and may therefore be an alternative to the more invasive and bothersome insulin regimen. Again, several lessons can be learned from this trial, which was the most expensive clinical trial project so far for Mukoviszidose e.V. with funds of approximately one million euros provided over a 10-year period: (1) The trial did not recruit well until MI took over sponsorship in 2007, thereby demonstrating the superiority of a well-organized research unit. (2) The trial was undertaken not only in Germany but also in France and Austria. This cross-border setting was successfully managed. (3) During the course of the trial improved processes helped in ensuring its successful completion.

A new era of research funding: the IMPACTT and VEMSE-CF projects

Traditionally, projects funded by Mukoviszidose e.V. were either solely or predominantly financed by the association's grants. Important exceptions were some clinical trials which were co-funded at least in part by the pharmaceutical industry directly, mostly by providing drug products. Public funding programs, however, were for a long time not part of the financing portfolio. This changed with two recently initiated research programs: IMPACTT and VEMSE-CF.

IMPACTT (for details see: http://www.impactt.eu) is a program mostly funded by the European Union's Seventh Framework Research Programme. A European consortium under the leadership of the University of Uppsala, jointly with MI, successfully applied for this project, which aims at establishing pre-clinical and clinical knowledge on the mode of action, safety and efficacy of anti-Pseudomonas-aeruginosa (PsA) IgY, an antibody derived from egg yolk, in preventing re-infection with PsA in CF patients aged 6 years or older. MI is heading up the work package on the clinical trial, which is the centerpiece of the project. 180 patients are being studied for an individual treatment time of 2 years. The trial is currently being conducted in four European countries (Sweden, Belgium, Italy, Germany) with a central lab in Copenhagen/DK. It will be further extended to Austria, Hungary, the Czech Republic, Poland, Spain and Ireland. With a total project volume of about 5.6 million euros, of which only 250,000 euros are provided from the association's funds, it is by far the largest and most leveraged project ever in the association's history. The complexity of this trial is a new challenge for MI, and so far the challenge is being met. The project commenced in 2011 and is likely to last until 2017.

VEMSE-CF is the name of a care-research project investigating the effectiveness of a comprehensive psychosocial intervention (i.e. a prospective integrated care model) compared to standard care in CF patients, as a role model for rare disease care in general. The project comprises 150 patients in the intervention group and 165 patients in the control group recruited in a cluster-randomized setting. 50 per cent of the 1.6 million euro budget is provided by the German Ministry of Health, and the remainder is mostly provided by Mukoviszidose e.V.

Discussion

When analyzing the research effort of Mukoviszidose e.V. and MI, critical success factors can be identified from the lessons learned in the past 15 years.

1. To avoid disappointed patients and frustrated donors, expectations should be managed as transparently and honestly as possible: research can never be predictable in outcome. We cannot guarantee results with a high patient impact, but we can strive to set up the right process to ensure that everything is done to achieve this ultimate goal as far as possible.
2. There is no perfect way to predict the scientific merit and patient impact of projects. The current peer review multi-step evaluation process, however, seems the best way to avoid biased judgments.
3. In general, scientists tend to be overoptimistic when estimating deadlines. Hence, both budget allocation and reporting must be adjusted to a realistic scenario taking likely delays into account.
4. Clinical trials are of particular complexity. They need very critical analysis of their feasibility to avoid bad recruitment, which is costly and may even bring the project to a premature end. Of course, good clinical practice standards must be applied as for every other clinical trial. Patients' safety must never be compromised. It is also highly unethical

in relation to patients at risk to conduct a poorly organized clinical trial that is unlikely to produce meaningful results. Non-profit sponsors such as MI must act at the same level of professionalism as commercial contract research organizations (CROs) or industry. They can and should, however, be more flexible when making decisions and finding innovative solutions. In particular, non-commercial sponsors are an ideal partner for investigator-initiated trials that may address clinically important questions that will never have a chance to be answered in a commercial setting because of a lack of intellectual property protection such as observational trials, trials testing non-pharmacological interventions (e.g. exercise, psychosocial) or trials investigating the effect of re-purposed drugs on a rare disease.

5. Dedicated and well-trained staff are an absolute pre-requisite for managing the research effort well and ensuring that funds are spent in the best way possible. This includes not only scientific but also administrative and accounting functions.
6. The organizational context must be prepared to carry out its research funding work as professionally as possible. It may be necessary to "re-invent" the organization or to set up a separate legal entity (such as MI). If clinical trials are officially sponsored, this is even a pre-requisite to avoid liability issues for the association. Obviously, professionalism and traditional patient support and advocacy structures may not be compatible with each other. In particular, typical German self-help associations tend to find it difficult to accept a change of context and to adapt to new demands. Organizations must therefore make an informed choice about which way to go. It will not be enough to repeat what has been done for many years. Sticking only to the same organizational routines is unlikely to help anybody, in particular patients demanding new therapeutic options.
7. Communication is instrumental for allowing patients, relatives, scientists and donors to participate in the processes and results of research funding and organization. It is an inherent danger for all expanding organizations that they may lose touch with their target audiences as a result of poor communication. However, only if they have a feeling of being part of a larger community will those audiences be prepared to support the process by providing time and effort, money or – in the case of patients – by becoming subjects in clinical trials.
8. Communicating regularly and thoughtfully is important not only to external audiences but also for internal audiences in the professional organization, in particular senior management, PR and fundraising functions. They need to understand why a certain research project is being undertaken and why it is in the interest of patients to spend the organization's funds on it.
9. A phenomenon common to research funding in many funding agencies is double funding and redundant research, i.e. projects that are

being undertaken by other groups elsewhere in parallel. Double funding should be avoided, for obvious reasons. MI requests applicants not only to declare any other sources of funding but also to allow third-party sponsors to disclose their records on that applicant. If undeclared third-party funding is detected, this constitutes a breach of contract with MI and provides grounds for termination without notice. Redundant research – if known from the literature or other sources of intelligence – may deliberately be accepted, as at the end of the day the results available to patients are in the main interest of the organization. This again is an important difference to commercial sponsors, who may terminate a project once they find out that competitors are ahead in development. To some extent redundant research and competition between different groups can help to achieve results, so competition effects should not be avoided *per se.*

10. Last but not least, research funding is a long term commitment that requires careful financial planning. Terminating projects because resources are no longer available is malpractice and must be avoided at all cost. While this is already true for non-clinical projects, in clinical trials this would become an ethical and even legal issue. It is irresponsible to commence a clinical trial without ensuring that the funds are available for the entire duration of the study. Hence, fundraising communications must stress the need for funds but must also take account of the fact that reserves for the project have already been built up. Donors – in particular if they provide substantial amounts of money – like the idea of leveraging their donation by multiplying the donated euros by money provided by third parties. These parties may be other non-profit organizations, industrial partners or public funders such as the EU or the German DFG.

Fostering patient-centered research with the objective of achieving patient impact is not at all a straightforward mission. It is quite difficult to prospectively estimate the potential impact a project might have if it is successfully completed. However, it has become apparent both in internal discussions with the board of directors and in discussions with colleagues from other funding organizations in the field of CF and other (rare) diseases that it is eventually the impact on patients that should govern the allocation of funds to research projects. Organizations should therefore make the effort needed to forecast that potential impact as precisely as possible.

When discussing the scope of the research funding with scientists within the organization, the question was raised whether scientific excellence and patient impact may be in conflict with each other. In other words, may there be situations where funds are better spent in scientifically excellent projects with moderate or even no patient impact rather than the other way round? It seems obvious that scientifically flawed projects may never have any patient impact, because they will either never come to a conclusion at all or that conclusion will be dubious because of the poor quality of research. However, this should not mean that projects should be funded that are unlikely to produce any impact on patients simply because they are not designed to do so, even if they are scientifically outstanding. The strategic approach must therefore be constantly challenged by patients and relatives as experts on their disease. They alone can tell what should be at the center of the research effort. It will then be up to the scientists to carry out sound research to achieve these objectives.

How transferable is this model of research funding to other (rare) diseases? The organizational prerequisites are described above. Along these lines, the effort can be scaled up or more likely be scaled down to meet the capabilities of the specific organization and the disease area. Elements of the entire process, i.e. the peer-reviewed evaluation, can be easily copied. However, a particular strength of Mukoviszidose e.V. is the combination of patients and their relatives with medical and scientific professionals in one organization. This kind of co-operation is not at all easy, and can be very bothersome at times. However, Mukoviszidose e.V. is a uniquely positioned organization with the capacity to make patient-centeredness work.

This having been said, that setting appears, unfortunately, to be a rare role model in the patient organization scene, at least in Germany. It is therefore important for other organizations without this setting to establish very close and reliable relations with their scientific counterparts without leaving the specific patient focus behind.

Eventually, by establishing MI, Mukoviszidose e.V. went beyond the classical patient-organization pathways as MI is applying a social entrepreneurship approach to solve as yet unaddressed medical and scientific issues. Combining the strengths of an idealistic non-profit background with the strengths of an entrepreneurial context designed to be flexible and outcome-oriented, we are well prepared to meet the needs of patients in Germany and elsewhere.

Notes

1 <www.cftr2.org> (accessed 30 July 2013).
2 See <www.ema.europa.eu/ema/index.jsp?curl=pages/medicines/human/orphans/2009/11/human_orphan_000623.jsp&mid=WC0b01ac058001d12b> (accessed 29 July 2013) for details.
3 See www.alltrials.net (accessed 29 July 2013) for details.

References

Griesenbach, Uta; Geddes, Duncan M. and Alton, Eric W. (2006) Gene therapy progress and prospects: Cystic fibrosis, *Gene Therapy*, 13(14), 1061–1067.

Griese, Matthias; Kappler, Matthias; Eismann, Claudia; Ballmann, Manfred; Junge, Sibylle; Rietschel, Ernst; van Koningsbruggen-Rietschel, Silke; Staab, Doris; Rolinck-Werninghaus, Claudia; Mellies, Uwe; Köhnlein, Thomas; Wagner,

Thomas; König, Susanne; Teschler, Helmut; Heuer, Hans-Eberhard; Kopp, Matthias; Heyder, Susanne; Hammermann, Jutta; Küster, Peter; Honer, Marguerite; Mansmann, Ulrich; Beck-Speier, Ingrid; Hartl, Dominik; Fuchs, Carola and Hector, Andreas (2013) Inhalation treatment with glutathione in patients with cystic fi brosis: A randomized clinical trial, *American Journal of Respiratory and Critical Care Medicine*, 188(1), 83–89.

Kerem, Eitan; Conway, Steven; Elborn, Stuart and Heijerman, Harry (2005) Standards of care for patients with cystic fibrosis: A European consensus, *Journal of Cystic Fibrosis*, 4(1), 7–26.

McPhail, Gary L. and Clancy, John P. (2013) Ivacaftor: The first therapy acting on the primary cause of cystic fibrosis, *Drugs of Today (Barcelona)*, 49(4), 253–260.

Parsons, David W. (2005) Airway gene therapy and cystic fibrosis, *Journal of Paediatrics and Child Health*, 41(3), 94–96.

Riordan, John R.; Rommens, Johanna M.; Kerem, Batsheva; Alon, Noa; Rozmahel, Richard; Grzelczak, Zbyszko; Zielinski, Julian; Lok, Si; Plavsic, Natasa; Chou, Jia-Ling et al. (1989) Identification of the cystic fibrosis gene: cloning and characterization of complementary DNA, *Science*, 245(4925), 1066–1073.

Schlangen, Miriam and Reimann, Andreas L. (2011a) Developing new products in cystic fibrosis: needs and obstacles for activities of small and middle-sized companies, *Journal of Cystic Fibrosis*, 10(2), S103–109.

—— (2011b) Medical needs of cystic fibrosis patients and policies for fair co-operation between small and middle-sized companies and patient organizations, *Journal of Cystic Fibrosis*, 10(2), 110–113.

Sens, Brigitte and Stern, Martin (2012) *Qualitätssicherung Mukoviszidose 2011*, Bad Honnef: Hippocampus Verlag KG.

3 EURORDIS

Empowering patients living with rare diseases to participate in biomedical knowledge production

Christel Nourissier, Monica Ensini and Maria Mavris

Introduction: EURORDIS and the world of rare diseases

This chapter will describe the role of EURORDIS (European Organization for Rare Diseases) in the field of medical research. EURORDIS is a non-governmental, patient-driven alliance of patients' organizations and individuals in Europe, representing the voice of people living with rare diseases.[1]

There are an estimated 5000–7000 rare diseases[2–3] (Stolk et al. 2006); a disease is considered to be rare when it affects no more than 5 in 10,000 citizens in the European Union. Although most rare diseases are of extremely low prevalence (affecting one in 100,000 citizens or less), an estimated total of 30 million individuals are affected in the European Union. Because of the relatively low numbers they receive very little attention. The characteristics of rare diseases, limited patient numbers and a scarcity of relevant knowledge and expertise, identify them as a unique domain of added value for action at the level of community.

Despite their diversity, rare diseases share some similarities: they are chronic, often progressive, life-threatening and/or seriously debilitating diseases.[4] The majority have already identified genetic origins, yet they differ regarding their clinical manifestations, their causes, the populations they affect, their severity, and the age of onset.

The greatest barrier to the prevention, diagnosis and treatment of rare diseases has been, and still is, insufficient knowledge of the mechanisms of pathogenesis and the natural history of the various diseases. In addition, there is little likelihood that a treatment exists for a particular disease and little chance that it is being researched anywhere. Millions of patients live with undiagnosed rare diseases and in most cases with no available treatment. Progress in research is their only hope.

EURORDIS' main activities and goals

Faced with the prospect of little hope for diagnosis or treatment, many patients and families decide to establish a patient group. This is an essential first step, along with the establishment of centres of expertise and data collection, toward progress. Progress in the form of empowered patients means recognition of the fact that they can act as full and equal partners, developers or funders of fundamental, translational and clinical research (Mavris and Le Cam 2012).

It is with this objective that EURORDIS was established in 1997 by four patient groups from different therapeutic fields: the Association Française contre les Myopathies (AFM) (French muscular dystrophy association), Vaincre la Mucoviscidose (cystic fibrosis), Ligue nationale contre le Cancer (LNCC), and AIDES Fédération. Today it is supported by its members and by the Association Française contre les Myopathies, AFM-Téléthon, the European Commission, corporate foundations and the health industry.

EURORDIS has a Board of Directors that is composed of 12 rare disease patient organization representatives from countries around Europe. The member organizations elect the Board at the Annual General Assembly from the full members of the Association for a period of three years. The Board of Directors retains powers to make, in the name of the Association, all decisions which are not exclusively reserved to the General Assembly.

With respect to the mission to build and empower a strong pan-European community of people living with rare diseases, and their organizations, and to promote research, EURORDIS has played an important role in:

a. encouraging research policies by advocating at European, national and international levels;
b. making the best use of new technologies to produce knowledge, in particular about living with largely unknown diseases: the online communities project – RareConnect;
c. conducting surveys with a high political impact on a large range of topics;
d. getting involved in science by supporting research infrastructures and networks;
e. empowering its nearly 600 member organizations to improve access to medical and social care, and to support the development of diagnosis, treatments and medicinal products.

Encouraging research policies

EURORDIS was established to advocate for a European Regulation on Orphan Medicinal Products,[4] similar to the FDA Orphan Drug Act in the USA (1983).[5] The regulation was adopted by the European Parliament in December 1999, and has proven to be an overwhelming success with 1184 medicinal products currently designated as orphan, and 82 authorized for marketing.[6] Further, EURORDIS successfully advocated for the adoption of the European Regulation on Medicinal Products for Paediatric Use in 2006,[7] and for the European Regulation for Advanced Therapies in 2007.[8]

The creation of a committee within the European Medicines Agency is one of the obligations under these Regulations. The Committee for Orphan Medicinal Products is the first committee where patients were included as full voting members, and each subsequent committee created has followed suit.

The active participation of patient representatives of rare diseases in the elaboration and advocating for the adoption of three European regulations was a first important step toward the recognition of rare diseases as a major public health issue. As most rare diseases are apparent at birth or in childhood, involvement in the Paediatric Committee (PDCO) was essential;[7] as with the Advanced Therapies regulation, the development of products for rare diseases will certainly be moving more towards this area and hence representation on the Committee for Advanced Therapies (CAT) was also important (Committee for Orphan Medicinal Products et al. 2011).

The development of treatments for rare diseases is the ultimate goal for patients. However, proper coding, classification and recognition of these diseases in the health and social care systems, and access to diagnosis and to adapted health and social care are absolute necessities on the way to adapted treatments.

The difficulty in obtaining the correct diagnosis is the first dramatic hurdle for rare disease patients. It may take years or even decades to overcome. The EurordisCare surveys (2003–2008) first investigated barriers in access to diagnosis, followed by an evaluation of the medical and social services for people living with rare diseases in Europe.[9] The surveys based on collected individual experiences of 12,000 patients and families provided, for the first time, quantitative evidence on delays in diagnosis and thoroughly investigated the main causes of such delays: lack of awareness of health professionals, complexity of the diseases, and misdiagnoses. Delayed diagnoses and inappropriate treatments have severe, irreversible, debilitating and life-threatening consequences. They result in additional physical, psychological and intellectual impairments, inadequate or even harmful treatments and loss of confidence in the health care system. Some rare diseases are compatible with a normal life if diagnosed in time and properly managed. The numerous consultations, examinations, tests and inefficient treatments represent a major financial burden. In addition, families endure lifelong feelings of guilt due to inappropriate behavior toward the affected person prior to diagnosis, in particular when the learning or behavioral problems of a child were misunderstood and adequate support for the child was not provided. Delayed diagnosis may also result in the birth of additional affected siblings.

The EurordisCare surveys also investigated various barriers including lack of scientific knowledge and organizational, financial and personal restrictions, all of which limit patient access to medical and social services. These surveys demonstrate that the services required by rare disease patients are often inadequately available and not adapted. National healthcare services in the EU for diagnosis, treatment and rehabilitation of people with rare diseases differ significantly, depending on their availability and quality.

In addition, no clinical guidelines exist for the vast majority of the diseases. The segmentation of medical specialties further impedes the organization of multidisciplinary care.

Collecting the voices of 12,000 patients in Europe has helped to shape policy. It was understood that the establishment of a comprehensive strategy for rare diseases at the European level was a necessary prerequisite for the development of new treatments, including diagnosis, medical and social care organization, raising awareness, informing and training patients and encouraging research. Stakeholders (patients' advocates, regulators, policy-makers, industry members) agreed that key solutions in addressing the unmet needs of patients were the establishment of centres of expertise hosting clinical research and clinical trials, linked to research centres, and the coordination of these centres through the establishment of European Reference Networks.[10-13] Thus EURORDIS requested and actively contributed to the Communication of the Commission "Rare diseases, Europe's challenge" (2008)[2] and to the Recommendation of the Council (2009) (Council of the European Union 2009). EURORDIS' members actively participated at all stages of the public consultation of the European Commission. Supported by a EURORDIS-wide awareness-raising campaign, the public consultation received many comments; this resulted in one of the most successful participation rates in the public health field. The European Commission received 584 contributions, including 197 from patient groups and 20 from National Alliances, making a total of 217 patient associations. The many other respondents to the consultation included 11 European countries, public and private bodies, pharmaceutical companies, and individual patients and their families. Following the adoption of the Recommendation of the Council, rare diseases have become a long-term public health and research priority both at European and national level, with the commitment of all Member States for National Plans and strategies for Rare Diseases to be implemented before the end of 2013.[14]

Patients have also participated in the definition of research priorities in the EU framework programs. They rely on widely disseminated common position papers and policy fact sheets.

The main priorities of people living with rare diseases (patients' advocates) until 2020 are:

- allocation of more funds to basic, translational and clinical research;
- development of disease registries and harmonization of data collection;
- setting-up of registries and biobanks-networks and their coordination;
- reinforcing multidisciplinary European Networks of Reference for Rare Diseases and Centres of Expertise, national experts, diagnostic and research laboratories and patient associations;
- fostering public–private partnerships;
- establishing training on rare diseases for researchers;
- exploring broad treatment strategy/protocol trials;
- developing research in social and human sciences.

Similarly, the European Commission has launched an International Rare Diseases Research Consortium (IRDiRC), an initiative for global cooperation on rare disease research that began in 2010 and ends in 2020.[15] The consortium aims at fostering transatlantic cooperation on rare disease research, which is of utmost importance for patients. IRDiRC brings together researchers, funders and other stakeholders with the proclaimed aim of delivering 200 new therapies for rare diseases and diagnostic tools for most rare diseases by 2020.

European rare diseases patients' representatives are involved in the IRDiRC executive committee and scientifi c committee on therapies via EURORDIS.

Making the best use of new technologies

In 2010, EURORDIS sealed a Strategic Partnership agreement with NORD (the US National Organization for Rare Disorders). The aim of the partnership is to bring patient advocates from Europe and the US closer and to promote rare disease research as an international public health priority.

Rare Connect is one of the joint collaboration projects and aims to create rare disease communities. These communities are an online social network for patients and families to connect with each other, to offer support and to share vital experiences on aspects of living with a rare disease. Organized into disease-specific communities, the platform also provides links to quality information and involves patient associations in the governance and growth of each community.[16]

The communities are organized into three sections: "Understand," "Meet," and "Learn." The "Understand" section features patient stories and blog-style updates from patients and patient organization representatives. The "Meet" section is a forum, moderated by volunteers, offering human translation services in five languages. Since patients and families are spread thinly across the globe, it is vital to create a space where information can be shared through the best possible translation. Finally, the "Learn" section is an information resource in the form of frequently asked questions, documents, recently published news and scientific articles, upcoming events, and patient organizations' contact information.

Patients are a source of knowledge and are prominent actors in research.

- Knowledge is generated via networks of patients' organizations, as well as through individual patients and their families using information technologies (e.g. online patient communities).
- Patients generate research questions (identification of needs). A direct dialogue amongst patients and between patients and researchers is emerging, thanks to the development of online patient communities and other supporting IT tools. From these exchanges, questions take shape that relate to health systems, health and social services,

their interrelations, etc. For example, how can disability policies and, more specifically, disability evaluation grids widely used by social services, based on the needs of elderly people or on the International Classification of Functioning (CIF), be better adapted to the specific needs of people living with rare diseases?

New technologies also offer EURORDIS opportunities to develop other networking and information projects, such as online learning services as part of EURORDIS' commitment to train patients' representatives to be empowered in the processes of medicines development.

There is of course a need for caution with all the communication technologies that exist, from the point of view of monitoring content for validity and protection of the information that patients choose to share. The current revision of the Data Protection Directive is one such example that needs to be considered for the protection of users of these technological tools.

Conducting surveys

EURORDIS has conducted many surveys, for instance:

- access to diagnosis, care and social services involving 200 patient groups in 23 countries ("The Voice of 12,000 Patients");
- access to orphan drugs in the EU and pharmaceutical companies' experience of compassionate use for orphan drugs (during the last three years);
- patient organizations and their involvement in research, in collaboration with the "Centre de sociologie de l'innovation" – Ecole des Mines, Paris, France (2009).[17]

The survey on patient organizations' involvement in research aimed at evaluating the support they provide to research activities by collecting their experiences of collaboration with researchers, as well as their opinion on priorities and obstacles for research on rare diseases.

An on-line questionnaire, available in six languages (English, French, German, Italian, Spanish, and Hungarian) was sent to 772 patient organizations, including both members and non-members. EURORDIS received 309 valid responses from members and non-members (a 40 percent response rate), representing 110 rare diseases (approximately 1.3 million patients) in 29 European countries. Diseases represented included multisystem, neurology, dermatology, musculoskeletal, ophthalmology, metabolic, neuromuscular, oncology, cardiovascular, and hematology.

Of the patient groups that responded, 37 percent stated that they are funding research. Of these, 77 percent have initiated and funded a specific research project, 75 percent have co-financed the operating budget for a project, 54 percent have funded the acquisition of specific research equipment, 47 percent are financing a fellowship for a young researcher, and 39 percent and 30 percent respectively are funding meetings of clinicians and researchers, and training.

An interesting finding was that patient organizations primarily fund basic research (81 percent), followed by research on therapeutics (57 percent), diagnosis (56 percent) and epidemiology/ natural history of their diseases (54 percent). They also fund research on assistance technology/daily life (24 percent), and research infrastructures (24 percent).

Interestingly, patient organizations also provide less visible, non-financial, but essential support to research by creating links between patients, researchers and physicians (76 percent), supporting clinical development such as helping identify patients to participate in clinical trials (57 percent), providing information and counseling to potential participants (49 percent), and collaborating in clinical trials design (45 percent). Some patient groups are also involved in campaigns for the collection of biological samples, or participate in scientifi c committees responsible for defining research orientations.

The 2009 survey demonstrated that patient organizations are a driving force for research on rare diseases, making unmet needs visible and disseminating research outcomes. Patient organizations demonstrate a high level of interest in all areas (i.e. basic, translational, therapeutic, human and social sciences), and great preparedness to collaborate with researchers. Relations between patients' groups and researchers are good, having developed and improved over the years. The long history of several organizations and their continuous commitment to basic research proves that they understand that research is a slow and long-term process that is worth their investment.

However, their budgets are limited. They can play a triggering role and momentarily "fi ll the gaps" by supporting types of research that are less attractive to the public or private sectors. They do not wish to (and they cannot) replace public or private research institutions, but rather collaborate with them, as fully recognized partners bringing important specific contributions.

Getting involved in science

In order to make high quality biological material of rare disease patients accessible to the whole scientific community, EURORDIS initiated in 2003, and then coordinated, EuroBioBank, the European network of DNA, Cell and Tissue Biological Resource Centres for Rare Diseases. Fifteen biobanks from eight European countries (France, Germany, Hungary, Italy, Malta, Slovenia, Spain and the United Kingdom, in addition to Israel and Canada) were brought together in the network. They all complied with a common charter.

A web-based catalog facilitated access to samples for researchers:[18] 440,000 samples were made available across the network. On average

13,000 samples were collected from rare disease patients and 7,000 samples were distributed to researchers each year. Since 2012, Eurobiobank has been coordinated by Telethon Italia and included in the larger BBMRI, Biobanking and Biomolecular Resources Research Infrastructure project.

Rare Disease Patient Registries represent a fundamental research effort upon which a number of critical activities are based. They constitute key instruments for increasing knowledge on rare diseases by pooling data for fundamental and clinical research, epidemiological research, and real-life post-marketing observational studies. EURORDIS is today a partner of EPIRARE (European Platform for Rare Disease Registries). This European project (co-funded by the EU Commission, DG Health and Consumers, from April 2011 to September 2013) aims at building consensus and synergies in order to address the regulatory, ethical and technical issues associated with the registration of rare disease patients in Europe, to explore the feasibility of an agreement on a minimum data set common to all rare diseases, and to prepare the feasibility of a future EU registry platform (legal basis, governance, options for sustainability, etc.)

EURORDIS is particularly responsible for the elaboration of policy scenarios on the scope, aims, governance and sustainability of a European policy regarding registration systems of patients living with rare diseases. In the project framework, EURORDIS has elaborated a survey addressing the experiences and expectations of patient organizations regarding patient registries run by academic groups, industry, or public administrations. The survey was conducted online in 11 European languages (English, French, German, Spanish, Italian Portuguese, Greek, Czech, Romanian, Danish, and Hungarian) and was accessed by more than four thousand respondents. The analysis of the survey data will feed into the process of elaboration of the EU registry platform, thus ensuring that patients' needs remain the priority.

Empowering nearly 600 member organizations

EURORDIS is the only patient organization in Europe with a coordinated team of volunteer representatives at the European Medicine Agency (EMA).[6] The legal role of the Agency, as per its website, is stated in the following terms: "The Agency provides the Member States and the institutions of the EU the best-possible scientific advice on any question relating to the evaluation of the quality, safety and effi cacy of medicinal products for human or veterinary use referred to it in accordance with the provisions of EU legislation relating to medicinal products."[19]

Seven scientifi c committees composed of members of all EU and European Economic Area and European Free trade Area states conduct the Agency's main scientific work in the field of medicines evaluation. Four of these committees include representatives of patients and healthcare professionals.

EURORDIS Patients' Representatives have been nominated to the following committees:

- Committee for Orphan Medicinal Products (COMP) – two members and one observer – since 2000; to date, the Vice-Chair of COMP has always been a patient and a member of EURORDIS;
- Paediatric Committee (PDCO) – one member and one alternate since 2008;
- Committee for Advanced Therapies (CAT) – one member and one alternate since 2009;
- Patients' and Consumers' Working Party (PCWP) – two members since 2006. The current co-chair is a EURORDIS volunteer;
- Involvement in Protocol Assistance (Scientific Advice), Risk Management Plans and Scientific Advisory Groups.

Other actions organized by EURORDIS to support patients' representatives in the above activities include the EURORDIS Summer School, a capacity building of patient representatives on clinical trials and EU regulatory process.

In order to support patients' representatives in activities related to medicines development, EURORDIS initiated a training forum entitled the EURORDIS Summer School in 2008. The principle idea of the Summer School is to empower rare disease patients' representatives by teaching them about the processes involved in clinical trials of a medicinal product and the EU regulatory pathways to bring this product to the market. Essential to this training is illustrating throughout the presentations where patients can be involved and make a difference.

All presentations are recorded and available online, and are available openly for participants to revise and refresh their knowledge, as well as providing a learning opportunity for all patient representatives to study a subject of their choice in more detail.[20]

In 2004, EURORDIS launched a Round Table of Companies, in order to establish a long-term educational relationship with companies with an interest in orphan medicines and treatments for people living with rare diseases.

In the context of the Round Table, EURORDIS organizes two workshops annually for informal exchanges on orphan medicines development and issues of access to these medicines between representatives of industry, regulatory agencies, patient groups, clinicians and academics. The topics are suggested by the participants themselves and include i) New Methodologies for Clinical Trials in Small Populations, ii) Rare Disease Patient Registries: a Fundamental Tool in the Development of Therapies? iii) Proof of Concept and Level of Evidence in Orphan Drug Development, iv) Significant Benefit of Orphan Drugs: Impact on Clinical Development and Assessment, v) Improving Access to Orphan Drugs for all Patients Affected by Rare Diseases in Europe: EU Assessment of Clinical Added-Value of Orphan Drugs (CAVOD) to name a few.[21]

EURORDIS also supports the establishment and development of European Federations of patient associations, networking with academics:

- partnerships in TREAT-NMD (Translational Research in Europe – Assessment and Treatment of Neuromuscular Diseases);[22]
- support for the establishment of 35 disease-specific European/international federations of patient associations networking with researchers and clinicians;
- exchange of best practices in the EURORDIS Council of European Federations.

EURORDIS organizes a large Membership Meeting every year, and, every second year since 2001 has organized a European Conference on Rare Diseases and Orphan Drugs (ECRD). This provides a unique platform for exchanges of experiences across all rare diseases and all European countries, bringing together all stakeholders, covering research, development of new treatments, health care, social care, information, public health and support at European, national, and regional levels. This event is synergistic with national and regional conferences. Step by step, partnerships have been established with the EU Committee of Experts on Rare Diseases (EUCERD), EMA-COMP, Orphanet, the European Society of Human Genetics, the European Federation of Internal Medicine, EBE EuropaBio, NORD and CORD, and with the DIA for the co-organization of the conference. The ECRD takes place in a different European city each year (Copenhagen, Paris, Luxembourg, Lisbon, Krakow, Brussels in 2012, and Berlin in 2014). Over 700 participants from 45 countries are expected in Berlin.[23]

Future challenges

Today, new challenges are being faced: to support the development and implementation of National Plans for Rare Diseases in all Member States, to contribute to the implementation of the Directive on cross border health care, and to take part in the revision of three European Directives, all with an important impact on patients. The Directive on data protection, the Directive on clinical trials to facilitate multicentric clinical trials across Europe, and the transparency Directive, to reduce delays for pricing and reimbursement, all improve transparency in decision making process and pricing of innovative medicinal products. Moreover, EURORDIS encourages patient-reported outcome records on adverse effects of orphan drugs, and has launched a first survey on off-label use of medicines.

EURORDIS is also promoting research on "protocols of care" ("strategy trials"), on the basis of the experience developed in the European Reference Networks of Centres of Expertise, and the collection of relevant information in patient registries aims to define "best clinical practices of care." Protocols of care cover a range of areas that are essential for patients' quality of life. They are comprehensive and should include (in addition to drug treatments) paramedical treatments, use of medical devices, physiotherapy, nutrition, as well as surgery and complementary treatments.

In addition, EURORDIS is promoting research on the burden of rare diseases: e.g. the impact of diseases, cost for families, costs for the national health and social systems. Rare diseases demonstrate the added value of exploring the links between public health and social policies. EURORDIS representatives in EUCERD actively participate in the Joint Action for Rare Diseases, a Joint Action co-funded by the European Commission, DG Health and Consumers, which includes healthcare and social policies.[24] In particular, work package (WP)6 aims to map "National initiatives addressing the quality of care in the field of RD," WP7 addresses "Specialised social services and integration of RD into social policies," and WP4 supports the development of National Plans on RD where social and healthcare policies should go hand in hand.

As mentioned, between 5000 and 7000 rare diseases have already been described. Thanks to the development of high-speed genome sequencing, thousands more will be identified in the near future, all affecting very small numbers of patients. Nevertheless they are models which will help us to better understand common diseases, to develop innovative treatments and therapies, and to promote an improved organization of coordinated care and social services for the benefit of all.

Acknowledgements

The authors would like to thank all the EURORDIS team, volunteers and staff, who together have built the organization and contributed to the improvement of patient's lives.

In particular François Faurisson (Institut national de la santé et de la recherche médicale – INSERM) who coordinated the EurordisCare and other EURORDIS surveys along with Fabrizia Bignami, Ariane Weinman, Yann Le Cam, and many dedicated volunteers in France and in Europe.

A special mention to the researchers of the Centre de Sociologie de l'Innovation, Ecole des Mines, Paris, France, for their invaluable support to EURORDIS surveys, and to Sarah MacKenzie for technical support.

Notes

1 EURORDIS website: <www.eurordis.org> (accessed 22 December 2013)

2 Commission of the European Communities (2008) Communication from the Commission to the European Parliament, the Council, the European Economic and Social Committee and the Committee of the Regions on Rare Diseases: Europe's challenges. Available online at: <http://ec.europa.eu/health/ph_threats/non_com/docs/rare_com_en.pdf> (accessed 22 December 2013).

3 Orphanet website: <www.orpha.net> (accessed 22 December 2013.

4 Regulation (EC) No 141/2000 of the European Parliament and of the Council of 16 December 1999 on orphan medicinal products. Available online at: <http://eur-lex.europa.eu/LexUriServ/LexUriServ.do?uri=CELEX:32000R0141:EN:HTML> (accessed 22 December 2013).

5 Orphan Drug Act of 1983. Available online at: <http://rarediseases.about.com/gi/o.htm?zi=1/XJ&zTi=1&sdn=rarediseases&cdn=health&tm=6&f=00&tt=2&bt=4&bts=76&zu=http%3A//www.fda.gov/orphan/oda.htm> (accessed 22 December 2013).

6 European Medicines Agency website: <www.ema.europa.eu> (accessed 22 December 2013).

7 Regulation (EC) No 1901/2006 of the European Parliament and of the Council of 12 December 2006 on medicinal products for paediatric use and amending Regulation (EEC) No 1768/92, Directive 2001/20/EC, Directive 2001/83/EC and Regulation (EC) No 726/2004. Available online at: <http://eur-lex.europa.eu/LexUriServ/LexUriServ.do?uri=CONSLEG:2006R1901:20070126:EN:PDF> (accessed 22 December 2013).

8 Regulation (EC) No 1394/2007 of the European Parliament and of the Council of 13 November 2007 on advanced therapy medicinal products and amending Directive 2001/83/EC and Regulation (EC) No 726/2004. Available online at: <http://ec.europa.eu/health/files/eudralex/vol-1/reg_2007_1394/reg_2007_1394_en.pdf> (accessed 22 December 2013).

9 EURORDS, Kole, Anna and Faurisson, François (2009) *The Voice of 12 000 Patients: Experience and Expectations of Rare Disease Patients on Diagnosis and Care in Europe.* Available online at: <www.eurordis.org/IMG/pdf/voice_12000_patients/EURORDISCARE_FULLBOOKr.pdf> (accessed 22 December 2013).

10 Centres of Reference for rare diseases in Europe: State-of-the-art in 2006 and recommendations of the Rare Diseases Task Force. Available online at: <http://ec.europa.eu/health/archive/ph_threats/non_com/docs/contribution_policy.pdf> (accessed 22 December 2013).

11 European Commission: European networks of reference for rare diseases. Available online at: <http://ec.europa.eu/health/rare_diseases/european_reference_networks/erf/index_en.htm> (accessed 22 December 2013).

12 Orphanet website: Expert Centres <http://www.orpha.net/consor/cgi-bin/Clinics.php?lng=EN> (accessed 22 December 2013).

13 EURORDIS website, Fact Sheets: <www.eurordis.org/sites/default/files/publications/factsheet_EuroRefNetworks.pdf> (accessed 22 December 2013).

14 EUROPLAN Project website: <www.europlanproject.eu/_newsite_986989/index.html> (accessed 22 December 2013).

15 International Rare Disease Research Consortium (IRDiRC) website: <http://ec.europa.eu/research/health/medical-research/rare-diseases/irdirc_en.html> (accessed 22 December 2013).

16 RareConnect website: Online communities <www.rareconnect.org/en> (accessed 22 December 2013).

17 EURORDIS website: Survey on "European Rare Disease Patient Groups in Research: Current role and priorities for the future" <www.eurordis.org/content/survey-patient-groups-research> (accessed 22 December 2013).

18 European Network of DNA, Cell and Tissue banks for Rare Diseases website: <www.eurobiobank.org> (accessed 22 December 2013).

19 European Medicines Agency website: Mission Statement <www.ema.europa.eu/ema/index.jsp?curl=pages/about_us/general/general_content_000106.jsp&mid=WC0b01ac0580028a44> (accessed 22 December 2013).

20 EURORDIS website: online Training Resources <www.eurordis.org/training-resources> (accessed 22 December 2013).

21 EURORDIS website: Round Table of Companies (ERTC) <www.eurordis.org/ertc> (accessed 22 December 2013).
22 Translational Research in Europe: Assessment and Treatment of Neuromuscular Diseases (TREAT-NMD) website: <www.treat-nmd.eu/> (accessed 22 December 2013).
23 The European Conference on Rare Diseases & Orphan Products (ECRD 2014) website: <www.rare-diseases.eu> (accessed 22 December 2013).
24 European Committee of Experts on Rare Diseases (EUCERD) website: <www.eucerd.eu> (accessed 22 December 2013).

References

Committee for Orphan Medicinal Products and the European Medicines Agency Scientific Secretariat (2011) European regulation on orphan medicinal products: 10 years of experience and future perspectives, *Nature Reviews Drug Discovery*, 10(1), 341–349.

Council of the European Union (2009) Council Recommendation of 8 June 2009 on an action in the field of rare diseases, *Official Journal of the European Union*, 7–10.

Mavris, Maria and Le Cam, Yann (2012) Involvement of patient organisations in research and development of orphan drugs for rare diseases in Europe, *Molecular Syndromology*. 3(5), 237–243.

Stolk, Pieter; Willemen, Marjolein J. C. and Leufkens, Hubert G. M. (2006) Rare essentials: drugs for rare diseases as essential medicines, *Bulletin of the World Health Organization*, 84(9), 745–751.

4 The entanglement of scientific and political claims

Towards a new form of patients' activism

Madeleine Akrich, Órla O'Donovan and Vololona Rabeharisoa

Introduction

Over the last few decades, social scientists have extensively studied the involvement of patients' organizations in biomedical research as illustrative of the upsurge of lay expertise and the democratization of science and technology (see for instance Brown et al. 2004; Epstein 1995; Rabeharisoa and Callon 1999). Biomedical research, however, is not the only research area in which patients' organizations invest. Blume's (2009) investigation of deaf communities offers a seminal example: he shows that rather than embracing a biomedical framing of and "solutions" to deafness, these communities turn to socio-linguistics with a view to asserting sign language as a language in its own right and as the pivotal ingredient of deaf culture. Blume's and other studies suggest that patients' organizations and groups of activists' engagement with certain bodies of knowledge should be examined in light of the causes they defend. This article pursues this line of reflection: it looks at how patients' organizations and groups of activists relate issues of knowledge to their politics of illness, and how this (potentially) impacts on the structuring of research policies on their conditions.

We draw on fieldwork we undertook in four condition areas, namely rare diseases, ADHD (Attention Defi cit Hyperactivity Disorder), childbirth in France, and Alzheimer's disease in Ireland. The choice of these four condition areas was motivated by concerned patients' organizations and groups of activists' contrasted positioning vis-à-vis biomedical research. French rare diseases patients' organizations massively engage with biomedical research to foster the development of cures, whereas the French group of parents of children with ADHD considers biomedical knowledge as one body of knowledge amongst many others able to contribute to a better understanding of the disorder. The French group of childbirth activists enters into the black box of medical evidence on certain birth practices to point to their limits and reveal their shadow zones, whereas the Alzheimer Society of

Ireland mobilizes social science methodologies in order to express patients' views and reflect on patient-centered care.

How to make sense of the variety of knowledge, and of knowledge-related activities, undertaken by the patients' organizations and groups of activists mentioned above? It may be argued that the conditions at stake and the national contexts play a determinant role. We take a different stance here. Rather than positing conditions and national contexts as givens, we look at how these groups problematize their conditions and picture the network of expertise and issues they deem relevant to target. Indeed, our fieldwork suggests that clarifying what their situations are, how these situations relate to their medical conditions (whose characteristics they actively explore), and what issues should be addressed at an individual and a collective level to improve these situations, constitutes the main preoccupation of these groups. This implies a radically different view of knowledge for these groups and for the social scientists who study them: rather than contemplating knowledge as a mere resource "out there" which patients' organizations and groups of activists rely on to defend their causes, knowledge (and what counts as such), should be considered as "something" to be produced and discussed. This article shows that patients' organizations and groups of activists collect and format[1] the experiences of the people concerned, in order to document what it is to have and to live with their conditions. They simultaneously identify pieces of academic knowledge on their conditions, and put them to trial with their own "experiential knowledge" (Arksey 1994; Borkman 1976). This work on and with academic and experiential knowledge contributes to sorting out, ordering, and articulating an understanding of their conditions and the problems they induce, for themselves and for specialists. This reconfigures the epistemic network they make themselves part of, and results in a politics of knowledge that eventually transforms the modalities of research and in the production of new evidence for grounding health policies in their condition areas. This is the reason why we suggest calling this form of patients' activism "evidence-based activism" (Rabeharisoa et al. 2014).

The following sections document and analyze these groups' "evidence-based activism", and the compound dynamic interplay between the politics of illness and politics of knowledge it entails in the four condition areas we studied. The first section looks at French rare diseases patient organizations' engagement with biomedical research. Thanks to a better understanding of their bioclinical profiles and improved care strategies, patients now experience the extension of their life expectancy and a series of problems similar to those with which patients with chronic illnesses are familiar. So much so that these organizations now embrace a diversified range of knowledge, and promote their articulation via interlinked platforms associating biologists, clinicians, health professionals and patients' groups. The second section on ADHD looks at how HyperSupers, the French group of parents, strive to make sense of their experience of the complex, variable and individual manifestations of the disorder, and to articulate a multidisciplinary network of expertise bringing together neuroscientists, geneticists, behavioral scientists, child psychiatrists, psychologists, educational scientists and pharmacologists on this confrontational condition. In doing so, the group intends to connect around ADHD different scientific communities which have so far kept their distance from each other. Departing from the classic picturing of childbirth activism as a feminist movement seeking to de-medicalize childbirth practices, the third section focuses on the strikingly intense and enduring effort of CIANE, the French group of childbirth activists, in the critical reading of medical evidence on certain birth practices, and, drawing on a series of surveys, its confrontation to women's experiences. This highly sophisticated work on and with various species of figures and statistics questions medical evidence from the inside as much as it challenges, from the outside, the range of relevant evidence on what "normal birth" should be. The last section looks at how the Alzheimer Society of Ireland reflects on the relevance of social science methodologies for collecting and expressing the views of people with dementia, and for putting them center-stage in the provision of services. Rather than simply mobilizing these methodologies, the organization's involvement in mutually informing the politics of illness, the politics of knowledge and the politics of identity has required it to renew them.

Reflecting on the similarities and differences between the four condition areas we explore, the concluding section offers a few thoughts on whether the intervention of patients' organizations and groups of activists in the fabrics of knowledge entails a process of co-optation and institutionalization of patients' activism. Does "evidence-based activism" put patients' organizations and groups of activists at risk of losing sight of their identity and oppositional power? Although we should avoid romanticizing "evidence-based activism," our analysis suggests that it brings in uncertainties about what exactly relevant and legitimate evidence is, and therefore introduces a form of collective reflexivity on the shaping of research policies.

The dual dynamics of research and issues: the transformation of rare diseases activism

On both sides of the Atlantic, patients' activism in the area of rare diseases was originally motivated by the absence of cures for these lethal conditions (Asbury 1985; Brewer 1983; Crompton 2007; Huyard 2011/2). In France, the AFM (*Association Française contre les Myopathies* – French Association against Myopathies), created in 1958 by a few parents of children with Duchenne de Boulogne dystrophy, has played a prominent role in relating this deficiency of the drug market to specialists' ignorance and lack of interest in these diseases because of their rareness, and to the need for patients' and parents' groups to actively engage with biomedical research. Aimed at "knowing the enemy [the disease] in order to combat it", as the former President of the AFM phrased the basis of the association, it articulates "therapeutic activism" (Epstein 1995) with "biomedical activism". Since the mid-1980s, the AFM has established partnerships with the biomedical community (Rabeharisoa 2003). In the absence of a robust corpus of credentialed knowledge on neuromuscular diseases, the AFM has introduced families' experiences to biomedical practitioners with a view to starting and sustaining the research process (Rabeharisoa and Callon 2004). It has provided financial support to research teams, and participated in the orientation of research policies on neuromuscular and other rare diseases in France through its annual call for research projects (Rabeharisoa and Callon 1999).

The model of engagement with biomedical research that the AFM has promoted has been adopted and adapted by a number of French rare disease patients' organizations. Drawing on interviews and ethnographic observations of 12 French rare diseases patients' organizations, all created after the AFM and contrasted in terms of their size, the nature and prevalence of their diseases, their resources and organizational features, we observed that even though these groups do not intervene directly in the definition and conduct of research activities as the AFM does, they nevertheless establish dialogue with researchers, scrutinize research hypothesis and findings, and circulate them to families and medical and health professionals. When asked about their motives for such an intensive acquisition and dissemination of scientific knowledge and enduring relationships with the biomedical community, they mention a series of interlinked problems which, according to patients and families, continue to hinder the "war on rare diseases": the scarcity of information available on these conditions, the low number of clinicians who can accurately diagnose their diseases and provide care to patients, the complexity of rare diseases and the need for long-term investment in research, and the need to ensure that the research teams they ally with explore the topics they deem important for a better understanding of their pathologies. As the patients' representatives we interviewed suggested, "war on diseases" is a multifaceted endeavor, implying a complex investigation with the goal of deciphering the diseases at stake and the problems to which they give rise, including those resulting from the perceived deficiencies of the market, the research system and the medical and health institutions when facing rare diseases. This problematization of rare diseases has multiple and interrelated consequences for the research policies and politics of knowledge in this area. Two of them are particularly worth highlighting.

First, for a number of rare diseases, the dialogue between patients' organizations and specialists, though sometimes confrontational, gives shape to epistemic communities which bring together patients, researchers and clinicians around the collective exploration of diseases, and within which experiential knowledge and academic knowledge together constitute a seamless web of knowledge. One remarkable feature of these communities is that their contours, as well as their epistemic focus, progressively evolve alongside the knowledge, problems and issues brought in by the different parties. To take but one example, *SolHand "Solidarité Handicap – Autour des Maladies Rares"* (Association on rare disabilities and diseases), formed in 2008, brings to the fore questions that its chairwoman qualifies as "medico-social" and on which no research has yet been undertaken. The formulation of these questions is partly enabled by the efforts that have been devoted to biological and clinical research. The results obtained have had the effect not of healing patients (cure remains rare), but of gradually adjusting the care they receive. The natural history of rare diseases has thus been altered. Some of them became chronic illnesses that generated unexpected problems, on the fringes of biomedicine. That is why *SolHand* insists on the need to mobilize rehabilitation therapists and researchers in human and social sciences in the production of knowledge focused on solutions to problems that patients encounter in their daily lives, such as chronic pain, fatigue, depression, disability, or inclusion in the job market.

Interestingly, this articulation of biomedical research with the production of knowledge on families' day-to-day preoccupations and the adjustment of care practices now stands at the core of research and public policies on rare diseases. In 2000, patients' organizations decided to join forces within the French Alliance on Rare Diseases and asked for the creation of centers of reference for diagnosis and care in various regions of France. This resulted in the launching of a National Plan for Rare Diseases by the French government in 2004, and the creation and provision of support to centers of reference which propose multidisciplinary consultations and bring together researchers, clinicians and care professionals, in order to ensure continuity from research to the clinic, from diagnosis to treatment, social care and information for patients and families. How exactly this articulation between biomedical research and healthcare is performed, and to what extent patients' organizations act as fully-fledged stakeholders in the functioning of these centers, remain to be explored. We can, however, say that these centers design innovative platforms for research and care policies, within which a variety of academic and experiential knowledge and know-how are supposed to be mutually nurtured. This also led the recently formed French Foundation on Rare Diseases, responsible for coordinating research efforts in this condition area, to include a social and human sciences chapter in its activities.

Second, the knowledge-related activities undertaken by patients' organizations profoundly transform the identification and specification of rare diseases and open discussion on their classification. To take but one example, *Génération 22*, concerned with the 22q11 deletion syndrome (DS), a complex syndrome involving heterogeneous disorders with multiple manifestations, has actively contributed to clarifying the clinical profiles of affected patients. In particular, drawing on families' observations, it pinned down the high prevalence of schizophrenia in these patients compared to the general population. While French specialists have long been reluctant to consider the extending range of manifestations and co-morbidities of this syndrome, *Génération 22* has recently secured collaboration with a psychiatric genetics team in Switzerland with the aim of exploring the psychiatric disorders that accompany 22q11 DS. Moreover, the association now suspects that this syndrome may be less rare than previously estimated, as certain persons with schizophrenia may carry the deletion. By entering into the black box of complex biological pathways and entities that are still to be explored, *Génération 22* contributes, as similar organizations do (Navon and Shwed 2012), to the emergence of an *ad hoc* disease category bringing together "developmental disorders and deformity syndromes", as French specialists provisionally term it.

Fighting reductionism: the politics of knowledge of an ADHD group

Parents of children with ADHD often start to mobilize to fight the lack of medical recognition of this disorder, and the stigmatization of children as "brats", notably because of parents'/mothers' supposedly bad parenting. Indeed, ADHD has long been, and still is, a contested condition. Neurobiologists, child psychiatrists and psychologists, to cite but a few specialties, hold different views on the causes and manifestations of this disorder (Rafalovich 2001). In France, certain child psychiatrists with a psychodynamics background even deny the existence of ADHD, arguing that observed symptoms may instead express a form of suffering or depression, or even epitomize "normal" child or adolescent evolution. Some of them worry about "over-diagnosis" of ADHD, which, from their point of view, is often a misdiagnosis (Garcin 2011). Social scientists have highlighted how biomedical practitioners, the pharmaceutical industry and parents' groups have promoted a biomedical framing of the disorder as a way of attesting to its "reality" against the prevarications of certain credentialed experts. Two phenomena are said to support this biomedicalization of ADHD: brain images which trace the dysfunction of certain neurotransmitters in children with ADHD, and the effi ciency of certain medications, namely Ritalin©, when prescribed for inattentive and/or hyperactive children. This biomedicalization of ADHD raises concerns about the risk of social normalization and control over behaviors considered as non-desirable in performance-oriented societies (Conrad 2007).

HyperSupers, the French parents' group on ADHD created in 2002 after the launching of an electronic discussion list, soon realized that biomedicalization is not the "one best way" of understanding the disorder and caring for their children. Although the group manifests its interest in the neurodevelopmental make-up of ADHD, as attested by a conference it organized on this topic following its 2010 general assembly of families, and is happy with the development of drugs, it tirelessly questions what exactly ADHD is and how to address the multifaceted problems which children and their parents face in their everyday life. Drawing on parents' testimonies, which point to the complex, variable and evolving manifestations of the disorder, HyperSupers steps back from any simple causal interpretation of the condition. Not only does it emphasize the multi-factorial nature of ADHD, it also casts doubt on the claim that the causes and consequences of the disorder can be easily sorted out. The president of HyperSupers, whom we interviewed a number of times, insisted that the neurodevelopmental, social and psychological aspects of ADHD are interwoven and impact on each other. From the outset, this politics of illness has gone hand in hand with the group's intensive efforts to collect and articulate a variety of bodies of academic knowledge with the aim of opening up discussion on the bio-psycho-social framing of the disorder.

HyperSupers' eclecticism and openness was recently seen in its launching of the *Journée Ribot-Dugas*, a one-day annual scientifi c symposium named after two French psychologists. What is remarkable with this *Journée* is that despite the reluctance of its scientific committee, HyperSupers has managed to gather specialists from very different backgrounds who are not used to engaging in dialogue with each other: neurobiology, cognitive sciences, education sciences, child psychiatry, psychology, pharmacology, epidemiology, and even psychodynamics. Issues as diverse as the neurological mechanisms implied in ADHD, the sleep disorders that sometimes occur, and even the role of Omega 3 fatty acids in alleviating certain "symptoms" have been put on the scientific agenda. Rather than taking the side of one or the other scientifi c community, the design of the *Journée* allows HyperSupers to shed light on the complexity and uncertainty of competing scientific understandings of ADHD. However, this does not mean that the association thinks anything goes: on this and other occasions, the president of HyperSupers has called for further clarification of the hypotheses and methodologies that underlie the research projects undertaken by different scientific communities. HyperSupers' epistemic efforts have had two main effects on the politics of knowledge in this condition area.

First, by confronting diverse scientifi c communities that more often than not turn a deaf ear to each other, HyperSupers clearly intends to give shape to a multidisciplinary network of expertise and issues on ADHD. Although the association has historically established close ties with a few specialists who are sympathetic to its cause, it nevertheless strives to expand the bodies of knowledge it deems relevant to assemble around families' experiences. It is too soon to tell whether this will renew research policies on ADHD, but one can fairly assume that the association is playing a crucial mediating role in the development of multidisciplinary approaches in this condition area. HyperSupers' numerous publications provide evidence of the association "shopping around" with concerned people's experiences as its compass. For example, the "Token economy method" it posted a few years ago on its website, advising parents to reward their children when they are doing well and to draw their attention to alternative small tasks when they are "going into a spin", was simultaneously nurtured by parents' experiences and by psychological theories which show that children with ADHD tend to lose self-esteem because of the constant denigration of their behavior. This does not prevent parents from considering other "solutions" to other problems posed by ADHD, such as neurofeedback for instance, a type of biofeedback which focuses on the brain and central nervous system: by placing sensors on a person's head, it provides a display of brain activity, or "brainwaves" that can be monitored and retrained. Though neurofeedback is not necessarily perceived as an evidence-based therapy by the wider medical community, and is much discussed within the association, it surfaces as one body of knowledge and practices at which the association is taking a close look.

Second, one major consequence that HyperSupers expects from its epistemic efforts is the shaping of what it calls a "multimodal cure and care strategy". As suggested by the examples mentioned, HyperSupers advocates a range of medications, parenting therapies, educational methods, and even psychotherapies, adjusted to each child's situation and its evolution. Such a strategy not only translates the association's politics of illness; it also enacts its politics of knowledge insofar as it implies a continuing exploration and weighing up of the evidence basis of various cure and care practices. Thus, the politics of illness, the politics of knowledge and the politics of care together constitute a threefold strategy towards the recognition of ADHD as a complex disorder that cannot be reduced to the biological, the social, or the psychological only.

Raising issues and unpacking evidence: the knowledge politics of a childbirth group

Childbirth activism displays a configuration which contrasts with the conditions we analyzed, as it has often been described as a de-medicalization movement: drawing upon a survey of 19 organizations in England, the Netherlands and Germany, Tyler (2002) points to the existence of shared views on pregnancy and childbirth seen as "natural physiological life events that should be as free as possible from medical intervention" and "the routine application of medical technology [experienced] as disempowering" (ibid.: 139). More recently, other contributions have stressed the emergence of a rhetoric of "choice" which should extend to the right to choose elective cesarean section (Beckett 2005). Much of the academic discussion revolves around the relationships between these movements and various waves of feminism (Annandale and Clark 1996; Reiger 1999, 2000): for some, technology supports obstetricians' control over women's bodies and is seen as alienating (Katz Rothman 1982; Murphy-Lawless 1998; Halfon 2010); for others, technology can contribute to women's empowerment by freeing them from biological determinism. Standard medical practices appear as external factors which obey their own logic: depending on their perspective, women demand the possibility to opt in or opt out. Recent contributions have criticized this view by stressing that the way women frame their choices is highly dependent on obstetrics itself, on its organization and on the knowledge it mobilizes to define appropriate practices (Crossley 2007; Donovan 2006; Spoel 2007). Our observations in four European countries (Akrich et al. 2014) led to the conclusion that childbirth organizations have indeed been taking this criticism as a point of departure for their activism: one can argue that, at least for the last decade, they have tried to transform obstetrics from within and that, to do so, they have drawn upon an extensive knowledge work seeking the integration of women's experiences as a challenging or complementing source of obstetric knowledge. Drawing upon the French case in the following section, we describe this knowledge work and its implications for both research policy and health policy.

Created in 2003, the *Collectif interassociatif autour de la naissance* (CIANE) is a collective of about 40 French childbirth organizations, local support groups and national organizations focusing on specific issues (cesarean section, homebirth, post-partum depression, etc.). Some of these organizations emerged in the early 2000s from internet discussion groups which developed a scientific expertise and a culture of discussion articulating this expertise with personal experiences (Akrich 2010) which has been crucial in the development of CIANE. The CIANE involvement in knowledge activities takes three forms, which we examine below.

First, they question current medical practices in the light of an analysis of the scientific literature and, among other actions, make it politically operative by participating in the elaboration of clinical guidelines organized by the HAS (High Authority of Health). They even take part in the determination of its work program by sending referrals on the issues they deem relevant. Drawing on its scientific expertise, CIANE has thus provoked and participated in the elaboration of guidelines on topics such as induction, episiotomy, fundal pressure, and indications for planned cesarean sections: the choice of the topics to be tackled was linked to the informal knowledge that they gathered on women's experiences, and especially on situations where women were confronted with professionals' decisions that they eventually found detrimental, and possibly made on disputable grounds. To a certain extent, the CIANE approach can be understood as a way of re-opening all these individual failed debates between professionals and women: thus, the aim is to set up a space for negotiation where the expectations of both parties can be framed in a stabilized and public way.

Second, they question the relevance of medical practices, authoritative discourse and credentialed knowledge from the perspectives opened by experiential knowledge: this strategy does not exclude the previous one, as is illustrated by the critical analysis produced by CIANE very early in its existence of the guidelines on episiotomy produced by the College of Obstetricians. This analysis was elaborated by drawing on existing internet discussion groups: the groups called for testimonies, used them to confront the academic literature, and pointed to several complications of episiotomy that have been neglected both by the literature and the guidelines but have severe consequences in women's everyday life; it ended up by reframing the problem not as "the prevention of episiotomy", an expression that naturalizes the intervention, but as "the prevention of perineal lacerations", which opens up a whole set of other policy options. Among these options, acting upon positions during labor seemed relevant, but CIANE pointed to another difficulty, the oversimplification associated with experimental protocols of research which exclude gathering data on situations where women are free to choose their position. The de-medicalization vocabulary is indeed useless to describe what is at stake here: the mobilization and production of experiential knowledge allowed the group to deconstruct both the framing of the issue and the legitimacy of credentialed knowledge; it led to propositions for amending the guidelines but also raised some issues as regards medical research, thus trying to influence both health policy and research policy.

Third, they put together existing but separate pieces of knowledge in an attempt to reframe the issues at stake: this might result in a questioning of research policy as well as of health policy, as can be seen in the following examples. In 2004, CIANE asked to review clinical guidelines on the prevention of post-partum hemorrhage (PPH), which appears to be involved in more than half maternal deaths. Again, they contested the use of the word "prevention", as the guidelines did not even mention the issue of what may cause PPH, with the exception of well-known risk factors that do not represent the majority of severe cases. CIANE put together, first, the fact that the prevalence of HPP was higher in France than in other countries and, second, the fact that some scarce publications, including publications by midwives, formulate hypotheses about the role of medical practices and the administration of oxytocin during labor in the occurrence of PPH: as this practice is more frequent in France than in most countries, it is possible to infer a correlation between the two facts. After months of work, they succeeded in convincing an administration to fund a research project which resulted in a first publication in 2011 in the BMJ, confirming the existence of a link between the administration of oxytocin and PPH. In this case the different pieces of knowledge were all medical, but in a more recent case the knowledge they put together was much more heterogeneous: they drew up a document developing a new approach as regards health professional insurance. Due to European legislation, midwives attending homebirths need to have professional insurance cover. In France insurers take as a reference the insurance premium paid by obstetricians, an amount which is not affordable for midwives. The CIANE analysis consists of a large diagram making visible the different kinds of risks, some specific to hospitals, some specific to homebirths, others common to both situations; the diagram is accompanied by a detailed argumentation based on medical knowledge but also on psychological or legal knowledge, as the risk at stake is a litigation risk which is not the same thing as a medical risk and depends upon a range of factors. This document has been endorsed by the National College of Midwives and three midwives' unions. It aims at re-opening the debate about the calculation of premiums, which has been closed unilaterally by insurers, not by providing the calculation key but by trying to demonstrate that the current one is neither adequate nor fair.

In all these actions, CIANE does not appear as driven by a normative perspective. It does not claim special rights for women or for midwives, it tries to build a users' perspective on obstetrics, its practices and its organization, borrowing obstetric language itself: by doing so, it opens up a space of discussion and negotiation with other stakeholders.

Shaping the concerned publics: social enquiry in an Alzheimer disease organization

Emerging in the late 1970s and early 1980s, European Alzheimer's disease patients' organizations resembled in many respects those in the US from where they were isomorphically imported. In both contexts, the cause around which Alzheimer's disease patients' organizations were initially mobilized was the need to provide support to carers of people diagnosed with the disease, not patients themselves who were deemed to have experienced a "loss of self" and thus to be liminal or non-persons (O'Donovan et al. 2013). However, there was a significant difference between the early US and European Alzheimer's disease patients' organizations in respect of their knowledge-related activities. The prioritization of proactive engagement in biomedical knowledge production in the quest for a cure that was a defining feature of US patients' organizations, as described by Patrick Fox (1989), was not replicated by the European organizations, including the Alzheimer Society of Ireland. Established in 1982, the Alzheimer Society of Ireland was the second Alzheimer's disease patients' organization to emerge in Europe, and similar to its British counterpart established three years previously, its chief preoccupation was service delivery. The organization has since become one of the largest service provision charities in Ireland; in 2011, 86 per cent of its €17 million budget, most of which came from State grants, was spent on service delivery (Alzheimer Society of Ireland 2012). Notwithstanding this prioritization of service provision, the Alzheimer Society of Ireland is now also engaged in intensive epistemic work producing and circulating facts and figures about dementia and its care, much of which is motivated by efforts to establish the condition as a national and European public health priority. The *Dementia Manifesto 2007–2009*, the "cornerstone of the Society's political lobbying campaign" (Alzheimer Society of Ireland 2007) serves as one example; it was a synthesis of knowledge about priority issues for people with dementia and their carers generated by a National Consumer Summit, consultation with "stakeholders" and the commissioning of a position paper by a health economist. The organization is enmeshed in networks of biomedical expertise, including those at European level through its strong links with the European coalition of patient organizations, Alzheimer

Europe, but engagement in biomedical research is just one feature of the organization's varied repertoire of knowledge-related activities.

Social research has featured prominently in the history of the Alzheimer Society of Ireland's epistemic work. Motives for considering this species of knowledge have included encoding and formalizing the experiential knowledge of carers and the "costs of caring". However, in recent years, moves to redefine Alzheimer's disease patienthood and recognize the fully-fledged personhood of those diagnosed with the disease have presented the organization with profound epistemic challenges; it relies upon social research to represent patients' experiential knowledge and perspectives, but is simultaneously confronted with the limitations of those very social science techniques and with the need to innovate methodologically. These epistemic challenges are intimately connected with the political challenge of social enfranchisement of people with dementia within the organization. To understand the distinctive features and challenges of this Alzheimer's disease evidence-based activism, it is important to appreciate the significant and hybridizing shift that has taken place in the "cause regime" of the organization, which has included an expansion of the constituency the organization claims to represent to include both carers and patients. Similar to Alzheimer's disease organizations elsewhere, the Alzheimer's Society of Ireland has been transformed from a carers' organization to a carers' and patients' organization.

The organization has made the "turn to personhood", which problematizes knowledge about the disease that understands it as inducing a "loss of self" form of patienthood, knowledge that it and other organizations in the international Alzheimer's disease movement played a crucial role in co-producing and circulating (Beard 2004). Much of the scholarship on what Nancy Scheper-Hughes and Margaret Lock (1986: 137) referred to as Alzheimer's disease's metaphoric "double", "the layers of stigma, rejection, fear and exclusion" attached to the disease, attributes blame primarily to its biomedical framing as a disease that gradually destroys the patient's brain and consequently their personhood (Basting 2003; Kitwood 1997). But equally, the more recent understanding of what it means to be diagnosed with dementia that recognizes the personhood of the patient tends to be attributed to the Alzheimer's disease biomedical enterprise's investments in new devices for early diagnosis and treatments aimed at delaying the progression of the disease (Moreira 2009).

The Alzheimer Society of Ireland's research on telecare – remote care providing the care and reassurance needed to allow patients to remain living in their own homes – provides an illustration of how the organization has co-produced and subsequently problematized the "loss of self" patient identity and confronted the epistemic challenge of representing the perspectives of people with dementia. In 2007, the organization instigated a pilot project of telecare as a technology of independent living. The research evaluating the project framed carers rather than people with dementia as the users of the telecare technologies and as the actors whose perspectives the research sought to ascertain. The social disenfranchisement of people with dementia through their exclusion from direct participation in the evaluative study was compounded by the exclusion of many of them from the decision to participate in the pilot project and the installation of the telecare devices (Alzheimer Society of Ireland 2010). A subsequent telecare project, the EU-funded INDEPENDENT – ICT Enabled Service Integration for Independent Living, is adopting a very different style of research by including people with dementia as research participants, rather than relying on their carers as proxies. Explaining the intention to use the technique of ethnographic interviewing to generate knowledge of patients' experiences of the impact of telecare on their quality of life, a researcher involved in the project explained:

> We will be doing a detailed assessment of the quality of life with people with dementia. Hopefully, we'll be working with them directly to understand their view of … what is important in quality of life for them and how telecare might impact that. Now obviously we can do that with people with mild to moderate dementia. We have to work really carefully with people who are further on in the disease to see what is the best way of communicating with them to get this information.
>
> (Delaney 2010)

Here we can see that social science techniques are not a given, but are to be explored as potential voicing devices that can make the experiential knowledge of people with dementia visible and meaningful. As we have discussed in more detail elsewhere (Moreira et al. 2014), the technique of the interview is embedded in a politics of subjectivity that views individuals as knowledgeable agents in their own social worlds. Such presuppositions may require revisiting the methodological innovations being crafted in this second telecare project of the Alzheimer Society of Ireland.

Conclusion

Through the variety of cases we have presented, our intention was to demonstrate that patients' and activists' involvement in knowledge activities is not restricted to a limited set of diseases (e.g. those for which biomedical research is considered as a priority), but extends to all kinds of conditions, including those which remain contested.

This involvement in knowledge stands at the core of patients' organizations' activities, and that is what we try to capture through the expression "evidence-based activism". First, this expression sheds light on how patients' organizations define the causes they engage in: even if patients' organizations come into being around a shared condition or experience, this does not necessarily imply a straightforward definition of their claims. Sometimes, as illustrated by the case of the French association on rare disabilities and diseases, what the "shared experience" consists of is not given once and for all but emerges and changes in the course of the on-going transformation of people's lives in which medicine itself plays a significant role. Thus, the transformation of individual complaints into collective claims involves the collective production of knowledge and analysis of individual situations and its articulation with the existing medical and care system: without the constitution of such expertise – which largely draws on, and even renews, as seen in the Alzheimer's disease case, social science techniques – patients' organizations would not be anything else than support groups.

Second, this entanglement between knowledge work and political work is also at stake in the engagement of patients' organizations in medical research: as demonstrated in the case of 22q11 DS and in the ADHD case, the active participation of patients' organizations in "research policy", or at least in the formulation of research issues they deem relevant, cannot be separated from their continuous effort to get a grip on their condition, i.e. to understand what it is and how and why it affects people's lives, which can eventually lead to a radical redefinition of diseases or the emergence of new nosographic categories.

Third, patients' organizations' engagement in science and in knowledge production is a key element in the building of relationships, even confrontational relationships, with a number of other actors, and especially professionals and researchers: being able to go back and forth between people's experiences and medical knowledge opens new capacities of action for patients' organizations. As mentioned above, participating in the medical definition of the condition is one of these capacities, as is participating in the elaboration of guidelines, in the setting up of centers of reference, or in the definition of care pathways: more generally, this engagement with knowledge opens up new spaces for discussion and negotiation with the actors involved and, in some cases, results in the building of epistemic communities.

Does our analysis suggest a move towards institutionalization of patients' organizations that would hinder their contestation power and "normalize" them as ordinary players in a game ruled by official authorities? Are patients' organizations instrumentalized as civil society representatives that give legitimacy to decisions still massively in the hands of the "real experts"? In other words, are such organizations losing their contestation power and autonomy?

On the one hand, it could be said that patients' organizations who engage in what we called evidence-based activism accept the language of "dominant" actors, and that should be considered a success for biomedicine and health professionals. In this process, patients' organizations may lose their capacity to mobilize around more overtly political slogans centered around rights for instance, and may contribute to the overshadowing of issues such as social health inequalities. On the other hand, we have tried to demonstrate that evidence-based activism constitutes a powerful leverage which allows patients' organizations to penetrate others' territories, to redefine borders, and to bring in new entities and new issues, so that the whole geography may be turned upside down in some cases. Research actions that some rare diseases organizations have undertaken were explicitly aimed at shaking the medical world, which thought there was nothing to be done; pushing Alzheimer's disease patients into the arena of discussion through the mediating tools of social research is not especially intended to please professionals or policy makers; criticizing the way obstetricians frame interventions and questioning research methodology is generally perceived as rather aggressive by the professionals; forcing various disciplines to discuss their understandings of ADHD is clearly to infringe on what researchers and clinicians consider as their prerogatives. So, evidence-based activism is not, in our view, a soft version of activism that would facilitate the instrumentalization of patients' organizations more than other forms of activism would do; on the contrary, it gives them quite effective tools with which they can contest both medical "paradigms" and the organization of care.

Note

1 The point here is that patients' organizations collect concerned people's experiences (e.g. through surveys or testimonies) and put them in a format which allows these experiences to be circulated. and worked upon as pieces of knowledge by different actors (medical experts, health professionals, policy-makers, but also patients and families).

References

Akrich, Madeleine (2010) From communities of practice to epistemic communities: Health mobilizations on the internet, *Sociological Research Online*, 15(2).

Akrich, Madeleine; Leane, Máire; Roberts, Celia and Arriscado Nunes, João (2014) Practising childbirth activism: A politics of evidence, *BioSocieties*, 9(2), 129–152.

Alzheimer Society of Ireland (2012) Annual Report 2011, Blackrock: Alzheimer Society of Ireland.

—— (2010) *Telecare Project: Interim Evaluation*, Blackrock: Alzheimer Society of Ireland.

—— (2007) *Dementia Manifesto* 2007–2009, Blackrock: Alzheimer Society of Ireland.

Annandale, Ellen and Clark, Judith (1996) What is gender? Feminist theory and the sociology of human reproduction, *Sociology of Health & Illness*, 18(1), 17–44.

Arksey, Hilary (1994) Expert and lay participation in the construction of medical knowledge, *Sociology of Health & Illness*, 16(4), 448–468.

Asbury, Carolyn H. (1985) *Orphan Drugs: Medical versus Market Value*, Lexington, MA: Lexington Books.

Basting, Anne D. (2003) Looking back from loss: Views of self in Alzheimer's disease, *Journal of Aging Studies*, 17(1), 87–99.

Beard, Renée L. (2004) Advocating voice: Organisational, historical and social milieux of the Alzheimer's disease movement, *Sociology of Health & Illness*, 26(6), 797–819.

Beckett, Katherine (2005) Choosing cesarean: Feminism and the politics of childbirth in the United States, *Feminist Theory*, 6(3), 251–275.

Blume, Stuart (2009) *The Artificial Ear: Cochlear Implants and the Culture of Deafness*, New Brunswick, NJ: Rutgers University Press.

Borkman, Thomasina (1976) Experiential knowledge: A new concept for the analysis of self-help groups, *The Social Service Review*, 50(3), 445–456.

Brewer, Georg J. (ed.) (1983) Orphan Drugs and Orphan Diseases: Clinical Realities and Public Policy. Proceedings of a conference held in Ann Arbor, Michigan, September 27–29, 1982, New York: Alan R. Liss.

Brown, Phil; Zavestoski, Stephen; McCormick, Sabrina; Mayer, Brian; Morello-Frosch, Rachel and Gasior Altman, Rebecca (2004) Embodied health movements: new approaches to social movements in health, *Sociology of Health & Illness*, 26(1), 50–80.

Conrad, Peter (2007) *The Medicalization of Society: On the Transformation of Human Conditions into Treatable Disorders*, Baltimore, MD: Johns Hopkins University Press.

Crompton, Helen (2007) Mode 2 knowledge production: Evidence from orphan drug networks, *Science and Public Policy*, 34(3), 199–211.

Crossley, Michele L. (2007) Childbirth, Complications and the Illusion of "Choice": A Case Study, *Feminism & Psychology*, 17(4), 543–563.

Delaney, Sarah (2010) Telecare and Dementia: The ASI experience. Paper presented at the Technology and Dementia Seminar, The Living with Dementia Programme, School of Social Work and Social Policy, Trinity College Dublin and the Dementia Services Information and Development Centre (DSIDC), St James' Hospital, Dublin, 28 October.

Donovan, Sarah (2006) Inescapable burden of choice? The impact of a culture of prenatal screening on women's experiences of pregnancy, *Health Sociology Review*, 15(4), 397–405.

Epstein, Steven (1995) The construction of lay expertise: AIDS activism and the forging of credibility in the reform of clinical trials, *Science, Technology & Human Values*, 20(4), 408–437.

Fox, Patrick (1989) From senility to Alzheimer's disease: The rise of the Alzheimer's disease movement, *The Milbank Quarterly*, 67(1), 58–102.

Garcin, Vincent (2011) Introduction de cadrage sur le processus de révision de la CIM-10 en pédopsychiatrie, *L'information psychiatrique*, 87(5), 355–357.

Halfon, Saul (2010) Encountering birth: Negotiating expertise, networks, and my STS self, *Science as Culture*, 19(1), 61–77.

Huyard, Caroline (2011/2) Quand la puissance publique fait surgir et équipe une mobilisation protestataire: L'invention des "maladies rares" aux Etats-Unis et en Europe, *Revue française de sciences politiques*, 61(2), 183–200.

Katz Rothman, Barbara (1982) *In Labor: Women and Power in the Birthplace*, New York: W.W. Norton.

Kitwood, Tom (1997) *Dementia Reconsidered: The Person Comes First*, Philadelphia, PA: Open University Press.

Moreira, Tiago (2009) Testing promises: Truth and hope in drug development and evaluation in Alzheimer's disease, in J. Ballenger, P. Whitehouse, C. Lyketsos, P. Rabins and J. Karlawish (eds) *Do We Have a Pill for That? Interdisciplinary Perspectives on the Development, Use and Evaluation of Drugs in the Treatment of Dementia*, Baltimore, MD: Johns Hopkins University Press.

Moreira, Tiago; O'Donovan, Órla and Howlett, Etaoine (2014) Assembling dementia care: Patient organisations and social research, *BioSocieties*, 9(2), 173–193.

Murphy-Lawless, Jo (1998) *Reading Birth and Death: A History of Obstetric Thinking*, Bloomington & Indianapolis, IN: Indiana University Press.

Navon, Daniel and Shwed, Uri (2012) The chromosome 22q11.2 deletion: From the unification of biomedical fields to a new kind of condition, *Social Science & Medicine*, 75(9), 1633–1641.

O'Donovan, Órla; Moreira Tiago and Howlett, Etaoine (2013) Tracking transformations in health movement organisations: Alzheimer's disease organisations and their changing "cause regimes", *Social Movements Studies: Journal of Social, Cultural and Political Protest*, 12(3), 316–334.

Rabeharisoa, Vololona (2003) The struggle against neuromuscular diseases in France and the emergence of the "partnership model" of patient organization, *Social Science & Medicine*, 57(11), 2127–2136.

Rabeharisoa, Vololona and Callon, Michel (1999) *Le pouvoir des malades: L'Association française contre les myopathies et la Recherche*, Paris: Presses de l'Ecole des mines.

—— (2004) Patients and scientists in French muscular dystrophy research, in S. Jasanoff (ed.) *States of Knowledge: The Co-Production of Science and Social Order*, London and New York: Routledge, 142–160.

Rabeharisoa, Vololona; Moreira, Tiago and Akrich, Madeleine (2014) Evidence-based activism: Patients', users' and activists' groups in knowledge society, *BioSocieties*, 9(2), 111–128.

Rafalovich, Adam (2001) Psychodynamic and neurological perspectives on ADHD: Exploring strategies for defi ning a phenomenon, *Journal for the Theory of Social Behaviour*, 31(4), 397–418.

Reiger, Kerreen (1999) Birthing in the postmodern moment: Struggles over defining maternity care needs, *Australian Feminist Studies*, 14(30), 387–404.

—— (2000) Reconceiving citizenship: The challenge of mothers as political activists, *Feminist Theory*, 1(3), 309–327.

Scheper-Hughes, Nancy and Lock, Margaret M. (1986) Speaking "truth" to illness: Metaphors, reification, and a pedagogy for patients, *Medical Anthropology Quarterly*, 17(5), 137–140.

Spoel, Philippa (2007) A feminist rhetorical perspective on informed choice in midwifery, *Rhetor: Journal of the Canadian Society for the Study of Rhetoric* 2, University of Regina, SK. Available online at: <http://ourspace.uregina.ca/bitstream/handle/10294/665/Vol2_art11_spoel.pdf> (accessed 9 August 2012).

Tyler, Suzanne (2002) Comparing the campaigning profile of maternity user groups in Europe: Can we learn anything useful? *Health Expectations*, 5(2), 136–147.

5 Obesity, the alternative food movement, and complete streets

New forms of "patient" activism and the evolution of health social movements

Mercedes C. Lyson and Stephen Zavestoski

Health social movements and the obesity epidemic

The study of health social movements, in the United States in particular, as a special category or class of social movements has matured over the last ten years. Spurred by theoretical and empirical advancements introduced by Brown University's Contested Illness Research Group (Brown et al. 2012), work in the field has drawn variously from the sociology of health and illness, social studies of science and, of course, social movements scholarship. Brown and colleagues initially focused on movements that arose to challenge dominant understandings of illnesses by insisting on greater attention to possible environmental causes. This research included analyses of activism around conditions such as asthma, breast cancer, and Gulf War Illnesses (Brown et al. 2003; McCormick et al. 2003; Zavestoski et al. 2002) while also developing a theoretical framework for "embodied health movements" using concepts such as the Dominant Epidemiological Paradigm (Brown et al. 2004; Zavestoski et al. 2004).

But Brown and colleagues also noted that while their framing of health social movements was new, organizing around health issues began as early as the Industrial Revolution, out of which emerged movements around industrial hygiene, urban poverty and occupational health (Waitzkin 2001). As discussed later in this chapter, such organizing around health issues, notably during the Progressive era, set the stage for activism with a decidedly "missionary" impulse. Such a strain of missionary zeal continues today, reflected in the framing of the alternative food and complete streets movements as, in part, movements to address the problem of obesity.

In contrast to the missionary-style of advocacy and activism, the women's health movement of the late twentieth century was organized by women who mobilized on their own behalf to challenge male-dominated approaches to medical practice. These efforts achieved a number of successes, including fundamental shifts in medical research practices (Ruzek 1978; Ruzek et al.

1997; Morgen 2002). Even more recently, AIDS activists demonstrated the power of health social movements by successfully securing funding for research and treatment and demanding shifts in protocols around clinical trials (Epstein 1996).

The Contested Illness Research Group and other health social movement scholars have evolved a body of research on health social movements that recognizes these early forms of health social movements while advancing our understanding of them by introducing theoretical frameworks and identifying new manifestations of health-related social movement organizing. Recent efforts have been made, for example, to expand beyond disease-specific research and into new domains of health and illness. The Contested Illness Research Group has expanded its scope to examine efforts to build coalitions between health- and environment-focused organizations and labor movements (Mayer 2008), new controversies around the "right-to-know" in toxic body burden studies (Morello-Frosch et al. 2009), challenges in deploying community-based participatory research in health social movements scholarship (Brown et al. 2012), and transnational health social movements (Zavestoski 2009). Yet, even while research on the causes of obesity is exploding, no attempts have been made to understand the escalating concern around obesity – a concern that extends from North America and parts of Europe to rapidly developing countries like India – from a health social movements perspective.

Obesity has arisen as a noteworthy public health concern over the past decade, mobilizing a plethora of actors from varying ideologies and sectors of society who strive to help people lead healthier lifestyles. From nutritionists to epidemiologists and from urban planners to transportation planners, strategies to address the obesity "epidemic" tend to coalesce around what people eat and how they move. We build on prior analyses of health social movements by examining how dynamics of race, class and power are implicated when advocacy is driven by one group of individuals acting on behalf of a "target population" such as those diagnosed as obese.

The chapter begins with a background and analysis on the role of the alternative food movement and the complete streets movement as potential remedies to the obesity epidemic. We draw on the theoretical framework of Health Social Movements to analyze the convoluted field of social movement actors aiming to define and redefine obesity. The conclusion explores whether activism around the obesity epidemic can usefully be considered a form of patient activism, and the kinds of advances analysis of such activism can make in our understanding of patient activism.

Emergence of an "obesity epidemic"

The field of social movement activism around obesity offers an excellent opportunity to expand the scope of health social movement research. But it is a complex field, muddied by the wide range of actors and agendas operating within it. Public health officials made the initial push for the medicalization of obesity, while the fat acceptance movement emerged to challenge the dominant epidemiological paradigm in which obesity is medicalized, where diet and exercise are seen as the solutions to a problem rejected by the fat acceptance movement. In turn, new movements with their own agendas entered the field intent on utilizing obesity's medicalization to achieve their own ends. The food justice and sovereignty movements and complete streets movement both see obesity as a symptom that their "solutions" can fix.

The notion of obesogenic neighborhoods – those neighborhoods characterized by lack of access to parks and open space, poor or nonexistent public transit, and high prevalence of fast food restaurants – implies that the link to obesity extends beyond access to healthy food to the built environment and municipal infrastructure. Advocates of urban reform, as a result, see the obesity epidemic as an opportunity to justify demands for walkable neighborhoods, pedestrian-oriented urban design, and greater investment in public spaces and transit: urban design characteristics that have come to be known as "complete streets."

While previous studies to date recognized a clear patient, or patient/activist, the current "moral panic" around the United States' obesity epidemic offers a complicated and novel health movement, with ambiguous agencies, and fraught power and class politics. Growing panic in the past decade over increasingly large waistlines has been accompanied by many public health interventions, state and municipal efforts at regulating food environments, and a popular discourse on healthy eating and physical activity. Indeed, efforts such as creating local food alternatives and reforming the built environment have begun to play a significant role in both discursively and practically encouraging citizens to lead "healthier lives" and ameliorate obesity.

Yet, despite many well-intentioned efforts at stemming the increasing weight of Americans, obesity continues to be seen as an "epidemic" with no end in sight. Guthman and DuPuis (2006) point out that in the contemporary neoliberal context of the past 25 years, characterized by "free" market capitalism and an accompanying reinforcing political ideology, there has been a shift in personhood from citizen to consumer which encourages overeating in an abundant food environment at the same time that the moral ethos of neoliberal individualism and self-discipline vilify it. From this perspective, ideal citizens are rational and self-disciplining, and can achieve thinness amidst plenty. Prior efforts at mitigating obesity have been unsuccessful because they are ultimately incomplete: the medicalization of obesity either shifts the locus of politics to medical science or depoliticizes the issue completely. Solutions to the problem inevitably circle back around to rest on personal lifestyle choice and responsibility. Eating has become the embodiment of what contemporary society values: consumption. The hypervigilance that surrounds personal control and deservingness creates divisions between active citizens (those who can manage their own risks) and "targeted populations" (those who require interventions to manage risks for them). The latter group is overwhelmingly the working poor, racial/ethnic minorities, and women (Boardman et al. 2005).

The growing body of literature on the "politics of obesity" (Gard and Wright 2005; Guthman and Dupuis 2006; Oliver 2006; Metzl and Kirkland 2010) forcefully argues that the "obesity epidemic" is nothing more than a medical construct, perpetuated by a symbiotic relationship between health researchers, government bureaucrats, and drug companies who all maintain a vested interest in obesity as a significant public health concern; this "health-industrial complex" (Oliver 2006) has actively campaigned to define the growing weight of Americans as an epidemic. In the process, arbitrary definitions of what is considered overweight and obese have taken hold. Researchers rely on the perpetuation of the obesity epidemic to secure large grant funds, government health agencies use the obesity epidemic as the rationale for increasing program and budget allocations, and pharmaceutical companies are constantly at work to find the next "quick fix" diet drug. An entire industry is devoted to dieting and weight-loss surgeries, an industry valued at $36 billion per year (McNamara 2009). Included in these numbers are ten major segments of the US diet industry: diet drugs, diet books and exercise videos, diet soft drinks, artificial sweeteners, diet dinner entrees and meal replacements, health clubs, diet websites, commercial chains, hospital/RD/MD-based programs, child weight loss camps, and bariatric surgeries. Diet soft drinks claim the largest share of the industry at 29.5 percent, being worth $19 billion in 2006 (Healthy Weight Network website).

Additionally, the argument goes that asking Americans to "eat less and exercise more" is fundamentally at odds with the dominant logic of American culture, and flies in the face of a consumer-oriented democracy that is constantly creating desire, and expanding personal choice and freedom. Moreover, Americans also have strong cultural biases against body fat and fat people, and fixating on obesity is a way for America's elite to express their own moral superiority and latent class snobbery and racism. In other words, it is the poor and minorities, with the highest obesity rates, who need to be "protected" from the fast food industry and a toxic food environment.

Yet, those in the medical and public health fields forcefully maintain that obesity is more than just a medical construct, and that there are serious health consequences associated with carrying excess weight, such as diabetes, heart disease, certain cancers, and other diseases and conditions (Chopra et al. 2002). In particular, a 2004 Centers for Disease Control and Prevention (CDC) study presented data to show that poor diet and lack of exercise was nearing tobacco as a primary cause of death, responsible for 400,000 deaths in 2000 (Mokdad et al. 2003). While Americans have indisputably gotten, on average, larger over the past 30 years, those who study the politics of the obesity epidemic are most interested in whether or not excess weight actually is correlated with increased morbidity/mortality, and whether these trends have affected everyone equally. Through various iterations of epidemiologic studies, results indicate that people who are modestly overweight actually have a lower risk of death than those at "normal" weight, suggesting a potential need to revise tools like the BMI (body mass index) calculator and its cut-off points. Further, obesity and ill health in general is strongly correlated with other demographic indicators like socioeconomic status/class, geography, and race. Such study results leave no doubt that obesity – as both a moral judgment as well as a real medical problem – does not affect everyone equally.

With the exception of the involvement of the fat acceptance movement, tension between the medicalization and demedicalization of obesity arises primarily from the roles public health experts, medical care providers, policymakers, and other professionals play in advocating on behalf of the target population of those medically defined as obese. This complicates somewhat the "embodied health movement" approach to understanding illness contestation (Brown et al. 2004). Some types of embodied health movements are formed by individuals with a subjective experience of illness who come to see themselves collectively as part of an illness group that must demand a label for a condition. Kroll-Smith and Floyd (1997) document such a group in their study of multiple chemical sensitivity and Zavestoski et al. (2002) characterize Gulf War veterans as such a group in their study of Gulf War Illness. In these instances, activists fight to gain legitimacy in the eyes of the medical profession. Less studied, but perhaps equally important, are efforts to shed disease or illness labels. Such movements are generally compelled by the desire to remove the stigma attached to particular disease definitions. Sometimes such movements aim to remove the stigma by shifting the disease definition, but there are also instances in which a movement may want to challenge the notion that a condition should be defined as a disease or illness at all. These efforts to "de-medicalize" (Conrad 2007) include the disability rights movement's attempts to reframe disability in terms of access and civil rights and gay and lesbian rights activists' efforts to demedicalize homosexuality. Other examples include the women's health movement's efforts to demedicalize menstruation, pregnancy, and menopause. Similar efforts can be seen in the loosely organized and primarily internet-based movement, evident in "pro-ana" (or pro-anorexia) websites. Pro-ana websites range from discussion forums for those attempting to recover from the illness to celebrations of anorexia-nervosa as a lifestyle choice that deny that it is a mental illness in need of treatment. A recent study found that 84 percent of pro-ana websites embrace anorexia as desirable (Borzekowski et al. 2010).

The fat acceptance movement, although at the opposite extreme of pro-ana websites, represents another attempt at demedicalizing obesity. Sometimes also referred to as the size acceptance, fat liberation, or fat power movement, the fat acceptance movement is growing fastest in the United States, United Kingdom, and Australia. Similarly concentrated on the internet, fat acceptance is sometimes characterized as resistance to the "war on obesity," in which obesity is medicalized through the body-mass index that sets weight-to-height ratios for optimum health. According to one fat acceptance blogger:

> When people talk about eliminating obesity, they typically mean eliminating people who are visibly fat. The war is not against a ratio of weight and height that's greater than 30, it's against people who don't fit the stereotype of beauty. And the front lines of this war are everywhere we look and listen – magazine covers, billboards, commercials, infomercials, ads on the internet, random strangers on the street, health care and wellness professionals, talk show hosts etc.
>
> (Chastain 2012)

The pro-ana and fat acceptance examples represent forms of "patient" activism in which semi-organized movements endeavor to destigmatize and demedicalize anorexia and obesity, respectively. Equally important is that they share a common underlying objective of destabilizing popular conceptions of normative/non-normative bodies. Alternative food and complete streets efforts, as movements advocating on behalf of a target population, fail to question critically cultural norms surrounding bodies. In shifting attention to food access or the "active transportation" options defined by the built environment, these advocates seem to challenge the attachment of moral responsibility to individuals for regulating bodies. Yet, as we will argue below, although they may shift the locus of responsibility from the individual to food, urban planning and transportation decision-makers, in continuing to medicalize obesity, these approaches embrace a "technical solutions" strategy that is all but blind to the underlying class politics. Furthermore, if addressing the problems of food access and built environment do not result in declines in obesity, these approaches simply revert to explanations of personal lifestyle choice and individual responsibility.

Battles to define obesity are no longer just in the doctor's office, but also in fast food restaurants, the grocery store, on neighborhood streets, in parks and recreation spaces, and in legislative offices. Activists in the food movement, whose diverse elements include not just organic and sustainable food advocates, but also advocates of food justice and food sovereignty, have begun to see the war on obesity as an opportunity to communicate concerns about lack of access to fresh and healthy food in some communities. Advocates for complete streets – which include accessible sidewalks, bicycle lanes and access to public transportation – have similarly latched onto alarm about the obesity epidemic as a way of advancing their agendas. In the remainder of this chapter, our aim is to advance our understanding of "patient" activism and health social movements by examining a health social movement arena in which the primary actors tend to focus on a target population – the obese – that is not only defined by a contested concept but also is made up largely of individuals who do not see themselves as patient activists or as part of a health social movement.

Obesity: a new form of "patient" activism?

Health-related issues have become a top priority in today's national funding climate. Driven by the empirical realities of mounting costs related to population health care management and the accompanying moral panics around lifestyle related illnesses, money available from the government and private foundations in competitive grants has largely focused on not just health-related endeavors, but specifically on creating and enacting policy change. Relatedly, efforts around local food, such as community gardens or participatory food councils often invoke an image of bringing people together, and representing an essential quality of individual and community life. In the world of grant-getting and community activism, linking these efforts explicitly with health has been an intentional discursive tactic, and an act that has turned the movement to fight obesity into a movement advocating for a target population rather than a patient movement.

There are several primary categories of strategies or mechanisms that are employed to both govern population health, as well as instill the cultural imperative to good health on an individual level, i.e., self-governmentality. Much has been written about the hyper-individualist focus in American culture (Brooks 2004; Cullen 2003; Derber 2000; McKibben 2007), and this is reflected in the near-dogmatic discourse of "individual choice" as the ultimate arbiter of good health for some, and ill health for others. Resolving the structural impediments to making "good choices" is one aspect most can agree on, but beyond this many will argue that people are not sufficiently "educated" on how to lead healthy lives. Indeed, there is a pervasive reliance on education as an integral precursor or accompaniment to individual choice as the ideal solution.

In spite of choice as the dominant discourse, there also exists a cultural history and contemporary activity that while not mutually exclusive from the individual choice ideal, sits ideologically and logistically separate from it. In recent years a number of government attempts have sought to regulate food environments on behalf of people. Examples include zoning against fast food franchises (Mair et al. 2005; Wood 2007), posting calorie counts in restaurants (Rosenbloom 2010), placing stipulations on eligible products under benefit programs like food stamps and WIC (Women, Infants, and Children) (Eng 2012; Whitefield 2012), and proposals to tax foods deemed "unhealthy" (Grynbaum 2012). Such a dichotomy, between individual choice and government intervention, often sparks quasi-political debates positing big government liberalism against strains of libertarianism. While many would argue that individuals need to be motivated to make the "right" choice, many seem to believe that not only would such "nanny state" efforts be unpalatable to people, but that they would not produce the intended outcome.

Who controls the obesity frame?

While the United States population enjoys high life expectancy rates, lifestyle-related chronic diseases – such as cancer, diabetes, and heart disease – have become critical public health concerns. One realm of health and illness that has recently gained public notoriety, and some might argue has spurned a moral panic, are "diet-related" illnesses, conditions for which being overweight or obese is a risk factor. In particular, there has been a heightened moral panic around childhood obesity, with First Lady Michelle Obama choosing "Let's Move" as one of her public initiatives focused on improving childhood wellbeing.

Within this context, the alternative food movement has purported the tangible health benefits to be derived for a more localized, participatory food system. Such a coupling between alternative food and health has also been the basis for a trend in government and private foundation funding streams toward non-profi t efforts focused on improving food environments, food access, and population health. Similarly, municipal governments and transportation agencies are increasingly turning to the CDC to fund "active transportation" programs. The CDC's Division of Nutrition, Physical Activity, and Obesity (DNPAO), for example, has supported the "Bike to Market Project" in Boston, Massachusetts, Missouri's "Livable Streets Project," and San Francisco's "Sunday Streets" events that close city streets to automobiles on select Sundays.

Whether linked to alternative food or complete streets efforts, a large portion of such activity focuses explicitly on social justice and equality through both education and policy efforts, seeking to remedy acute and structural causes of health disparities along race and class lines. Yet, the class politics embedded in the relations of power between the well-intentioned food activists/advocates, and the "targeted populations" has opened up new spaces to regulate health, and sparked new iterations of social and policy debates surrounding individual liberties and the public good. While not new concerns, the way these issues are playing out within the realm of the alternative food and complete streets movements in the context of contemporary public health problems in a neoliberally structured context is a new realm of governance, with an accompanying set of evolving class politics.

Perhaps the biggest critique to be made of the public health establishment and accompanying state intervention or prevention programs is the dominant framing of the discourse and problems associated with overweight and obesity, along with the tools used to both defi ne and seek remedies to the problem (BMI as a metric, built environment, behavior change). Contemporary ideas about fatness and non-normative bodies are couched within a language of health, which legitimizes the role these state government programs play. Yet as Guthman has extensively argued (2006, 2008, 2011), using health to talk about non-normative bodies serves to work against social justice, as it effectively diverts attention away from base inequalities in society, born out through the life course. The realm of health/health care has become a "scientific" and ostensibly value-free way to talk about non-normativity, yet still remains plagued by deeply rooted cultural preoccupations with morality, and drawing boundaries among social groups.

The United States is a unique case in the way that notions of healthism/health-seeking articulate with health care management. There has been a devolution in health responsibility from the state/public sphere to the individual/private sphere, whereas this transition was incomplete in nations where a national healthcare system was maintained. Yet, as this detailing of state government programs demonstrates, the state still takes on some responsibility for (re)shaping environments that lead to the realization of personal health achievement. Many public health programs are rooted in the "obesogenic environment" thesis, meaning that where one lives has a strong impact on health. While this is indeed born out in research, the correlation is spurious at best. What may be "predicting" obesity prevalence or other ill health outcomes in particular localities is more likely a reflection of class and race, with features of the built environment being an effect of this spatial patterning, rather than a cause (Guthman 2011).

Food environments and the alternative food movement

As obesity has fimly become the persona non grata of the public health establishment in the twenty-first century, a number of different actors have pursued multiple avenues for its amelioration. Indeed, the alternative food movement has become a "master frame" to address an entire host of social issues, including public health concerns about general health status and an obesity epidemic, environmental degradation, regional economic revitalization, the loss of the family farm, and farmworker rights. Yet, as with other social movements, the alternative food movement is characterized by differing agendas and schisms between actors. A common critique of the alternative food movement is that many of its recommended practices (shopping at farmer's markets or participating in community-supported agriculture shares, for example) are a luxury of middle- and upper-class educated people, who not only have the necessary income, but also the time, knowledge, and identity politics that contribute to their participation in these alternative food spheres.

To provide a brief grounding in understanding the current public embracing of alternative ways of producing and consuming food, there are two main ways to tell the story of the shift in the US food system and agriculture during the course of the twentieth century. The first is the civic agriculture perspective (Lyson 2004), which advocates for a relocalization of food production that is tightly linked to a community's social and economic development. This includes activities such as farmers' markets, community gardens, community-supported agriculture, farm-to-school programs, roadside fruit and vegetable stands, urban gardens, and community kitchens. They represent a counter-voice, in social movement form, to the conventional paradigm of food production and consumption. As Lyson contends:

> These new organizational forms have the potential to nurture local economic development, maintain diversity and quality in products, and provide forums where producers and consumers can come together to solidify bonds of local identity and solidarity. By rebuilding linkages between farmers and consumers wherever possible, communities throughout the United States will establish a foundation for a more socially and environmentally integrated food system.
>
> (Lyson 2004: 7)

The second discourse comes from an urban theory perspective, understanding that as the United States industrialized, people actually desired to leave small-town agrarian life, and were drawn to the emancipatory potential of newly developing cities. Food systems research lays out the most salient trends that have impacted how Americans produce and consume food, namely the steady decrease in the number of farms (from 6.4 million farms in 1910 to fewer than 2 million farms today), the consolidation and hyper-concentration of "agricultural pockets" of production (e.g. California, and the Midwestern "bread basket"), increasing specialization (most farms produce only one or two crops, versus more diversified farms of the past), and the nearly complete severing between local food production and local food consumption in most American communities (Lyson 2004: 30–31). Yet, what seems to be often missing from such discussions of a changing American agriculture is how these shifts articulate with broader historical economic and labor shifts happening concurrently. Industrialization and urbanization processes, which also ushered in the era of automobile-dominated urban planning against which the complete streets movement is a reaction, drew people away from the family-farm rural agrarian model of life, often by choice and with the promise of new opportunities.

The Chicago School of urban sociology theorists posited these changes in a largely positive light (Wirth 1938; Fischer 1995). Thus, while the shift from agrarian to urban lifestyles could be viewed positively from an individualistic, capitalistic perspective, such shifts were not without unintended consequences for social organization and relationships. It is no coincidence that we see the same impulses that spurred urbanization – impulses towards individualism and the casting off of the restraints of traditional "community," which in turn shifts the locus of morality from community to the individual – invoked more than 100 years later in the context of the obesity epidemic. The continued presence of these impulses places the efforts of alternative food movement advocates, including those embracing the civic agriculture discourse, in a difficult position. On one hand, they can invoke romantic notions of the very "community" from which urbanization provided an escape. On the other hand, they can accept the cultural biases towards individualism and personal moral responsibility for regulating bodies with the consequence of glossing over the complex racial and class implications of such a position.

As the alternative food movement has gained traction and become more mainstream (in its current iteration) in the past decade, there has been a notable bifurcation with respect to how issues of class, race, and gender are accounted for in civic agriculture activities. With the acknowledgement that the production and consumption of food is severely stratified by race, class, and gender (Kwate 2007; Boardman et al. 2005) the concepts of food justice and food sovereignty have been born out of the environmental justice tradition which originally sought to address issues of disproportionate exposure to toxic environmental burdens.[1] To this end, food systems researchers have increasingly been calling attention to these clear schisms within the alternative/local food movement (known colloquially as "locavores"[2]), with respect to who is setting the agenda and participating in such alternatives, and who is truly benefiting (in terms of health, economics, community engagement, and so on) from the alternative food movement.

At the same time as the emergence of this lifestyle-based embracing of food alternatives, there has been a concurrent development of very different health-related food initiatives geared towards the working poor and lower-class Americans. These include efforts taken by all levels of government to regulate food environments on behalf of poor and minority citizens who either lack the structural access to procuring healthy affordable food, or are not sufficiently "educated" on the benefits of alternative food options. As previously mentioned, some examples of this are zoning against fast food franchises, posting calorie counts in restaurants, placing restrictions on what benefit programs like food stamps and WIC can buy, and proposals to tax foods deemed "unhealthy". Whereas the approaches that emerged out of the environmental justice movement aim to address race, class, and gender dimensions of the food system head on, the policy approaches shaped by the political elite continue to embrace the personal responsibility approach by imposing restrictions where it is perceived that people cannot exercise self-restraint.

Drawing on these parallel efforts, local food activism discourse and practice can be understood as part of a larger governmentality framework. Governmentality refers to the ways that societies both practice governance and employ "technologies" that generate forms of self-government. Notions of health governmentality (Foucault 1978; Armstrong 1995) and "body policing" are useful theoretical frameworks because they emphasize how it is one's personal responsibility to maintain a healthy body. Within the realm of individual bodies, citizens are constantly implored to be purposeful and conscientious about maintaining their health, even amidst environments that are not conducive to such action. Despite the fact that the alternative food movement ostensibly seeks to remedy this disjuncture, there has been mounting criticism that the reality has not lived up to the ideals. In other words, people continue to be left out of enjoying improved health status and food access vis-à-vis local food alternatives.

Beyond this, the alternative food movement itself utilizes its own set of governmentality mechanisms to educate low-income and minority citizens about the benefits of "healthy living" and how they can attempt to comply with the cultural imperative to good health. While civic agriculture (Lyson 2004) or a food justice framework (Williams 2005; Alkon 2008) represent a way for those citizens less able to comply with the individual imperative to good health to achieve healthy bodies despite being at a social and material disadvantage, these activities have simultaneously opened up new spaces and methods of governing individuals, particularly with respect to their health and their bodies. Beyond the political economy of food and agriculture, the reductionist mentality that connects food with health is also part of the more overarching cultural Cartesian dualist mindset with respect to medicine, health, and the body. This same mindset shapes the approaches taken to the problem of mobility, or the lack thereof, that the complete streets movement aims to address.

Complete streets and obesity

> Complete Streets are streets for everyone. They are designed and operated to enable safe access for all users. People of all ages and abilities are able to safely move along and across streets in a community, regardless of how they are traveling. Complete Streets make it easy to cross the street, walk to shops, and bicycle to work. They allow buses to run on time and make it safe for people to walk to and from train stations.
>
> (National Complete Streets Coalition 2013a)

Since its first usage in 2003, the concept of "complete streets" has risen to prominence in the parlance of urban planners, architects, engineers, and, perhaps most importantly, policymakers. In the US, the concept is now institutionalized in the National Complete Streets Coalition, which is comprised of non-profit organizations and private entities, and overseen by a steering committee of a number of professional associations.[3] The mission of the National Complete Streets Coalition is to work "for the adoption and effective implementation of Complete Streets policies at the local, state and federal levels."

Couched within the broader movement for "livable cities" and "cities for people," complete streets as a concept and movement has exploded across the urban planning, transportation planning, environmental policy, sustainable communities, and other scenes. Organizations like National Complete Streets Coalition, Streetsblog, Transportation Alternatives, and 8-80 Cities have aided in the formation and growth of the complete streets movement in North America, while Living Streets in the UK, the Bicycling Empowerment Network in South Africa, Walk2,1 and Embarq are international examples.

The primary evidence of the movement's growth and strength is the number of municipal "complete streets" policies that have been implemented in the US in the last year alone. More than 25 percent of the 488 complete streets policies existing at municipal, county and state levels in the US were passed in 2012 alone. The number of policies in the US now exceeds 500, a milestone celebrated by the National Complete Streets Coalition on August 14, 2013 when it recognized Memphis, Tennessee and the 499 other "communities across the United States that have made their streets safer and more accessible for everyone who uses them" (National Complete Streets Coalition 2013b).

The term was originally introduced in 2003 by a staff member of the advocacy organization America Bikes and provided a stroke of marketing genius for advocates who had been using the term "routine accommodation" which was derived from federal policy aimed at promoting the "routine accommodation of bicyclists, pedestrians and persons with disabilities in all transportation projects" and "the regular inclusion of non-motorized transportation improvements in both new and rehabilitation project planning, design, funding, and construction" (Metropolitan Transportation Commission 2006: 6). Passed in 1990, the Americans with Disabilities Act (ADA) was being taken seriously by the early 2000s, in part due to several successful legal actions to force implementation. Municipal, regional and state governments found themselves compelled to design and construct roads and sidewalks, among other facilities, to be usable by persons with disabilities without restrictions. Meanwhile, 1998's Transportation Equity Act of the 21st Century (TEA-21) called for consideration of bicycle and pedestrian facilities whenever new construction or reconstruction of transportation facilities were being undertaken. These changes were followed by a significant increase in the availability of federal funds for non-motorized projects.

Despite these significant policy events, complete streets advocates were still fighting an uphill battle against powerful automobile industry and other stakeholders invested in maintaining transportation engineering practices aimed at maximizing "Level of Service," a measure most commonly applied to assess the flow of automobile traffic on roadways. But the year 2000 saw a significant landmark. For the first time the number of overweight adults exceeded the number of underweight adults (Gardner and Halweil 2000). In the US, the media began reporting an obesity epidemic around the same time, following a 1999 Journal of the American Medical Association (JAMA) article titled "The Spread of the Obesity Epidemic in the United States, 1991–1998," (Mokdad et al. 1999). By 2010, the CDC (CDC 2010) reported that none of the 50 states met the Healthy People 2010 target of less than 15 percent obesity prevalence, while nine states surpassed a 30 percent rate of obesity prevalence (up from zero states in 2000). Media coverage points to the period between 2003 and 2007 as the pinnacle of concern with childhood obesity (Barry et al. 2011), with news stories more consistently mentioning individual behavioral changes than system-level changes as a solution.

These trends opened the door for advocates to frame complete streets policies as one type of measure to address the growing concerns over obesity rates. Shortly thereafter, research examining the influence of built environments on physical activity levels and, in turn obesity – what is known as the obesogenic environments thesis – began to accumulate. Egger and Swinburn launched the field of study by pointing out "that there is a major deficiency in research into the 'obesogenic' environment and potential interventions" (1997: 479), opening the floodgates for later studies with titles like "The built environment and obesity" (Papas et al. 2007) and "Obesogenic environments: Exploring the built and food environments" (Lake and Townshend 2006). Soon to follow were a bevy of studies adapting the obesogenic environments hypothesis to explain higher rates of obesity among the poor and people of color (Burdette and Whitaker 2004; Lovasi et al. 2009; Casagrande et al. 2009). The backlash was soon to follow, with Evans, Crookes and Coaffee maintaining that "While recent policy has called for urban design and planning professionals to eradicate obesity there is, however, significant uncertainty in the science surrounding the relationship between body size, urban design and health and little definitive evidence about what works" (Evans et al. 2012: 100).

Despite mixed evidence for the obesogenic environments hypothesis, complete streets advocates continue to frame the advantages of complete streets policies in terms of health benefits that result from increased physical activity. As with alternative food movement activists whose embrace of a civic agriculture model depoliticizes the structural factors shaping food access and food sovereignty, complete streets advocates proclaiming the health benefits of complete streets tend to obscure the underlying politics of space that shape not just streets themselves, but also who uses them and how.

What complete streets advocates see as benign efforts to locate "beneficial amenities" in traditionally disadvantaged neighborhoods might be seen by residents of those neighborhoods as part of a privileged narrative. For example, bicycle lanes represent to some opportunities for active transportation while for others they may signal a gentrification process that will eventually exclude people from the neighborhood they call home. Furthermore, when residents of traditionally disadvantaged neighborhoods are not involved in the decision-making that brings amenities such as bicycle lanes into their communities, they may be understandably resentful. In short, unless complete streets policies are developed and implemented in democratic ways that give voice to the traditionally underrepresented members of a city or neighborhood, they will become nothing more than a practice of governmentality with complete streets elements such as curb bulb-outs, the "technologies" that generate forms of self-government. If mobility is restrained by (in)complete streets, so the reasoning goes, then complete streets policies will clear the obstacles and in turn allow individuals to make the correct, moral choices about physical activity.

Conclusion

In their attempts to redesign the food system and redesign our streets, the alternative food and complete streets movements have become attempts to "design out obesity." As Evans et al. (2012: 106) argue,

> Given that planners are increasingly being expected to act as "health experts" despite uncertain knowledges about what works, there is a clear need for critical work to become central to education, training and professional development in order to support urban design professionals who are called upon to respond to such policy imperatives.

Similarly, public health professionals are increasingly being asked to serve as urban planners who can design civic agriculture into the food systems of cities. But there are significant dangers in this possibility for planning and public health professionals, much less alternative food and complete streets advocates, to push forward their agendas under the guise of health social movements. Too easily the target populations are objectified and patronized, their voices ignored, and the deeper race, class, and gender dynamics at play become glossed over in favor of technical fixes that perpetuate traditions of individualism and personal moral responsibility for maintaining a healthy body.

The alternative food and complete streets movements, while not exactly forms of "patient activism," can be understood as forms of health social movements. Diverse actors – ranging from urban planners to food justice organizations and from fat acceptance activists to First Lady Michelle Obama – are contesting not just how we define obesity, but more importantly how we respond culturally, politically, and even technologically to the perceived problem of excessive obesity in society. A health social movements framework can help us better understand how dominant epidemiological paradigms form around a condition like obesity and how stakeholders, especially those in positions of power, utilize their positions to advance particular agendas. With respect to obesity, we have an opportunity to expand the health social movement framework to movements that are driven primarily by special interests acting on behalf of a target population with a contested condition. As long as the practice of governmentality continues, we can expect to see more of these types of movements.

Notes

1 We do not mean to conflate the concept of civic agriculture as an alternative food production framework – with other concepts that seek to incorporate social justice ideologies, such as the food justice movement, food democracy, and food citizenship.

2 The term "locavore" was first used in 2005 by Jessica Prentice (chef, writer, and co-founder of a community-supported kitchen cooperative in Berkeley, California).

3 Such as Trust for America's Health, Sierra Club, and Active Transportation Alliance, along with private entities such as Alta Planning + Design firm and transportation planning fi rm Nelson\Nygaard. The steering committee includes among others the AARP (formerly known as American Association of Retired Persons), National Association of Realtors, the American Public Transportation Association, Alliance for Biking and Walking, Institute of Transportation Engineers, the National Association of City Transportation Officials, and the Association of Pedestrian and Bicycle Professionals.

References

Alkon, Alison (2008) Paradise or pavement: The social constructions of the environment in two urban farmers' markets and their implications for environmental justice and sustainability, *Local Environment*, 13(3), 271–289.

Armstrong, David (1995) The rise of surveillance medicine, *Sociology of Health and Illness*, 17(3), 393–404.

Barry, Colleen L.; Jarlenski, Marian; Grob, Rachel; Schlesinger, Mark and Gollust, Sarah E. (2011) News media framing of childhood obesity in the United States from 2000 to 2009, *Pediatrics*, 128, 132–145.

Boardman, Jason D.; Saint Onge, Jarron M.; Rogers, Richard G. and Denney, Justin T. (2005) Race differentials in obesity: The impact of place, *Journal of Health and Social Behavior*, 46(3), 229–243.

Borzekowski, Dina; Schenk, Summer; Wilson, Jenny and Peebles, Rebecka (2010) e-Ana and e-Mia: A content analysis of pro-eating disorder web sites, *American Journal of Public Health*, 100(8), 1526–1534.

Brooks, David (2004) *On Paradise Drive: How We Live Now (And Always Have) in the Future Tense*, New York: Simon & Schuster.

Brown, Phil; Zavestoski, Stephen; Luebke, Theo; Mandelbaum, Joshua; McCormick, Sabrina and Mayer, Brian (2003) The health politics of asthma: Environmental justice and collective illness experience in the United States, *Social Science and Medicine*, 57(3), 453–464.

Brown, Phil; Zavestoski, Stephen; McCormick, Sabrina; Mayer, Brian; Morello-Frosch, Rachel and Gasior Altman, Rebecca (2004) Embodied health movements: New approaches to social movements in health, *Sociology of Health and Illness*, 26(1), 50–80.

Brown, Phil; Morello-Frosch, Rachel; Brody, Julia Green; Gasior Altman, Rebecca; Rudel, Ruthann A.; Senier, Laura; Pérez, Carla and Simpson, Ruth (2012) IRB challenges in community-based participatory research on human exposure to environmental toxins: A case study, in P. Brown, R. Morello-Frosch and S. Zavestoski (eds) *Contested Illnesses: Citizens, Science, and Health Social Movements*, Berkeley, CA: University of California Press, 245–260.

Brown, Phil; Morello-Frosch, Rachel; Zavestoski, Stephen and the Contested Illnesses Research Group (2012) *Contested Illnesses: Citizens, Science, and Health Social Movements*, Berkeley, CA: University of California Press.

Burdette, Hillary L. and Whitaker, Robert C. (2004) Neighborhood playgrounds, fast food restaurants, and crime: Relationships to overweight in low-income preschool children, *Preventive Medicine*, 38(1), 57–63.

Casagrande, Sarah S.; Whitt-Glover, Melicia C.; Lancaster, Kristie J.; Odoms-Young, Angela M. and Gary, Tiffany L. (2009) Built environment and health behaviors among African Americans: A systematic review, *American Journal of Preventive Medicine*, 36(2), 174–181.

Centers for Disease Control (CDC) (2010) Vital signs: State-specific obesity prevalence among adults – United States, 2009, *Morbidity and Mortality Weekly Report*, 59(30), 951–955. Available online at: <www.cdc.gov/mmwr/preview/mmwrhtml/mm5930a4.htm?s_cid=mm5930a4_w> (accessed 25 November 2013).

Chastain, Ragen (2012) Nobody wants to eliminate obesity, *Dances with Fat*. Available online at: <http://danceswithfat.wordpress.com/2012/08/07/nobody-wants-to-eliminate-obesity> (accessed 5 October 2012).

Chopra, M.; Galbraith, Sarah and Darnton-Hill, Ian (2002) A global response to a global problem: The epidemic of overnutrition, *Bulletin of the World Health Organization*, 80(12), 952–958.

Conrad, Peter (2007) *The Medicalization of Society: On the Transformation of Human Conditions into Treatable Disorders*, Baltimore, MD: Johns Hopkins University Press.

Cullen, Jim (2003) *The American Dream: A Short History of an Idea that Shaped a Nation*, Oxford and New York: Oxford University Press.

Derber, Charles (2000) *The Pursuit of Attention: Power and Ego in Everyday Life*, 2nd edition, Oxford and New York: Oxford University Press.

Egger, Garry and Swinburn, Boyd (1997) An "ecological" approach to the obesity pandemic, *BMJ: British Medical Journal*, 315(7106): 477–480.

Eng, Monica (2012) Politicians, health advocates seek transparency, restrictions in food stamp program, *The Chicago Tribune*, 20 June.

Evans, Bethan; Crookes, Lee and Coaffee, Jon (2012) Obesity/fatness and the city: critical urban geographies, *Geography Compass*, 6(2): 100–110.

Epstein, Steven (1996) *Impure Science: AIDS, Activism, and the Politics of Knowledge*, Berkeley, CA: University of California Press.

Fischer, Claude (1995) The subcultural theory of urbanism: A twentieth year assessment; *American Journal of Sociology*, 101(3), 543–577.

Foucault, Michel (1977–1978) *Security, Territory and Population: Lectures at the Collège De France*, New York: Palgrave Macmillan.

—— (1978–1979) *The Birth of Biopolitics: Lectures at the Collège De France*, New York: Palgrave Macmillan.

Gard, Michael and Wright, Jan (2005) *The Obesity Epidemic: Science, Morality, and Ideology*, Routledge: New York.

Gardner, Gary and Halweil, Brian (2000) Underfed and Overfed: The Global Epidemic of Malnutrition, Worldwatch paper no. 150, Washington, DC: Worldwatch Institute.

Grynbaum, Michael (2012) Health panel approves restriction on sale of large sugary drinks, *The New York Times*, 13 September.

Guthman, Julie (2008) Bringing good food to others: Investigating the subjects of alternative food practice, *Cultural Geographies*, 15(4), 431–447.

—— (2011) *Weighing In: Obesity, Food Justice, and the Limits of Capitalism*, Berkeley, Los Angeles, CA and London: University of California Press.

Guthman, Julie and DuPuis, Melanie (2006) Embodying neoliberalism: Economy, culture, and the politics of fat, *Environment and Planning D: Society and Space*, 24(3), 427–448.

Healthy Weight Network News Briefs: Statistics/Trends. Available online at: <www.healthyweight.net/trends.htm#9> (accessed 26 March 2013).

Kroll-Smith, Steve and Floyd, Hugh (1997) *Bodies in Protest: Environmental Illness and the Struggle over Medical Knowledge*, New York: NYU Press.

Kwate, Naa Oyo A. (2007) Fried Chicken and fresh apples: Racial segregation as a fundamental cause of fast food density in black neighborhoods, *Health & Place*, 14, 32–44.

Lake, Amelia and Townshend, Tim (2006) Obesogenic environments: Exploring the built and food environments, *The Journal of the Royal Society for the Promotion of Health*, 126(6), 262–267.

Lovasi, Gina S.; Hutson, Malo A.; Guerra, Monica and Neckerman, Kathryn M. (2009) Built environments and obesity in disadvantaged populations, *Epidemiologic Reviews*, 31(1), 7–20.

Lyson, Thomas A. (2004) *Civic Agriculture: Reconnecting Farm, Food, and Community*, Medford, MA: Tufts University Press.

Mair, Julie S; Pierce, Matthew W. and Teret, Stephen P. (2005) *The Use of Zoning to Restrict Fast Food Outlets: A Potential Strategy to Combat Obesity*, Baltimore, MD and Washington, DC: The Center for Law and the Public's Health at Johns Hopkins & Georgetown Universities.

Mayer, Brian (2008) *Blue-Green Coalitions: Fighting for Safe Workplaces and Healthy Communities*, Ithaca, NY: Cornell University Press.

McCormick, Sabrina; Brown, Phil and Zavestoski, Stephen (2003) The personal is scientifi c, the scientifi c is political: The public paradigm of the environmental breast cancer movement, *Sociological Forum*, 18(4), 545–576.

McKibben, Bill (2007) *Deep Economy: Economics as if the World Mattered*, London: Oneworld.

McNamara, Melissa (2009) Diet Industry is Big Business, 1 December. Available online at: <www.cbsnews.com/8301-18563162-2222867.html> (accessed 26 March 2013).

Metropolitan Transportation Commission (2006) Routine Accommodation of Pedestrians and Bicyclists in the Bay Area: Results from Interviews with Transportation Professionals and Recommendations to Encourage Routine Accommodation, Oakland, CA: MTC. Available online at: <http://apps.mtc.ca.gov/meeting_packet_documents/agenda_668/Routine_Accommodation_Ped_Bike_Study_6-06.pdf> (accessed 25 November 2013).

Metzl, Johnathan M. and Kirkland, Anna (eds) (2010) *Against Health: How Health Became the New Morality*, New York and London: New York University Press.

Mokdad, Ali H.; Serdula, Mary K.; Dietz, William H.; Bowman, Barbara A.; Marks, James S. and Koplan, Jeffrey P. (1999) The spread of the obesity epidemic in the United States, 1991–1998, *JAMA*, 282(16), 1519–1522.

Mokdad, Ali H.; Ford, Earl S.; Bowman, Barbara A.; Dietz, William H.; Vinicor, Frank; Bales Virginia S. and Marks, James S. (2003) Prevalence of obesity, diabetes, and obesity-related health risk factors, 2001 *JAMA*, 289(1): 76–79.

Morello-Frosch, Rachel; Brody, Julia G.; Brown, Phil; Gasior Altman, Rebecca; Rudel, Ruthann and Pérez, Carla (2009) Toxic ignorance and right-to-know in biomonitoring results communication: A survey of scientists and study participants, *Environmental Health*, 8(6). Available online at: <www.biomedcentral.com/content/pdf/1476-069X-8-6.pdf> (accessed 25 November 2013).

Morgen, Sandra (2002) *Into Our Own Hands: The Women's Health Movement in the United States, 1969–1990*, New Brunswick, NJ: Rutgers University Press.

National Complete Streets Coalition (2013a) Fundamentals. Available online at: <www.smartgrowthamerica.org/complete-streets/complete-streets-fundamentals> (accessed 25 November 2013).

___ (2013b) Complete Streets leaders celebrate 500 policies and look forward to the movement's future. Available online at: <www.smartgrowthamerica.org/2013/08/15/complete-streets-leaders-celebrate-500-policies-and-look-forward-to-the-movements-future> (accessed 25 November 2013).

Oliver, J. Eric (2006) *Fat Politics: The Real Story Behind America's Obesity Epidemic*, New York: Oxford University Press.

Papas, Mia A.; Alberg, Anthony J.; Ewing, Reid; Helzlsouer, Kathy J.; Gary, Tiffany L. and Klassen, Ann C. (2007) The built environment and obesity, *Epidemiologic Reviews*, 29(1), 129–143.

Rosenbloom, Stephanie (2010) Calorie data to be posted at most chains, *The New York Times*, 23 March.

Ruzek, Sheryl Burt (1978) *The Women's Health Movement: Feminist Alternatives to Medical Control*, New York: Praeger.

Ruzek, Sheryl Burt; Olesen, Virginia L. and Clarke, Adele E. (eds) (1997) *Women's Health: Complexities and Differences*, Columbus, OH: Ohio State University Press.

Saelens, Brian E.; Sallis, James F.; Frank, Lawrence D.; Couch, Sarah C.; Zhou, Chuan; Colburn, Trina; Cain, Kelli L.; Chapman, James and Glanz, Karen (2012) Obesogenic neighborhood environments, child and parent obesity: The neighborhood impact on kids study, *American Journal of Preventive Medicine*, 42(5), e57–64.

Waitzkin, Howard (2001) *At the Front Lines of Medicine: How the Health Care System Alienates Doctors and Mistreats Patients*, Lanham, MD: Rowman & Littlefield.

Whitefield, Paul (2012) Food stamps and Fanta shouldn't mix, *Los Angeles Times*, 19 September.

Williams, Orrin (2005) Food and justice: The critical link to health communities, in D. Pellow and R. Brulle (eds) *Power, Justice, and the Environment: A Critical Appraisal of the Environmental Justice Movement*, Cambridge and London: MIT Press, 117–130.

Wirth, Louis (1938) Urbanism as a way of life, *American Journal of Sociology*, 44(1), 1–24.

Wood, Daniel B. (2007) Diet-conscious Los Angeles eyes moratorium on fast-food outlets, *The Christian Science Monitor*, 13 September.

Zavestoski, Stephen (2009) The struggle for justice in Bhopal: A new/old breed of transnational social movement, *Global Social Policy*, 9(3), 383–407.

Zavestoski, Stephen; Brown, Phil; Linder, Meadow; Mayer, Bryan and McCormick, Sabrina (2002) Science, policy, activism, and war: Defining the health of Gulf War veterans, *Science, Technology, and Human Values*, 27(2), 171–205.

Zavestoski, Stephen; Morello-Frosch, Rachel; Brown, Phil; Mayer, Brian; McCormick, Sabrina and Gasior-Altman, Rebecca (2004) Embodied Health Social Movements and the Challenges to the Dominant Epidemiological Paradigm, in D. Myers and D. Cress (eds) *Authority in Contention: Research in Social Movements, Conflict and Change*, Oxford: Elsevier JAI, 253–278.

Zavestoski, Stephen; McCormick, Sabrina and Brown, Phil (2005) Gender, embodiment and disease: Environmental breast cancer activists' challenge to science, the biomedical model, and policy, *Science as Culture*, 13(4), 563–586.

Part II

Shifting contexts and new challenges

6 Autism, the Internet, and medicalization

Peter Conrad and Catherine Tan

The "autism epidemic"

According to the Centers for Disease Control and Prevention (CDC), data from the Autism and Developmental Disabilities Monitoring (ADDM) Network suggests that in 2012, the prevalence of autism was one in 68 children – a significant jump from the 2004 estimates of one in 150 children (Centers for Disease Control and Prevention 2012a). Others have suggested there is a 600 percent increase in autism diagnosis in the past two decades (Autism Speaks 2010). This rise in Autism Spectrum Disorder (ASD) diagnoses is often referred to as the "autism epidemic," a term popularized around 1999 (Grinker 2008). Currently, the etiology of autism is unknown (although that is contested by some) and there are no cures or sure treatments (Centers for Disease Control and Prevention: 2012b). It is unclear whether this is an epidemic change in condition or whether this is an increase in identifi cation and diagnosis of already existing conditions as autism or some combination of both. Sociological studies on the purported "epidemic" have identified social influence, diagnostic changes, and institutional change as possible causes for the drastic increase in cases.

In *The Autism Matrix*, Gil Eyal and his colleagues (2010) reason that new institutional conditions and changes about how society perceives and addresses disorders account for the growing autism diagnosis. For instance, conditions that previously were diagnosed and treated as mental retardation (MR) might now be diagnosed on the autism spectrum. While mental retardation is conceptualized as a life sentence, autism is believed to be a preferable diagnosis – affected children can potentially be rehabilitated. Thus, with these notions in mind, the diagnostic trend is affected by diagnostic substitution; children who would have been previously diagnosed with MR are now diagnosed with autism. This may also account for some of the rise in autism prevalence. As others have shown, the change in diagnostic criteria accounts for the rise in autism cases. As Marissa King and Peter Bearman (2009) note, in the period of diagnostic change, the odds of receiving an autism diagnosis increase. Children who would have otherwise been diagnosed with MR receive an autism diagnosis.

Peter Bearman and his colleagues, Ka-Yuet Liu and Marissa King (Liu et al. 2010) contend that the seemingly epidemic nature of autism can be in part accounted for by social influence and connection. Examining spatial clusterings of autism diagnoses, they find that when a child diagnosed with autism moves into a new community, neighboring children have a greater chance of being diagnosed as well. Another aspect of the Bearman research suggests that one of the best predictors of whether a child will be diagnosed with autism is whether the parents know a family where there is a child diagnosed with autism. This network factor explains 16 percent of the variance, a considerable influence. Living in proximity and interacting with another family with an autistic child may sensitize parents to defining certain behaviors as symptoms of autism and lead them to seek a diagnosis. In California, where Bearman and his colleagues conducted their study, a diagnosis of autism has certain advantages, i.e., it "buys" you something; special education, independent evaluations, individual professional attention etc. Thus, if a child exhibits certain symptoms, living in close proximity to an autism-diagnosed child will increase his/her chances of being diagnosed with autism.

There is no doubt that there has been a significant rise in the number of autism diagnoses in the past two decades. There is considerable debate about whether this is an epidemic representing an increase in the symptoms of the condition or whether it is an epidemic based on greater recognition and identification of extant symptoms that leads to an increase in diagnoses. What is clear, however, is that there is a sharp increase in the number of children diagnosed with autism. This has resulted in a number of social responses that are reflected in various aspects of society, including various support and advocacy groups on the Internet.

The Internet, the experience of illness, and patient activism

Until the past two decades, illness was largely an isolating experience. Most individuals, even those with chronic illnesses, did not know others with the same ailment and only on rare occasions communicated with others about their illness experience. While there were occasionally studies of patient subcultures in hospitals (e.g., Goffman 1961; Roth 1963), this was limited to a few illnesses and generally in hospital situations. Parsons and Fox (1952: 37) noted "illness usually prevents a patient from attaching himself to a solidary subculture of similarly oriented individuals." In rare circumstances, such as in the early days of end-stage renal disease (ESRD), there was enough interaction to sustain some kind of illness subculture (e.g., Kutner 1987), but for the most part patients remained individuals who were treated separately and lived their illness as a private individual experience. Patients talked to their doctor, family, and perhaps a few friends about their illness experience but not with fellow sufferers. Except for a few self-help groups, which were utilized by only a tiny fraction of those with illnesses, there was no possibility for patients to interact with others who shared their illness. For example, Schneider and Conrad (1983) interviewed 80 individuals with epilepsy, and found that no more than five respondents had ever spoken to another person with epilepsy. While there certainly was some patient interaction in the early days of the HIV/AIDS epidemic, largely because of the pre-existing gay and lesbian subculture, this was an unusual case. For the most part, illness remained a private experience and most individuals with illness did not interact with other sufferers in any meaningful way. This is no longer the case.

The Internet has fundamentally changed the experience of illness for many people. The thousands of websites, bulletin boards, chat rooms, and social media sites have created a myriad of vehicles for individuals with illness to communicate with others who have the same ailment (Conrad and Stults 2010). There are now several web or social media sites where individuals with illnesses can contact and exchange information with others suffering from the same illness. For some illnesses there are multiple sites where individuals can get information and interact with each other, each of these sites representing different experiences, views, or positions about the illness. These can be termed collectively as electronic support groups (ESG). Some of these web groups require users to sign up or join, but many are open to everyone and thus are available to anyone who wants to participate or just observe the online activity ("lurk"). There is no doubt these sites develop into social subcultures, something that would have been virtually unimaginable prior to the onset of the Internet. Billions of individuals use the Internet and there are thousands, probably tens of thousands, of sites focusing on nearly any kind of illness one can imagine.

One particular use of Internet has been to represent different views about an illness and even take advocacy stances concerning issues like diagnosis, treatment, etiology, prognosis, and illness management and experience. Different sites on the Internet have taken different positions and allowed for a certain kind of advocacy and activism (Conrad and Rondini 2010). The Internet has allowed the development of virtual patient organizations promoting particular viewpoints about an illness, making claims for legitimizing some perspectives on an illness while discrediting others, presenting alternative perspectives, making demands on the medical system, and promoting the salience of experiential knowledge about an illness (e.g., Barker 2008). The Internet has become a vehicle to present many voices and positions about any illness and its treatment.

The Internet can also facilitate the formation of advocacy groups for how and whether a particular disorder can or should be medicalized. Numerous social and medical analysts in recent years have written about the increasing medicalization of society (Clarke et al. 2003; Conrad 2007), i.e., how an increasing number of human conditions have become defined as medical problems, usually as a diagnosis or a disorder. The Internet has become a terrain where some of the debates over whether or not a particular condition is a disorder, and what kind of disorder it might be, take place. We have seen patient groups who want to medicalize fi bromyalgia (Barker 2008), who want to demedicalize anorexia (Conrad and Rondini 2010), and advocates who want to legitimize unknown illnesses like Morgellons disease (Fair 2010). The Internet has become a territory where different views of illness are presented and even advocated, including in some cases how a particular illness should or should not be medicalized.

The remainder of this chapter will take a look at three Internet presentations of autism and how these relate to an expanding or contracting medicalization of autism. These include: (1) Autism is a medical disease and needs more research into its etiology and treatment; (2) Autism is caused by environmental toxins (related to vaccines) and needs to be prevented by reducing exposure to toxins; and (3) autism is not a disease but rather one end of the human continuum and part of a normal range of neurodiversity. We will examine all three perspectives and analyze how these perspectives relate to the current medicalization of autism.

To achieve this analysis, we examined a range of websites for each of the three orientations (pro-medicalization, public health/vaccine toxins, and neurodiversity) and compared the presentation and concerns discussed on each website. By searching various combinations of key terms, we created a selection of websites that appeared regularly. Presumably, these websites are the ones most often accessed based on their ranking in the search results. All selected websites are publicly accessible. While this is not an in-depth study, from the websites we selected, we were able to illustrate a general picture of how each orientation is represented online.

Calling for more medicalization: medical research, treatment, and care

The first orientation toward autism found online argues for more and continued medicalization, which is typical for advocacy groups for specific diseases and illnesses. Approaching autism as a developmental disorder, this orientation calls for further biomedical research on etiology, prevention, treatment, and cures. The medicalization of autism characterizes the condition as an illness or developmental disorder. Unlike the other two orientations, which we will discuss below, the medicalization approach is institutionalized – the disorder is recognized in the DSM (Diagnostic and Statistical Manual of Mental Disorders), medical professionals offer the diagnosis, and biomedical science is researching the underlying cause. On websites such as *Autism Speaks*, *Autism Link*, *Operation Autism Online*, and *Defeat Autism Now!* the medicalization discourse is prevalent. Adopting the "epidemic" rhetoric, these websites promote further medicalization of autism by pushing for more awareness and research funding.

The mission of most pro-medicalization oriented websites is to provide support, educate, collect donations[1], and create a sense of community

(Autism Speaks 2013a; National Autism Association 2013a): "Our mission is to provide opportunities for inclusion, information, and support; to keep parents, family members of individuals with autism spectrum disorders and autistic individuals apprised of news and information, help them in their quest for services, and also in their quest for camaraderie with others in the autism community" (Autism Link 2013). These websites, which (based on the rhetoric) primarily target parents and families[2] of autistic children, offer users access to autism-related information on research, family services, conferences, local resources, education, etc.

Medicalization advocacy websites usually feature an "about autism" page, which defines autism as a spectral disorder and a "complex" developmental disability (Autism Society 2013a; Autism Speaks 2013d; Defeat Autism Now! 2013a). Taking a medical stance, these sites describe the diagnostic criteria (as specified in the DSM) and report statistics on prevalence:

> Autism is a complex developmental disability that typically appears during the first three years of life and affects a person's ability to communicate and interact with others. Autism is defined by a certain set of behaviors and is a "spectrum disorder" that affects individuals differently and to varying degrees. There is no known single cause of autism, but increased awareness and funding can help families today.
>
> (Autism Society 2013a)

> Autism statistics from the U.S. Centers for Disease Control and Prevention (CDC) identify around one in 68 American children as on the autism spectrum – a ten-fold increase in prevalence in 40 years. Careful research shows that this increase is only partly explained by improved diagnosis and awareness. Studies also show that autism is four to five times more common among boys than girls. An estimated 1 out of 54 boys and one in 252 girls are diagnosed with autism in the United States.
>
> (Autism Speaks 2013d)

These sites incontrovertibly frame autism as being a medical disorder. Although the causes are unknown (Centers for Disease Control and Prevention 2012b) and the diagnostic criteria vague, autism is consistently presented as being concrete and unquestionably a medically "real" disorder.

Approaching the condition as an epidemic and disorder, these websites emphasize the pressing need to stop the spread of autism by increasing medical research and knowledge. For example, the following mission statement is from *Autism Speaks*:

> Autism Speaks aims to bring the autism community together as one strong voice to urge the government and private sector to listen to our concerns and take action to address this urgent global health crisis.

> It is our firm belief that, working together, we will find the missing pieces of the puzzle.
>
> (Autism Speaks 2013a)

In this statement, autism is compared to a puzzle, which so happens to be the symbol for autism awareness. If autism is a puzzle, this implicates that the disorder is an enigma, that understanding is currently incomplete and complex, and that autism is a problem to be solved (and quickly, as it is a "global health crisis"). These websites advocate for more medicalization and the expansion of medical knowledge. Within this framework, autism is conceptualized as a medical issue, which requires medical intervention.

Currently, there is no definitive cure or treatment for autism (Centers for Disease Control and Prevention 2013). However, pro-medicalization websites usually list a range of treatment options that purportedly help with symptoms, such as Applied Behavior Analysis (ABA), Developmental, Individual Difference, Relationship-based/Floortime therapy (DIR/Floortime), Pivotal Response Therapy (PRT), Relationship Development Intervention (RDI), etc. (Autism Speaks 2013b). While none of these interventions are proven to be widely effective, some interventions are more often featured than others – for instance, ABA and DIR/Floortime (Autism Speaks 2013b; National Autism Association 2013b). At the same time, websites also list interventions that are more experimental and potentially harmful. On the *Defeat Autism Now!* website, underneath a short disclaimer[3], contested therapies such as "chelation"[4] and "virus elimination"[5] are listed alongside occupational therapy and music therapy (Defeat Autism Now 2013b). In support of autism cures and treatments, pro-medicalization websites include multiple intervention options for users; yet, some of these options have not been tested or researched for safety (requiring users to be extra discerning and critical of the information they receive).

One of the frequently iterated goals on pro-medicalization websites is building a sense of community: "The purpose of the Autism Speaks Web community is to provide a safe place for people on the autism spectrum and others affected by autism to connect, share stories, support each other and build lasting friendships" (Autism Speaks 2013c). Pro-medicalization websites offer information and access to local events, support groups, national conference registration, research participation opportunities, social networking pages, blog posts, and moderated chat rooms (Autism Society 2013b; Autism Speaks 2013c; National Autism Association 2013a). Despite the emphasis on fostering a sense of community, popular pro-medicalization websites do not often host open discussion forums. For instance, the *National Autism Association* links out to discussion groups hosted by Yahoo, *Autism Speaks* directs users to their accounts on Facebook, Twitter, Pinterest, Google+, and other social networking websites, and *Autism Society* provides a space where users can submit personal stories.

In the minority, *Autism Support Network* does host online chat rooms, which are organized by separate, themed groups and a general one that one can enter at any time. The process in which users (specifically, parents/guardians and service providers) form a community through these websites remains unexplored.

Having reviewed what these websites provide, further sociological research is required to understand how users interact with pro-medicalization website content. Since autism is understood as a "spectral" disorder – with no two cases exactly the same – parents and families of children with autism are can be seen as being part of a community and, at the same time, alone. If one of the major goals of pro-medicalization websites is to provide support and foster community, how then is this achieved? How do pro-medicalization website users find support and navigate online materials? In addition to building a community, these websites become patient-oriented organizations who advocate more medical research and support – including genetics, pharmacology, and different kinds of neurological treatments.

Pro-medicalization websites generally offer users similar resources and information about autism, which are fundamentally grounded in the idea that autism is an epidemic disorder and demands research on its causes, treatment, and cure. For many readers, this attitude toward autism aligns with the mainstream view of autism as a medical developmental disorder stemming from myriad (mostly unknown) causes. The answer here is for the community to come together to demand and support further medical research. However, as we explore the competing perspectives, we will show that the autism debate is quite contentious. Competing perspectives offer different understandings about the fundamentals of autism, and concomitantly suggest different strategies in approaching and managing the condition.

A quasi-public health approach: preventing autism by limiting vaccines

In the past few decades activists have claimed that toxins in the environment have been responsible for a range of illnesses including various forms of cancer, asthma, and gulf war syndrome. As Phil Brown (2007) has shown, coalitions of activists, patients, and scientists have contested the standard medical depictions of disease causation and showed how environmental factors, especially toxic substances, were implicated in disease causation. This has spurred both more research on toxins in the environment and new calls by laypeople and professionals for environmental research and interventions to prevent particular diseases.

In the 1990s, some physicians and autism activists began to raise the issue about whether vaccines (particularly against measles, mumps and rubella or MMR) given to children were a toxic cause of autism. Some suggested it was thimerosal (a mercury based preservative) in the vaccine that was a cause of autism, while others suggested it was the MMR vaccine itself that was toxic to some children in the doses administered. In 1998 UK physician Dr. Andrew Wakefield and colleagues (Wakefield et al. 1998) published an article in *The Lancet* connecting vaccines to gastrointestinal (GI) inflammation and to 12 cases of childhood autism. Even before this was published, parents of five of the children studied were seeking litigation against the companies producing MMR vaccine. This publication spurred controversy among physicians and in autism parent groups. While Wakefield's findings received a little medical support, his research findings generated a lot of publicity. Parents of autistic children began to form support and advocacy groups implicating vaccines as the cause of autism, calling for more research on the impact of vaccines on the onset of autism in children. For example, Safe Minds was formed in 2000 and used the Freedom of Information Act to obtain documents allegedly connecting symptoms of mercury poisoning with autism. This group attempted to refute medical critiques and highlight what they deemed as flawed medical studies (Jake Crosby – personal communication with Peter Conrad in 2010). Most mainstream medical sources found no significant connections between vaccines and the onset of autism (IOM 2004).

Beginning in the late 1990s a large number of what could be called "anti-vaccination groups" emerged, especially on the Internet. Andrew Wakefield became a spokesman and hero to the environmental/anti-vaccine advocates. Public figures like model and TV personality Jenny McCarthy and comedian Jim Carrey became advocates for the "vaccines are toxic" approach. McCarthy popularized an organization called Generation Rescue whose central belief was that vaccines cause autism or at the very least, there was not adequate research to declare that vaccines were safe. This approach, which we can generously call a public health approach, would be to ban or remove the "toxins," i.e., stop prescribing these vaccines. As it turns out, there is virtually no scientific evidence supporting the "vaccines cause autism" claim (IOM 2004). In 2008 the original paper that fueled this claim was found to be based on fraudulent and biased, or manipulated, data. In this context, *The Lancet* took the unusual move of retracting the original Wakefield paper, the British General Council investigated Dr. Wakefield and found misconduct and essentially removed his license to practice medicine in the UK (Harris 2010). One might think that such a repudiation of the vaccine hypothesis would have dissuaded supporters from continuing the anti-vaccine movement, but this was not the case. Internet groups attracted thousands to the anti-vaccine sites and advocates like Jenny McCarthy stayed the anti-vaccine course. Despite the scientific repudiation of the "vaccines cause autism" claims, the anti-vaccine movement continued to grow, calling for a ban on the current practice of vaccine usage, and short of that, more research on vaccine safety.

For a few of the anti-vaccination autism advocacy groups, the toxic vaccine suspicion expanded beyond the autism-MMR link to include the hepatitis B vaccine, Gardasil, the flu vaccine, and the diphtheria, pertussis, and tetanus vaccine (DPT) as potential causes of harm (Focus Autism 2012; Age of Autism 2012). These groups continued to draw attention to the detrimental effects of vaccination, questioning the safety of the vaccination schedule (McCarthy 2011) and suspecting conspiracy within science and between government agencies and pharmaceutical companies (Bearman 2010; Kata 2010; Russell and Kelly 2011). While their agenda has shifted to focus on environmental factors and vaccination as a choice, anti-vaccination activism has inspired concern among public health professionals. According to medical professionals, the anti-vaccination movement poses a threat to public health, weakening herd immunity and bringing back vaccine-preventable diseases (VPD) (Shetty 2010). Online anti-vaccination groups provide users with information on vaccine dangers and other autism-inducing toxins, personal stories of "vaccine injury," and treatment options for "recovery" (Age of Autism 2012; Generation Rescue 2012; Focus Autism 2012). Though these groups see themselves as adopting a "protect the public health from toxins" approach, this particular attitude toward autism actually conflicts with broader public health goals, as it perpetuates an immunization scare and promotes an understanding of the disorder that compromises disease prevention efforts. For example, comparing 2011 to 2012, pertussis cases ("whooping cough") have increased by 1,300 percent, in the state of Washington reaching rates similar to those of 1942 (CDC 2012c). With this rise, some argue that the growing anti-vaccination movement is to blame (Salzberg 2012).

The anti-vaccination movement in the United States is not new, dating back to 1879 with the Anti-Vaccination Society of America (Kaufman 1967). As Stuart Blume (2006) notes, the early movement represented conflicting ideas of "good citizenship." While immunization advocates defined "good citizenship" in terms of duty to public health, anti-vaccinationists contended that "good citizenship" is respect for individual bodies (Blume 2006). Current anti-vaccinationists make similar appeals as their late nineteenth-century counterparts, asserting that vaccination should be an informed choice (Generation Rescue 2012; Focus Autism 2012). One popular argument explicates that the return of anti-vaccination sentiments is attributable to vaccines' enormous success. Since the efficacy of vaccines is not overtly visible, its value has weakened over time, drawing attention to purported adverse reactions (Andre 2003; Poland and Jacobson 2001).

Although the autism-vaccine link has been scientifically discredited, many parents maintain their suspicions. Compared to the general public, parents of autistic children are more likely to omit or delay vaccinations for the younger siblings. The odds of omission and delay are higher if parents believe that their child's autism was caused by vaccination. (Rosenberg et al. 2013). This demonstrates that despite the medically proven safety of vaccines, many continue to harbor doubt. As we have found, anti-vaccination discourse persists on websites like *Generation Rescue*, *Focus Autism*, and *Age of*

Autism. On these websites, the anti-vaccination discourse supports an environmental-cause approach and emphasizes parents' rights to critically assess vaccine safety.

The environmental-cause approach extends beyond the effects of the MMR vaccine studied by Wakefield et al. to include warning against other vaccines, toxins, and unhealthy dietary habits. For instance, *Focus Autism* questions the safety of other immunizations, providing its visitors "stories of vaccine injury," such as this short anecdote about "Patrick":

> Patrick had two regressions: 1st he received the MMR, DTaP, and Hib on one day. Within 24–36 hours [he] seemed out of it, within a week, he was perseverating on things (he had just seen George of the Jungle and started running into trees) and all his language went from natural to scripted. Three months later, he had his chicken pox vaccine; within 24 hours of having this vaccine he started having severe, chronic diarrhea that lasted for over a year (until we got the secretin shot); his language deteriorated to all but 2 words (he had 150–200 words at the time)…he has never been the same.
>
> (Focus Autism 2012)

The story of Patrick highlights causation: after receiving three immunizations during a doctor's visit, Patrick develops autistic behaviors and loses communication skills; after another vaccination, Patrick experiences chronic diarrhea and his communication skills further diminish. The majority of immunization stories on *Focus Autism* and similar websites follow this narrative of cause and effect, of vaccination and harm. Peter Bearman refers to the perception of causation as "temporal confusion." Temporal confusion occurs when one looks for a "single-bullet" explanation and mistakes the *correlation* of vaccination time and autism onset for vaccination as *cause* (Bearman 2010). Broadening caution, these narratives warn visitors of the potential dangers of vaccination in general.

The websites do not specifically define themselves as anti-vaccine. *Age of Autism* (2012) states:

> We are published to give voice to those who believe autism is an environmentally induced illness, that it is treatable, and that children can recover. […] We believe that autism is the defining disorder of our age, man-made and therefore preventable.

Autism, then, is perceived as being within the realm of control – created by society, thus preventable by society. While these anti-vaccination websites claim that they do not oppose vaccinations, "[w]e are not in any way against vaccines, but we would like to see a great improvement in the safety of administering vaccines in addition to the vaccines themselves" (Focus Autism 2012), the harm-prevention strategies and information they offer visitors suggest otherwise. Visitors are told they should stay informed, but the information on immunization harms promulgated on these websites reinforces vaccine-scare. By omitting, or minimizing, the good of immunizations to public and individual health, anti-vaccination websites emphasize a risk assessment that favors individual protection.

While these websites represent the "vaccines are toxic" viewpoint, they regularly call out for more research that would show that the vaccines are safe for children; they emphasize their largely anecdotal perspective as evidence and discount the scientifi c data as biased or inadequate. These advocates say they would like a medical/scientifi c approach to show the impact of vaccines on autism but reject the current scientific evidence that does not find a link between vaccines and autism.

Autism as neurodiversity: a challenge toward demedicalization

Neurodiversity, a self-advocacy movement, contends that autism and other neurological, cognitive, and developmental conditions are *differences* in "brain wiring" (Blume 1998; Harmon 2004). Proponents argue that such conditions are considered disorders because of exclusionary definitions of normality. Jim Sinclair, Autism Network International (ANI) coordinator, stated in his 1993 address: "The tragedy is not that we're here, but that your world has no place for us to be" (Sinclair 1993). As a self-advocacy movement, neurodiversity groups push for acceptance of neurological variation, challenging medical expertise with experiential knowledge (Brownlow and O'Dell 2006). This particular orientation toward autism promotes a change in discourses on health and treatment. Instead of "treating" or "curing" the individual, the neurodiverse perspective advocates changing the medical definitions of autism. Others have pointed out, however, that wide adoption of this perspective is unfair to those who want a cure and may not be physically capable of voicing opposition (Rubin 2005; Ortega 2009). Unlike the two other orientations, which propose different approaches to medical intervention, neurodiversity demands that medical and scientific institutions cease involvement. Encouraging acceptance and social measures to support the participation of neurodiverse people, online neurodiversity groups essentially state that neurodiversity is part of the "normal spectrum" and essentially demand demedicalization. These neurodiversity websites provide visitors a range of information (for finding support groups, autism research, conferences etc.), involvement resources (mailing lists, local groups, retreats), and social networking tools (chat rooms/discussion forums).

The term "neurodiversity" was coined by Judy Singer, an Australian mother with autism whose child is also autistic (Solomon 2008). At the start of the movement, advocates were mainly comprised of parents (Solomon 2008). Since then, neurodiversity has developed into self-advocacy, declaring that "The best advocates for autistic people are autistic people themselves" (Sinclair 2012). With mottos like "nothing about us, without us" (Autistic Self Advocacy Network 2013) and claims that Silicon Valley is full of successful neurodiverse individuals (Buchen 2011), the movement represents a collective endeavor to seize control of definition rights. Neurodiversity aims to give autistics the power to shape autism discourse – to shape the way society discusses and conceptualizes their condition.

Although neurodiversity is dominated by high functioning people with autism and Asperger's Syndrome (Ortega 2009), the movement also includes those affected by Attention Deficit Hyperactivity Disorder (ADHD), bipolar disorder, dyslexia, Tourette's Syndrome, and dyspraxia (Fenton and Krahn 2007; Boundy 2008: 3; DANDA 2012). Perhaps due to the social and communication limitations of many neurodiverse advocates, the movement did not emerge until the early 1990s with the growing access to the Internet. The Internet, having been compared to braille for autistics (Blume 1997), is an invaluable facilitator of social interaction (Davidson 2008; Jordan 2010) and positive identity construction (Brownlow and O'Dell 2006).

Neurodiversity websites propagate a constructivist approach to autism, asserting that it is not autism but society that needs to be treated (Boundy 2008). As various neurodiversity groups indicate, with integrative accommodations, autistic individuals would be able to fully participate in society. This position is reminiscent of Susan Wendell's argument, which claims that disability is a product of exclusionary social arrangements. According to her, disabled individuals can live productive and independent lives if provided integrative programs (Wendell 1989). Pushing this perspective further, neurodiversity advocates contend that society loses potential contributions from autistics because of narrow definitions of normality – or favoritism of one particular kind of neurological processing over another: "Neurodiversity may be every bit as crucial for the human race as biodiversity is for life in general. Who can say what form of wiring will prove best at any given moment?" (Blume 1998) By framing autism and related conditions as natural differences, online advocacy groups note that the solution is not to change these differences but to change social norms. The claims include the position that research into the "disease" of autism may be largely unnecessary; rather research should be focused on how society can better accept and integrate neurodiverse individuals.

Neurodiversity websites, such as *Wrong Planet*, *Autistic Self Advocacy Network* (ASAN), *Autism Network International* (ANI), *Neurodiversity*, *Developmental Adult Neuro-Diversity Association* (DANDA), and *Aspies for Freedom* (AFF), proffer an ideology of neurological, cognitive, and developmental difference and acceptance. The difference in "brain wiring" (Blume 1998; Harmon 2004) is claimed to be another political category comparable to race, class, and gender (Jaarsma and Welin 2012; Singer 1999). Most websites provide self-advocacy resources and information, and a few feature additional interactive tools, like discussion forums and chat rooms. The mission and goals of these websites are more or less the same: to expand disability rights, form community, increase social participation, and above all, challenge the perception of autism (and related conditions) as disability (DANDA 2012; Sinclair 2012; AFF 2013). For instance, the philosophy and goals of ANI focus on social acceptance and accommodation of difference:

> Autistic lives are meaningful and worthwhile lives. … Supports for autistic people should be aimed at helping them to compensate, navigate, and function in the world, not at changing them into non-autistic people or isolating them from the world. … Autistic people of all ages and all levels of ability and skill are entitled to adequate and appropriate support services. … Autistic people have characteristically autistic styles of relating to others, which should be respected and appreciated rather than modified to make them "fit in." … In addition to promoting self-advocacy for autistic adults who are able to participate independently, ANI also works to improve the lives of autistic people who, whether because they are too young, or because they do not have adequate communication skills, are not able to advocate for themselves.
>
> (Sinclair 2012)

Certain websites, such as AFF, have more specific agendas that reflect the ideologies of neurodiversity:

> To prevent eugenic elimination of autistic people by opposing pre-natal testing for autism. … To oppose physically or mentally harmful "treatments" targeting autistic people. … To [emphasize] the "spectrum" view of autism, and de-[emphasize] the differences between the various autistic spectrum labels. …To oppose the idea of an autism "cure."… To evaluate alleged treatments for ethical approaches. … To increase funding for, and access to, autistic support services and ethical forms of treatment. … To oppose negative publicity campaigns against autistic people as a group. … To help promote an accurate yet positive image of autism. … To oppose all forms of prejudice and bigotry.
>
> (AFF 2013)

As illustrated in the AFF mission statement above, these specific goals translate abstract philosophies into concrete plans of action toward the institutionalization of neurodiversity. These online communities not only promulgate the movement's fundamental ideas and perspectives but organize action.

The culture and missions of online communities have efficacy in non-virtual society (Davidson 2008). Not only a medium to spread ideas, neurodiversity websites such as ASAN and DANDA serve as virtual recruitment space, offering visitors opportunities to participate in research, local projects, and offline events (DANDA 2012; Sinclair 2013; ASAN 2013). Some neurodiversity websites facilitate offline communities. The ANI website, as an example, features information about neurodiversity and links to other autism-related websites. In addition to online-content, ANI hosts an annual "Autreat," an offline neurodiversity retreat and conference, which "focuses on positive living with autism, NOT on causes, cures, or ways to make us more normal" (Sinclair 2013 – original emphasis). These retreats aim to bring together neurodiverse individuals and supporters. Unlike other autism conferences, Autreat claims to be for individuals with autism and other developmental differences (as opposed to service providers and researchers): "Family members and professionals are welcome to attend, but the structure and content of this event are determined by the interests and sensibilities of autistic people" (Sinclair 2013).

Aside from offline retreats, conferences, and local events, neurodiversity websites often include discussion forums and chat rooms, which connect neurodiverse proponents virtually. In Chloe Jordan's (2008) study of autism and Internet use, she argues that the online discussion boards enable autistic individuals to socially engage with others. With computer screens mediating interactions, social anxieties characteristic of autism are reduced (Jordan 2008; American Psychiatric Association 2013). Discussion topics on neurodiversity sites are not limited to autism or difference-related issues; rather, the forums extensively cover everything from politics to entertainment to personal dilemmas (AFF 2013; Wrong Planet 2013). Illustrating the diversity of discussion topics, on the *Wrong Planet* website, the top three discussion categories with the greatest number of posts are: "General Autism Discussion," "Random Discussion," and "Off the Wall: Forum games, Quizzes, Roleplaying, etc." In the case of discussion forums and chat rooms, neurodiversity is the common denominator that unites individuals. The views and political agenda of neurodiversity are not at the forefront of discussion, as individuals participating on the discussion forums already share these ideas.

Neurodiversity websites offer visitors resources that iterate the idea of "difference" and the goal of "acceptance." From our brief discussion above, it is clear that the neurodiversity movement is much more complex than seeking tolerance. These online groups demand demedicalization – with treatment being optional for those who want it (Boundy 2008), control over the definition of their group identity, and a broader normative understanding of neurological functioning/health. However, this orientation to autism conflicts with the disorder discourse held by many parents and medical professionals. In addition, the truly silent population of autistic people, those who are unable to communicate, cannot speak up against or for this movement. As some fear, the popularization of neurodiversity might deny treatment to those who want to be cured (Rubin 2005).

Autism and the internet: patient organizations and medicalization

In the past three decades autism has gone from a rare affliction to one that is as common as one in 68 individuals (CDC 2012a). While the actual underpinnings of this growth remain a mystery, it seems clear that at least part of the increase is explained by the changing definition of which behaviors should be diagnosed as autism (Eyal et al. 2010). As Peter Bearman and his colleagues have pointed out, there are also other factors, such as residence location and networks, which may also play an important part in coming to an autism diagnosis. The result is that we now have a range of individuals diagnosed, from high functioning individuals (e.g., those designated with Asperger's Syndrome) to those so severely affected that they are essentially non-verbal and profoundly disabled. Some of this may change with the new DSM-V diagnoses which have removed the separate Asperger's Syndrome as part of what serves as a diagnosis of autism (Wallis 2009). The impact of that change may reshape the Internet world of autism, but as of 2013, the three perspectives presented in this chapter are representative of the autism world on the Internet.

With the increase in autism diagnoses, it is not surprising that there are dozens of websites about autism. Many of these are patient or parent driven organizations that both serve the "autism community" and take different viewpoints in advocating for autism. In this paper we have described three different orientations of Internet websites, all of which are in their own way advocates for autism and suggest a different kind of research. What is particularly interesting to us is that in their advocacy for autism, each perspective has a different relationship to medicalization. There seems to be little question that the behaviors that make up the autism diagnosis have both had a lower threshold for diagnosis and become more well known to physicians and the public in recent years. Thus we have seen an increasing medicalization of autism in the past three decades, as more behaviors have come under the diagnostic umbrella of autism. It seems clear that the medicalized views of autistic behavior have led to the diagnosis of numerous children as autistic that previously might have been seen as vaguely developmentally disabled, just "a little odd," or somewhat asocial.

The dominant view of autism, then, has become a medicalized view and we have found this viewpoint very well represented on the Internet. These websites advocate for further medical research, emphasizing research on etiology, treatment and cure of what they generally see as an unabashedly medical disorder. According to this perspective, the more medicalization the better; research needs to result in better treatment and eventually a cure.

Another view of autism we call the "quasi-public health viewpoint" on autism, although many others would call this perspective the "anti-vaccine advocates." The supporters of these websites have their roots in a variety of purported "studies" that claim that the preservative in children's vaccines, or the treatment schedules of the vaccination, have, in their view, "without a doubt" been a major factor in the causes of the autism epidemic. These groups have been very successful in obtaining the public's attention and have created an even broader anti-vaccine backlash (Offit 2011) despite the fact that there is no scientific evidence linking vaccines to the onset of autism

(IOM 2004). Yet there are a plethora of patient and parent-driven organizations that are "absolutely sure" that vaccines are implicated in this rise of autism. Their view is to oppose vaccinations in children until these vaccines are "proven safe." Accordingly, they also take a medical view of autism, seeing it as caused by toxins, but their view is aimed largely at the prevention of what they see as toxic vaccines, rather than focusing primarily on treatment and cure. At the moment, they remain a group with little influence on medicine but a significant influence on some aspects of the public view of autism.

While the first two perspectives both call for some kind of medicalized response to autism, and could be seen as agents of medicalization, the third perspective essentially calls for a demedicalization of at least some aspects of autism. Those who support the neurodiversity websites claim that what is often diagnosed as autism is not a disease at all but rather one aspect of a continuum of normal and expected human behavior. This perspective suggests that most of us are "neurotypicals" who do not have the same characteristics as the neurodiverse and generally do not see the strengths of neurodiversity. They suggest that the neurodiverse have certain characteristics that include hyperfocus, seeing the world in patterns, imaging the world in pictures and shapes rather than words, and sensory processing differences, all of which are very valuable in their own right. The assumption here is that neurotypicals stigmatize and pathologize the behaviors of the neurodiverse, medicalizing those behaviors they deem as inappropriate. What the neurodiverse want is acceptance for who they are, equal rights, accommodations, and a demedicalization of the diagnosis that labels them as having a disorder.

Therefore, if one looks for patient organizations related to autism on the Internet, one finds at least three distinctive and active types of patient advocacy organizations. Each calls for a different kind of scientific research to support their perspective: the medicalized organizations want more biomedical research into cause, cure, and treatment; the quasi-public health/anti-vaccine groups want more research into the impact of vaccines, and believe they will be vindicated by the results; and the neurodiversity groups eschew medical research into their "condition" but call for research that would eliminate what they see as discrimination against them. There is relatively little overlap in what each group advocates, but all would see themselves as advocacy organizations for autism.

Notes

1 Autism Society: "Your gift will help support, autism education, awareness, advocacy, research, and most importantly, enable us to assist families living with autism" (Autism Society, 2013b).

2 On Fourth of July, the main page of Autism Speaks featured a Q&A titled, "Tips for an Autism-Friendly Fourth of July," which gave parents tips on how to help their autistic children enjoy the festivities (Elder 2013).

3 "Please note that these are types of therapies out there for children with autism. Not all therapies are the same. Please consult with your Doctor first before considering these types of therapies. These are just a few of the therapies out there, explore options that best meet your child's needs" (Defeat Autism Now 2013b).
4 "CHELATION: Dangerous heavy metals, such as mercury, lead, aluminum, cadmium, and arsenic can also be removed from the body with chelation treatment. The Greek word for "claw" is used to derive chelation (key-la-shun). Chelation side effects are minimal, but you will need a good mineral supplement to replace lost minerals" (Defeat Autism Now 2013b).
5 "VIRUS ELIMINATION: Occult (hidden) viral infections have been theorized for autism. Colloidal silver is particularly effective for its healing properties. Colostrum improves the immune response to viral infections. Echinacea also strengthens the immune system and detoxifies the lymphatic system. A Chinese herbal combination (capsule and liquid) creates an unfavorable environment for viruses and a great tasting chewable elderberry tablet can stimulate the immune system" (Defeat Autism Now 2013b).

References

Age of Autism (2012) *Age of Autism*. Available online at: <www.ageofautism.com/a-welcome-from-dan-olmste.html> (accessed 27 November 2013).
American Psychiatric Association (2013) *Diagnostic and Statistical Manual of Mental Disorders*, fifth edition, Arlington, VA: American Psychiatric Publishing.
Armstrong, Thomas (2011) *Neurodiversity: Discovering the Extraordinary Gifts of Autism ADHD, Dyslexia and other Brain Differences*, Cambridge, MA: Da Capo Press.
Andre, Francis E. (2003) Vaccinology: Past Achievements, Present Roadblocks and Future Promises, *Vaccine*, 21(7–8), 593–595.
Aspies for Freedom (AFF) (2013) *Welcome to AFF*. Available online at: <www.aspies-forfreedom.com> (accessed 3 July 2013).
Autism Link (2013) *About Us*. Available online at: <www.autismlink.com/about-us> (accessed 27 November 2013).
Autism Speaks (2010) What is Causing the Increase in Autism Prevalence? *Autism Speaks Official Blog*, 22 October 2010. Available online at: <http://blog.autism-speaks.org/2010/10/22/got-questions-answers-to-your-questions-from-the-autism-speaks%E2%80%99-science-staff-2> (accessed 9 July 2013).
—— (2013a) *Mission*. Available online at: <www.autismspeaks.org/about-us/mission> (accessed 3 July 2013).
—— (2013b) *Treatment and Therapies*. Available online at: <www.autismspeaks.org/family-services/tool-kits/100-day-kit/treatments-therapies> (accessed 3 July 2013).
—— (2013c) *Web Community Guidelines*. Available online at: <www.autismspeaks.org/about-us/web-community-guidelines> (accessed 3 July 2013).
—— (2013d) *What is Autism?* Available online at <www.autismspeaks.org/what-autism> (accessed 3 July 2013).
Autism Society (2013a) *About Autism*. Available online at: <www.autism-society.org/about-autism> (accessed 3 July 2013).
—— (2013b) *Get involved*. Available online at: <www.autism-society.org/get-involved/donate> (accessed 4 July 2013).
Autistic Self Advocacy Network (ASAN) (2013) *Autistic Self Advocacy Network*. Available online at: <http://autisticadvocacy.org> (accessed 3 July 2013).
Barker, Kristin K. (2008) Electronic Support Groups, Patient-consumers, and Medicalization, *Journal of Health and Social Behavior*, 49(1), 20–36.

Bearman, Peter (2010) Just-so Stories: Vaccines, Autism, and the Single-bullet Disorder, *Social Psychology Quarterly*, 73(2), 112–115.

Blume, Harvey (1997) "Autism & the Internet" or "It's the Wiring, Stupid," *MIT Communications Forums*. Available online at: <http://web.mit.edu/comm-forum/papers/blume.html> (accessed 5 May 2012).

—— (1998) Neurodiversity, *The Atlantic*, 30 September. Available online at: <www.theatlantic.com/magazine/archive/1998/09/neurodiversity/5909> (accessed 6 May 2012).

Blume, Stuart (2006) Anti-vaccination Movements and their Interpretations, *Social Science & Medicine*, 62(3), 628–642.

Boundy, Kathryn (2008) "Are You Sure, Sweetheart, That You Want to be Well?" An Exploration of The Neurodiversity Movement, *Radical Psychology*, 7(Summer), 1–20.

Bowker, Natilene and Tuffin, Keith (2002) Disability Discourses for Online Identities. *Disability & Society*, 17(3), 327–344.

Brown, Phil (2007) *Toxic Exposures: Contested Illnesses and the Environmental Health Movement*, New York: Columbia University Press.

Brownlow, Charlotte and O'Dell, Lindsay (2006) Constructing an Autistic Identity: AS Voices Online, *Mental Retardation*, 44(5), 315–321.

Buchen, Lizzie (2011) Scientists and Autism: When Geeks Meet, *Nature*, 479, 25–27. Available online at: <www.nature.com/news/2011/111102/full/479025a.html> (accessed 9 July 2013).

Centers for Disease Control and Prevention (CDC) (2012a) *Autism Spectrum Disorder (ASD): Data and Statistics*. Available online at: <www.cdc.gov/ncbddd/autism/data.html> (accessed 27 November 2013).

—— (2012b) *Autism Spectrum Disorder (ASD): Facts about ASDs*. Available online at: <www.cdc.gov/ncbddd/autism/facts.html> (accessed 29 April 2012).

—— (2012c) Pertussis Epidemic – Washington, 2012, *Morbidity and Mortality Weekly Report (MMWR)*. Available online at: <www.cdc.gov/mmwr/preview/mmwrhtml/mm6128a1.htm> (accessed 3 January 2014).

—— (2013) *Autism Spectrum Disorder (ASD): Treatment*. Available online at: <www.cdc.gov/ncbddd/autism/treatment.html> (accessed 3 July 2013).

Clarke, Adele; Mamo, Laura; Fishman, Jennifer R.; Shim, Janet K. and Fosket, Jennifer R. (2003) Biomedicalization: Technoscientific Transformations of Health, Illness, and U.S. Biomedicine, *American Sociological Review*, 68(2), 161–194.

Conrad, Peter (2007) *The Medicalization of Society: The Transformation of Human Conditions into Treatable Disorders*, Baltimore, MD: Johns Hopkins University Press.

Conrad, Peter and Rondini, Ashley (2010) The Internet and Medicalization: Reshaping the Global Body and Illness, in E. Ettorre (ed.) *Culture, Bodies and the Sociology of Health*, Burlington, VT and Farnham: Ashgate, 107–120.

Conrad, Peter and Stults, Cheryl (2010) The Internet and the Experience of Illness, in C. Bird, P. Conrad, A.M. Fremont and S. Timmermans (eds) *The Handbook of Medical Sociology*, sixth edition, Nashville, TN: Vanderbilt University Press, 179–190.

DANDA (2012) *About DANDA*. Available online at: <www.danda.org.uk> (accessed 12 April 2012).

Davidson, Joyce (2008) Autistic culture online: Virtual Communication and Cultural Expression on the Spectrum, *Social & Cultural Geography*, 9(7), 791–806.

Defeat Autism Now! (2013a) *Defeat Autism Now!* Available online at: <www.defeatautismnow.net> (accessed 3 July 2013).

___ (2013b) *Therapy*. Available online at: <www.defeatautismnow.net> (accessed 3 July 2013).

Elder, Lauren (2013) Tips for an Autism-Friendly Fourth of July, *Autism Speaks*, July 2. Available online at: <www.autismspeaks.org/blog/2013/07/02/tips-autism-friendly-fourth-july> (accessed 4 July 2013).

Eyal, Gil; Hart, Brendan; Onculer, Emine; Oren, Neta and Rossi, Natasha (2010) *The Autism Matrix: The Social Origins of the Autism Epidemic*, Cambridge and Malden, MA: Polity Press.

Fair, Brian (2010) Morgellons: Contested Illness, Diagnostic Compromise, and Medicalization, *Sociology of Health and Illness*, 32(4), 597–612.

Fenton, Andrew and Krahn, Tim (2007) Autism, Neurodiversity and Equality Beyond the "Normal," *Journal of Ethics in Mental Health*, 2(2), 1–6.

Focus Autism (2012) *Focus Autism*. Available online at: <http://focusautisminc.org> (accessed 27 November 2013).

Generation Rescue (2012) *Background*. Available online at: <www.generationrescue.org/about/background> (accessed 28 November 2013).

Goffman, Erving (1961) *Asylums: Essays on the Social Situation of Mental Patients and Other Inmates*, New York: Doubleday.

Grinker, Roy R. (2008) *Unstrange Minds: Remapping the World of Autism*, New York: Basic Books.

Harmon, Amy (2004) Neurodiversity Forever: The Disability Movement Turns to Brains. *The New York Times*, 9 May. Available online at: <www.nytimes.com/2004/05/09/weekinreview/neurodiversity-forever-the-disability-movement-turns-to-brains.html?pagewanted=all&src=pm)> (accessed 4 March 2012).

Harris, Gardiner (2010) Journal Retracts 1998 Paper Linking Autism to Vaccines, *New York Times*, 2 February. Available online at: <www.nytimes.com/2010/02/03/health/research/03lancet.html?_r=0> (accessed 9 July 2013).

Institute of Medicine (IOM) (2004) *Immunization and Safety Review: Vaccines and Autism*, Washington DC: National Academies Press.

Jaarsma, Pier and Welin, Stellan (2012) Autism as a Natural Human Variation: Reflections on the Claims of the Neurodiversity Movement, *Health Care Analysis*, 20(1), 20–30.

Jordan, Chloe J. (2010) Evolution of Autism Support and Understanding via the World Wide Web, *Intellectual and Developmental Disabilities*, 48(3), 220–227.

Kata, Anna (2010) A Postmodern Pandora's Box: Anti-vaccination Misinformation on the Internet, *Vaccine*, 28(7), 1709–1716.

Kaufman, Martin (1967) The American Anti-Vaccinationists and their Arguments, *Bulletin of the History of Medicine*, 41(5), 463–478.

King, Marissa and Bearman, Peter (2009) Diagnostic Change and the Increased Prevalence of Autism, *International Journal of Epidemiology*, 38(5), 1224–1234.

Kutner, Nancy (1987) Social Worlds and Identity in End Stage Renal Disease (ESRD), in J. Roth and P. Conrad (eds), *Research in the Sociology of Health Care*, Vol. 6. *The Experience and Management of Chronic Illness*, Greenwich, CT: JAI Press, 33–71.

Liu, Ka-Yuet; King, Marissa and Bearman, Peter (2010) Social Influence and the Autism Epidemic, *American Journal of Sociology*, 115(5), 1387–1434.

McCarthy, Jenny (2011) In the Vaccine-Autism Debate, What Can Parents Believe? *The Huffington Post*, 10 January. Available online at: <www.huffingtonpost.com/jenny-mccarthy/vaccine-autism-debate_b_806857.htm> (accessed 29 October 2012).

National Autism Association (2013a) *Mission Statement*. Available online at: <http://nationalautismassociation.org/about-naa/mission-statement> (accessed 3 July 2013).

—— (2013b) *Therapies*. Available online at: <http://nationalautismassociation.org/autism-treatment-2/therapies> (accessed 3 July 2013).

Offit, Paul A (2011) *Deadly Choices: How the Anti-Vaccine Movement Threatens Us All*, New York: Basic Books.

Ortega, Francisco (2009) The Cerebral Subject and the Challenge of Neurodiversity, *BioSocieties*, 4(4), 425–445.

Parsons, Talcott and Fox, Renée (1952) Illness, Therapy and the Modern Urban American Family, *Journal of Social Issues*, 8(4), 31–44.

Poland, Gregory A. and Jacobson, Robert M (2001) Understanding Those Who Do Not Understand: A Brief Review of the Anti-vaccine Movement, *Vaccine*, 19(17–19), 2440–2445.

Rosenberg, Rebecca E.; Law, J. Kiely; Anderson, Connie; Samango-Sprouse, Carole; Law, Paul A. (2013) Survey of Vaccine Beliefs and Practices Among Families Affected by Autism Spectrum Disorders, *Clinical Pediatrics*, 52(9), 871–874.

Roth, Julius (1963) *Timetables: Structuring the Passage of Time in Hospital Treatment and Other Careers*, Indianapolis, IN: Bobbs Merrill.

Rubin, Sue (2005) Acceptance versus cure, *Cable News Network* (CNN). Available online at: <www.cgi.cnn.com/CNN/Programs/presents/shows/autism.world/notebooks/sue/notebook.html> (accessed 6 April 2012).

Russell, Ginny and Kelly, Susan (2011) Looking Beyond Risk: A Study of Lay Epidemiology of Childhood Disorders, *Health, Risk & Society*, 13(2), 129–145.

Salzberg, Steven (2012) Anti-Vaccine Movement Causes the Worst Whooping Cough Epidemic in 70 Years. Forbes, July 23. Available online at: <www.forbes.com/sites/stevensalzberg/2012/07/23/anti-vaccine-movement-causes-the-worst-whooping-cough-epidemic-in-70-years> (accessed 31 October 2012).

Schneider, Joseph W. and Conrad, Peter (1983) *Having Epilepsy: The Experience and Control of Illness*, Philadelphia, PA: Temple University Press.

Shetty, Priya (2010) Experts concerned about vaccination backlash, *The Lancet*, 375(9719), 970–971.

Sinclair, Jim (1993) Don't Mourn For Us, *Our Voice*, 1(3), 16 March. Available online at: <www.autreat.com/dont_mourn.html> (accessed 27 November 2013).

—— (2012) Introducing ANI, *Autism Network International*, 9 April 2012. Available online at: <www.autreat.com/intro.html> (accessed 27 November 2013).

—— (2013) *Autism Network International*. Available online at: <www.autreat.com> (accessed 3 July 2013).

Singer, Judy (1999) "Why Can't You Be Normal For Once In Your Life?" From a "Problem With No Name" to the Emergence of a New Category of Difference, in M. Corker and S. French (eds) *Disability Discourse*, Buckingham and Philadelphia, PA: Open University Press.

Solomon, Andrew (2008) The Autism Rights Movement, *New York Magazine*, 25 May. Available online at: <http://nymag.com/news/features/47225> (accessed 23 March 2012).

Wakefield, Andrew; Murch, Simon H.; Anthony, A.; Linnell, J.; Casson, D. M.; Malik, M.; Berelowitz, M.; Dhillon, A. P.; Thomson, M. A.; Harvey, P.; Valentine, A.; Davies, S. E. and Walker-Smith, John A. (1998) Ileal-Lymphoid-Nodular Hyperplasia, Non-specifi c Colitis, and Pervasive Developmental Disorder in Children, *The Lancet*, 351(9103), 637–641.

Wallis, Claudia (2009) The Vanishing Diagnosis for Asperger's Syndrome, *New York Times*, 9 November. Available online at: <www.nytimes.com/2009/11/03/health/03asperger.html?pagewanted=all&_r=0> (accessed 7 July 2013).

Wendell, Susan (1989) Toward a Feminist Theory of Disability, *Hypatia*. 4(2), 104–124.

Wrong Planet (2013) *Community Discussion Forum*. Available online at: <www.wrongplanet.net/forums.html> (accessed 3 July 2013).

7 A community fractured

Canada's breast cancer movement, pharmaceutical company funding, and science-related advocacy[1]

Sharon Batt

Canada's breast cancer movement is now more than two decades old. During that time, breast cancer groups have successfully fought for a say in the official breast cancer research agenda; they have also undertaken research themselves, either independently or in collaboration with other players in the system. At the same time, government practices for funding grass-roots organizations have changed dramatically and the groups have gradually come to rely on the pharmaceutical industry as a source of funding.

Based on ethnographic research undertaken in Canada's women's health and breast cancer movements, I examine this realignment in the light of the parallel struggle for lay publics to participate in research decision-making. I argue that if patients' organizations are to make meaningful contributions to the research community they need to develop and sustain robust, independent communities; and further, that neoliberal governments in Canada have instituted practices that undermine these capacities. I begin by describing welfare state structures and policies that enabled the women's health movement to bring health research in line with women's needs while pushing science to a higher standard. The main sections of the chapter discuss policy changes that radically altered the environment in which health advocacy groups function, creating turmoil within the newly formed breast cancer movement and disrupting the essential connection between the patient community's grass roots members and its advocacy voice.

Health activism in Canada's welfare state era

From the mid-1940s to the mid-1970s, successive Canadian governments put in place and actively maintained a series of universal social programs. During this period of nation-building, postwar governments provided financial support to equality-seeking civil society groups representing marginalized communities, based on the conviction that they could broaden democratic participation and improve the process of public policy. These organizations clarified the needs of particular communities, channelled information, and lent legitimacy both to citizen's demands and to policy-making agencies (Pross 1992).

Federal and provincial governments recognized by the late 1960s that the women's movement expressed widespread concerns. A sub-movement, focused on women's health, challenged both the elitism and the research model of the medical establishment. These health activists claimed women's right to knowledge about their own bodies. They contested much in the medical and societal canon about women's bodies as based on myth and argued that lay women possess valuable self-knowledge (Morrow 2007). This discourse emboldened women to research and produce their own health publications.

Feminist health research relied on a critical reading of scientific literature measured against lay experiential knowledge, the community's values, and observations of research gaps, or what has recently been called "undone science" (Hess 2009). Feminists contributed to the *Birth Control Handbook*, (Cherniak and Feingold 1968, 1970) produced by students at McGill University in 1968, when providing contraceptive information was still illegal in Canada (Sethna 2006),[2] and in 1978 launched *Healthsharing*, a quarterly Toronto-based feminist health magazine published for 15 years. A newsletter, *A Friend Indeed*, contested the dominant medical paradigm for menopause, including hormone manufacturers' claims about the benefits of hormonal drugs.

By the 1980s, government funding supported a cross-Canada network of 100 women's centres which provided a range of alternative approaches to care, moved feminist discourses to the community level, and became sites for analyzing the social roots of women's health problems (Morrow 2007). The control that pharmaceutical companies exercised over women was a central point of concern within this critical discourse. From the 1950s to the 1980s, a series of pharmaceutical disasters involving women, among them thalidomide, diethylstilbestrol (DES), addictive psychotropic drugs, Depo-Provera and the Dalkon Shield, formed the basis of a feminist critique of the pharmaceutical industry. Women who had been harmed by drugs and medical devices mobilized to form grass-roots women's groups like DES Action Canada and Dalkon Shield Action Canada. Collaborative projects included a play, *Side Effects*, based on women's own stories about the harmful effects of pharmaceuticals, which toured Canada in 1985 (Tudiver 1994), and a book, *Adverse Effects: Women and the pharmaceutical industry* (McDonnell 1986).

The women's health movement's critiques of the dominant biomedical model received both moral backing and evidence-based support from researchers in the Canadian health policy and health research communities (e.g., Cooperstock and Lennard 1979; Lexchin 1984; Harding 1986). Further support came from government policy reports. The Canadian government positioned itself as a leader in developing policies that emphasized a broad range of social determinants beyond the biological that contribute to health, including gender, poverty and physical environments (Lalonde 1974; Epp 1986; WHO 1986). After the 1961 thalidomide tragedy, Canada amended its Food and Drugs Act to make approval for marketing a drug conditional on clinical trial results providing "substantial evidence" that the drug was both safe and effective in recommended clinical use (Carter 1999: 220). In 1969, the federal government instituted a legislated system of compulsory licensing to hold drug prices in check so that pharmaceuticals could be made available to all who need them. It overruled patent protection of pharmaceuticals, allowing Canadian generic companies to manufacture and import drugs that were still under patent on the condition that the company pay a royalty to the patent-holder (Lang 1974). Health and consumer advocacy groups were among the structural factors that strengthened the Canadian government's hand on the contentious price control issue.

The advent of neoliberalism

By the mid-1980s, a newly-elected conservative government began to soften its stance towards the pharmaceutical industry and reverse supportive policies towards civil society groups that challenged corporate power. In 1988, under Brian Mulroney's centre-right Progressive Conservative Party, Canada and the United States signed the Free Trade Agreement which was expanded in 1994 to include Mexico as the North American Free Trade Agreement (NAFTA). Canada's pharmaceutical policies were a key negotiating point for both treaties (McMahon 1996/7). In a series of concessions between 1987 and 1993, Canada abolished compulsory licensing and extended patent protection of brand name drugs (Cohen 2003/4). In return, the industry promised to invest at least $400 million or 10 per cent of its Canadian sales in research and development by the end of 1996. In a parallel transformation, the system to regulate drug safety became more oriented towards marketing and economic growth by speeding drug approvals. The number of staff responsible for enforcing drug safety standards was cut (Regush 1993) and user fees from the pharmaceutical industry were introduced to help cover the cost of improving drug review times (Lexchin 2008).

As the country gradually adopted the trappings of a neoliberal state, politicians discursively redefined social justice advocacy organizations as "special interest groups" (Jenson and Phillips 1996) and began to withdraw government support for them. One activist who worked with a women's health collective in the 1980s, recalled being "one hundred per cent funded by the provincial government and then we moved, in a day, to zero funding" (Interview with *Margaret* 2007).[3] Desperate for operating funds, some groups began to look to the pharmaceutical industry.

Activists in the women's health movement viewed these new funding arrangements with alarm. When a Canadian support group for infertile couples began to take money from Serono, the manufacturer of a drug associated with in-vitro fertilization, one concerned activist conducted a content analysis of the group's newsletter from 1985 to 1991. She concluded reproductive techniques were increasingly framed as "signs of hope" (Rochon Ford 1993: 85). The argument that risky medical interventions are justified because they provide patients with hope was at odds with analyses developed within the women's health movement but was embedded in many aspects of medical culture. In the United States, particularly, aggressive treatments often trumped scientifi c evidence (Payer 1988). In drug research circles, a "regime of truth" acknowledged the frequent failure of drugs to improve patients' health and co-existed in tension with a "regime of hope," a belief that failures could be overcome and propel research towards new discoveries (Moreira 2009). In oncology, the "message of hope" (Patterson 1987) or the "discourse of hope" (Delvecchio Good et al. 1990) was used to counter the popular belief that cancer was always fatal. Because clinical trials of cancer drugs rarely show evidence of extended life, drug regulators invoked the hope imperative to rationalize adopting the use of surrogate endpoints (such as tumour shrinkage) rather than a true endpoint (longer life) as the standard of efficacy for the approval of cancer drugs (Löwy 2000).

The early breast cancer movement: research concerns and an ideological split

During the transitional period of the late 1980s and early 1990s, women in Canadian communities around Toronto and Montreal spontaneously formed small, locally-based patient-run breast cancer groups. The women who started the groups and individual activists also began to speak on breast cancer policy questions in the media, expressing profound dissatisfaction with various aspects of the status quo in breast cancer: lack of information on which to make treatment decisions (McPherson 1992), inadequate emotional supports (Kelly 1991; McPherson 1992), harsh and often ineffective treatments (Batt 1989, 1994; Kelly 1991; MacPhee 1994), perceived paternalism on the part of physicians, researchers, and cancer charities (MacLeod 1990; Kelly 1991; Tardif 1992), cultural insensitivity (Amesbury 1995) and shock at learning that breast cancer rates were rising for reasons that were still largely unknown (Batt 1989; McPherson 1992).

While the breast cancer movement had echoes of the women's health movement, it had differences as well. Similarities included the assumptions that lay publics had the right to information about scientific innovations that affected them, and the knowledge to contribute to, and challenge, scientific evidence on which public policy was based. One marked difference, however, was the perspective on medications among members within the two movements. Protests over the medicalization of normal body processes were a hallmark of the women's health movement, which had focused on reproductive health issues and rarely on life-threatening health problems (Waserman 1997). In contrast, while breast cancer activists were critical of the medical establishment's record on breast cancer, many saw medical research as the main hope to improve breast cancer survival rates (ibid.; Kaufert 1998).

From the beginning, however, the Canadian breast cancer movement was heterogeneous. Several early support groups were modeled on the American self-help group Y-Me, a "relatively conservative" (Kaufert 1998: 296) organization which focused on the physician-patient encounter. A smaller, more radical network of explicitly feminist groups took the women's health and AIDS movements as its models and "moved protest out of the clinic and into the public domain" (ibid.: 297). Their members were "concerned that so much effort was directed to drug trials and so little to understanding the cause of the dramatic increase in rates" (Interview with *Christine* 2009); they pushed for research on the connections between environmental contaminants and breast cancer. A national breast implant advocacy network, *Je sais*/I know, demanded stricter regulations governing implant safety, action to halt pharmaceutical companies from misrepresenting their products, and sanctions for physicians who failed to inform women of the implants' risks (Tardif 1992).

These small, local organizations began to coalesce as a movement in the fall of 1991 when an all-party sub-committee of female Parliamentarians launched a study of breast cancer and breast implants. Representatives from the groups were among the 48 individuals called as witnesses.[4] Collectively, their testimony emphasized the gulf between what patients' needed to know and what the other witnesses – researchers, physicians, and the professionalized charitable organizations serving patients – were providing. The hearings put breast cancer on the federal government's policy agenda and moved patient participation to the forefront. Activists who came before the sub-committee built the case that their organizations should be consulted on matters which had been the exclusive domain of professionals. The sub-committee's report, *Breast Cancer: Unanswered Questions*, concurred, stating that the "experience and expertise" of support, advocacy and consumer group members should be included in cancer decision-making bodies (Greene 1992: xv). To this end, the sub-committee's members recommended government support to assist the development of a national network of local breast cancer survivor groups (ibid.: 42) and a national consensus conference, the National Forum on Breast Cancer. The latter was hailed as a "watershed event" because patients participated fully in the planning and round-table discussions (Mickleburgh 1993). New patient-led groups developed in communities across the country, aided by federal government funding to create a formal national network with a provincial/regional structure. Pharmaceutical companies were not part of the National Forum. Judith Erola, the President of the Pharmaceutical Manufacturers' Association of Canada at the time and a former Liberal cabinet minister, told me in an interview: "No one invited us – we were careful not to go in where it would be an intrusion"; nor, to my knowledge, did the industry provide funding for any of these early groups.

Health Canada (the federal department of health) also provided $20 million over five years as seed money to establish a dedicated breast cancer research fund, the Canadian Breast Cancer Research Initiative (CBCRI), to be targeted exclusively to breast cancer research. The five-year mandate was renewed several times and over the years and the fund became the Canadian Breast Cancer Research Alliance (CBCRA), with seven partners: two federal government departments, four cancer charities, and the national patients' network (again, no pharmaceutical companies were partners). Cancer researchers initially saw the specification of research areas and demands for lay participation as a threat to their autonomy and to the peer review process (Waller and Batt 1995); but the fund eventually incorporated lay participants on all of its four decision-making structures (CBCRA 2007). Although the lion's share of the awards went to basic and treatment research (ibid.)[5], the CBCRA responded to patients' demands and funded research on alternative therapies and toxic chemicals as potential risk factors, areas that were virtually absent from the pre-movement research agenda (Kaufert 1998).

Reaction in the scientifi c community was mixed. When the *Canadian Medical Association Journal* (*CMAJ*) published a series of six commissioned papers to evaluate unconventional therapies for cancer, along with a patient's guide to making decisions about such therapies (Kaegi 1998a to 1998g), two researchers asked, "What should we look for next? The *CMAJ* guide to Canadian witch doctors?" (Tannock and Warr 1998: 802). Patients, they argued, should confine their involvement to providing "much needed support and additional funding for research" (ibid.: 802). The journal's editor responded that evaluations of alternative therapies were needed and that the public should help set research agendas: "It is their disease and their money" (Hoey 1998: 804).

Within their own groups, early Canadian breast cancer activists undertook a range of activities that expressed their priorities about breast cancer research. First Nations groups promoted spiritual values through traditional ceremonies like the sweat lodge (Amesbury 1995). A group based in Kingston, Ontario launched a series of bi-annual international breast cancer conferences under the banner of the World Breast Cancer Conference. Although popular with women – up to 1,000 delegates from 55 countries attended each of the first two meetings – segments of the press and the research community dismissed them as "a forum for the disenfranchised" spreading "misinformation" (Sibbald 1999: 584). Groups in Montreal and Toronto sponsored events to encourage critical debate about a clinical trial to test the drug tamoxifen as a preventative (Breast Cancer Prevention Panel 1993)[6] while, in Vancouver, women joined with university researchers to form the first breast cancer dragon boat team, challenging the myth that upper body exercise would promote postoperative lymphedema (McKenzie 1998). A Nova Scotia organization launched an online breast cancer discussion group which went international (Radin 2006). One woman used the site to disseminate a survey she had designed herself to poll others taking the drug tamoxifen about whether they had been prepared for its side effects. Two hundred women responded, many of whom felt their physicians had not adequately informed them about potential problems (Radcliffe 1999).

Like the women's health movement, then, the early breast cancer movement spawned projects with a critical edge, grounded in the experiences and priorities of its members, including the excessive control of physicians over patients and the secondary role accorded to research on cancer prevention and quality of life. Despite establishment push-back, the movements' leaders began to form alliances with sympathetic, reform-minded physicians, researchers and policy makers, while federal and provincial agencies looked to the groups for policy input and provided funding to support regional and national networks.

From the outset, however, some advocates and organizations put a high priority on finding a medical cure and gaining access to expensive new treatments. One of the first was Sylvia Morrison, a woman who spoke before the Parliamentary sub-committee. In riveting testimony, she described the rapid advance of her cancer and her decision to go to the Sloan-Kettering Cancer Institute in New York to obtain a risky and expensive procedure unavailable in Canada, high-dose chemotherapy with stem cell rescue (Morrison 1991: 48). Members of the sub-committee wrote sympathetically that Ms. Morrison was luckier than most to have access to "cutting edge" treatment options (Greene 1992: 36). Two witnesses from the lobby organization for the pharmaceutical industry (the Pharmaceutical Manufacturers' Association of Canada) and a physician-researcher group, the Society for Clinical Investigation, echoed Morrison's lament that Canada lagged in its approval of new drug treatments (ibid.: 36).

In 1999, data collected in four international clinical trials showed that the procedure offered no survival advantage over standard-dose chemotherapy (Lerner 2001: 255). Shortly thereafter, sensational revelations published in *The Lancet* exposed the only clinical trials demonstrating benefit, conducted by a team in South Africa, to be fraudulent (Weiss et al. 2000). Although in Canada, and most other countries, the procedure had been restricted to clinical trials, in the United States "high-dose chemo" was offered to women with advanced breast cancer for a decade.

The perspective that access to new treatments should be restricted until evidence shows a true benefit was difficult for advocates to adopt when they knew women who were dying. Indeed, even some advocacy groups that remained wary of commercial interests fought for access to new drugs. From the perspective of the community, it was a way to rally support for members in need. One such group spearheaded Ontario's fi rst breast cancer drug access lobby, demanding that the province add the drug Taxol® to its formulary. *Virginia*, who was on the board of that organization in 1994, explained that the group mobilized when a board member who had liver metastasis gained access to the drug:

> [It] broke some barriers for women living with metastatic disease. … It was certainly easier to tolerate than Adriamycin®. … We then became really pissed off that only a certain number of women were able to get

> access to this drug because it was only being funded through certain [research] protocols.
>
> (Interview with *Virginia 2008*)

With experience, some seasoned advocates modified their stance on the access issue. Following the revelations of fraud in the research on bone marrow transplants, the American breast cancer advocate Musa Mayer reflected on the dynamics that drove Americans (including her) to embrace access to that procedure as an advocacy cause:

> [W]ishful thinking on the part of patients and oncologists, public pressure, heart-wrenching media stories of desperately ill young mothers, political and legislative mandates for insurance coverage, personal reputations of researchers, and profit margins of hospitals with transplant beds to fill all managed to widely promote a toxic and expensive treatment before there was sufficient evidence of its safety or efficacy.
>
> (Mayer 2005)

Patricia Kaufert cites class bias as another factor shaping the goals of early advocates: "above all they wanted a cure and they expected it would come through medical research" (Kaufert 1998: 303). This "middle-class faith in the power of scientific knowledge, an assumption that should a cure be found it would be available to them, and the luxury of taking access for granted" (ibid.: 303) contrasted with the (largely absent) voices of poor women. In the United States, particularly, the poor did not have access to basic medical care, let alone any hope of obtaining the latest treatments. In Canada, where the medical system aims to provide basic care to all, middle-class assumptions obscured a different understanding: that the country's universal system of care, vitally important to the poor, could not be sustained under the pressure of ever-more costly medical treatments with modest or non-existent benefits. Over the next 15 years, drug access lobbies became the type of advocacy for which the patients' movement is best known, a shift that coincided with an increase in alliances between groups and the pharmaceutical industry.

The later breast cancer movement: funding from pharma and revised research priorities

The centrist Liberal party regained power in Canada in 1993 and implemented its own version of a neo-liberal agenda. The country was deeply in debt and the federal government responded, in part, by cutting its financial contributions to the health care system, which is administered provincially. Patients were sent home from hospital sooner to be cared for by unpaid family members; news stories about hospital deficits reinforced the belief that health care institutions should adopt a privatized business model, despite repeated studies showing the single-payer system to be more economical (Armstrong et al. 1994). The government invoked traditional ideals of volunteerism to shift the burden of support, care, and fundraising onto community organizations, businesses, families, and individuals (ibid.).

Groups that maintained an advocacy identity risked losing two key sources of funding – government grants and tax-exempt donations to registered charities. Civil society groups complained they had "more responsibility and no voice" (Floyd 1996). Within the breast cancer community, groups were advised their funding would be phased out and they should become self-sufficient. The groups, however, were growing in number and in the range of services they were expected to shoulder. *Jenny*, who worked in the office of a regional breast cancer group, recalls her astonishment when she learned of the federal strategy of cutting funding to the groups to promote self-sufficiency:

> Yes, yes! That's why they cut the money. It's an "incentive". It was the incentive to find money elsewhere! [laughs] And it … had exactly the opposite effect. All of these projects all over the country just ceased to be; because, really, there is no other money out there [for a support network].
>
> (Interview with *Jenny*, 2007)

About this time, leaders within the groups began receiving overtures from drug companies. *Virginia* recalled the group's public panel discussion in April 1993 as her first contact with the pharmaceutical industry. "I was approached by a pharma rep at that event. I remember her giving me a card and saying, 'we would like to help you.'" The success of the Forum, six months later, accelerated the process, said *Eve*, another activist. Although the offers were relatively small, intended for one-off events or projects, they touched off intense debates within the boards. Often the tension was between "high powered women with connections" who had been brought onto the boards to raise money and saw all sources as acceptable, and volunteers who worked directly with patients and who worried about compromising the group's reputation, or the quality of the information they were able to provide. Said one: "There was a lot of concern about it because we thought we might need to say things the company didn't like. … It was the advocacy we worried about, that we would look tainted if we took it" (interview with *Sara*).

These internal debates splintered several groups. Members opposed to pharma funding argued that they needed to be, and to be seen, as unbiased, particularly with any statements concerning drug treatments. Others insisted the funds were given as unconditional educational grants and were therefore strings-free.

Struggles over the pharma funding issue within and among the groups continued between 1996 and 2000 and eventually the pro-pharma camp gained dominance. One turning point was an advocacy conference, primarily for patients, held in late 1996 and funded almost entirely by pharmaceutical companies. At one session of the conference, forming good working partnerships with drug companies was framed as a positive goal (Kelly et al. 1997). At another session, an oncologist weighed in on the debate over treatments. Citing Canada–U.S. disparities in breast cancer survival rates, he argued that a rapid uptake of new, aggressive treatments available in the United States but not in Canada (including bone marrow transplant) was the key to improving the survival of Canadian cancer patients. He identified governments as the central problem because, he said, they stood in the way of rapid access to new, lifesaving interventions (ibid.).

This meeting laid the groundwork for different type of cancer patient organization: pharma funded, divorced from community service and devoted entirely to advocacy, particularly for access to new drugs. The first such group, launched in 2000, caused a national media sensation with its claim that state-by-state and province-by-province Canadian cancer patients had worse outcomes than US citizens because they lacked access to lifesaving treatments. Cancer epidemiologists immediately challenged the assertion that under-spending on cancer treatments was at the root of regional differences in cancer mortality rates; they accused the group of ignoring incidence rates, cherry picking data and otherwise misrepresenting the science (Bramswell 2000; Buist 2000; Murray 2000). Nonetheless, the claim that hope for cancer patients' lay in rapid access to new treatments gained wide exposure.

Gradually, patient group alliances with the industry became normalized around a central discourse that claimed the two parties had a common interest in rapid access to new treatments. Formal structures evolved to address ethical concerns, including written agreements and rules of practice (for example, that the group would not promote a specific drug). Public relations companies, whose services were paid for by the drug companies, became useful intermediaries, putting their communications skills at the service of the groups and providing a buffer between group members and the companies. Meanwhile, the composition and identities of patients' groups began to change. Several high profile activists left organizations they had worked to build when they concluded their battle against pharma funding was lost. The president of one national organization resigned when a biotechnology company presented her with a contract that would require reciprocal benefits in return for three years of funding for advocacy (Nebenzahl 2003). *Virginia*, who remained active for almost a decade in a large group with both a volunteer board and paid staff, said that over time, and with increased pressure to raise funds, the board became dominated by women from the corporate world whose values differed from those of the group's founders and from the women who volunteered at the community level. "It was the two things happening," she explained. "The pharmaceuticals were always knocking at the door but the door was being answered now by people who didn't see anything wrong with that."

By 2000, pharmaceutical companies had become a staple source of funding. Industry discourse, found in marketing publications and presentations at trade meetings, tied partnerships with patients' groups to business objectives with the claim that patients and the industry shared a common goal: rapid regulatory approval of new treatments and their placement on provincial drug insurance formularies (Rule and Chapman 1999). Pharmaceutical company funding was allocated primarily to groups engaged in advocacy, and particularly for projects that would encourage rapid access to new drugs. A new national advocacy coalition of patients' groups representing a range of diseases formed in 1999 with major funding from the industry, promoted access to new medications as its central goal (Best Medicines Coalition 2013).

A few groups resisted. One closed its doors, rather than accept funding from big pharma (Interview with *Virginia* 2007); another scaled back its activities to focus on environmental causes of cancer and adopted a corporate donations policy that ruled out funding from the pharmaceutical industry (Breast Cancer Action Montreal 2001). One effect within the community was, in the words of one activist, "a huge war" between "the pharma-takers and the sanctimonious ones on the other side" (Interview with *Jillian* 2008). This division became public in 2000, when a national consumer rights television program advanced the position that patients' groups were being used to market drugs (Johnson 2000). Two months later, leaders in a half-dozen national patients' organizations vigorously rebutted these claims in a national newspaper: "The money has to come from somewhere," said the president of a colorectal cancer group, "And thank God it's coming from these [pharmaceutical] companies because it's not coming from anywhere else" (Picard 2001: A8).

Funding from the pharmaceutical industry brought with it a new type of patient-group research – projects carried out under the auspices of the cancer patient movement with study results announced in press releases and published in slick, professional publications and/or online. In interviews, group members say the sponsoring companies never interfere in any way with these projects. Nonetheless, the results of the studies align with the goals of the pharmaceutical industry – privatized health care, rapid drug approvals and formulary acceptance of new cancer drugs.

Few remaining breast cancer groups had the critical perspective and the independent resources to challenge such claims. One woman who had worked (without regrets) in several pharma-funded cancer advocacy organizations acknowledged this. "There's a huge gap in the critical spectrum. Where are the patients who are standing up lobbying for lower drug costs?" (*Jillian* 2008). Meanwhile, a few groups and activists from the early breast cancer movement continued to work in the tradition of the women's health movement. They promoted the precautionary principle and non-pharmaceutical disease prevention (Ley 2009: 91–95) and pushed to have toxic products removed from cosmetics and personal care products (FemmeToxique 2012). Community-based research documented unmet support needs of marginalized groups of patients (e.g., Sinding et al. 2004). Just before losing their federal funding, several women's health organizations collaborated with epidemiologists and unions to conduct research on breast cancer rates among women exposed to toxic chemicals in plastics and automotive parts industries (Brophy et al. 2012; DeMatteo et al. 2012; Smith 2012).

The offi cial breast cancer research agenda also underwent change. In March 2010, having awarded more than Can. $197 million for 583 research grants over 17 years, the Canadian Breast Cancer Research Alliance disbanded (CBCRA 2007). In its newsletter, one breast cancer organization called the announcement "a bombshell" (Brown 2012), particularly because it came on the heels of an exhaustive review process that created a National Breast Cancer Research Framework to guide the Alliance on a future of high-impact research (NBCRF 2009). The review recommended that more funding go towards targeted research, particularly studies of early detection and etiology (National Breast Cancer Research Framework 2009: 15, note 14) The breast cancer group's newsletter report called the fund's closure both a mystery ("former members are reluctant to say why they chose to disband" (Brown 2012)) and regrettable, because the proposed new funding in research on etiology resonated with the group's focus on environmental causes of breast cancer. Two years after the announcement, no new structure had replaced the defunct body (ibid.).

Canada's breast cancer movement and democratic participation in science

Vibrant, healthy organizations that represent the diversity of experiences and opinions within a patients' community have the potential to benefit science in numerous ways. The Canadian women's health movement and the early breast cancer movement productively pushed the boundaries of research through the mechanism of collectively analyzing experiential knowledge and forming alliances with researchers willing to systematically test the resulting insights. Supportive government policies enabled this pattern of discovery, serving the early breast cancer movement as well. Since the late 1990s, however, the movement has responded to radical changes in the political landscape and has lost much of its diverse character.

Kelly Moore and colleagues, recognizing the influence of neoliberalism on national and global economies and public policies, have called for explorations that identify new patterns in the interrelationships among industry, science, and social movements (Moore et al. 2011). Of particular interest are conflicts arising from countervailing pressures, "from industry and the 'right hand' of the state on one side … and from civil society and the 'left hand' of the state on the other side" (ibid.: 527). In my assessment, the majority of members of the now-fractured Canadian breast cancer movement are now aligned with industry and the state's right hand, that is, the agencies within government that promote markets and trade as the means of solving social problems. The withdrawal of government support from civil society advocacy left a void the pharmaceutical industry has willingly filled; indeed partnerships that provide matching funds are now a requirement for some government grant programs for health movement and patients' organizations (Public Health Agency of Canada 2013).

Although state funding for civil society groups in Canada's welfare state era was a practice with recognized pitfalls, a political analyst who studied them concluded that governments in Canada had little choice but to fund certain advocacy groups if challenges to well-resourced commercial interests were to be possible. The real issue, he argued, was to ensure all elements of the community have an opportunity to be heard in public debate through structured processes designed to minimize "the dangers of intimidation, favouritism and manipulations" (Pross 1992: 209). Neoliberal governments have destabilized the balance that their predecessors worked to create. Furthermore, the delinking of community service from advocacy has fostered industry-funded advocacy groups that have patients or former patients as spokespeople but lack a community membership structure and provide no services in the community. The basis on which these groups claim a right to speak for patients is far from clear.

Admittedly, the truth/hope balance is not an easy one for patients. The myth of the imminent cure has a powerful emotional resonance, particularly when prospects are dire; however, the claim that hope for patients resides in access to novel drugs distorts the evidence, obscures choices that are not drug-related and puts the democratic ideals of the health system at risk. Drug treatments can reduce quality of life, shorten life, or both, while equating hope to an unproven drug commodifies a yearning that is essentially spiritual. As one ethicist has argued, a more rewarding approach (especially for patients for whom a cure is not imminent) is to discover hope in ways that are "potentially achievable, sustainable, or acceptable" (Simpson 2004: 249). And while an individual patient will rightly focus on his or her own situation, patients' organizations have a responsibility to take a larger view. Demands for costly drugs whose demonstrated benefits are minimal, hypothetical, or non-existent draw scarce resources from the healthcare system, threatening the fair distribution of medicine's benefits for current and future patients.

Researchers and health professionals are now approaching consensus on the misalignment between drug costs and their benefits, calling the industry's pricing practices excessive, unsustainable and morally indefensible (Experts in chronic myeloid leukemia 2013). In this climate, patients' groups that single-mindedly advocate for rapid access to these treatments while accepting industry largesse must do more than merely protest that they are immune to influence. Alternatives to corporate funding of patients' groups have been proposed (Rochon Ford 1998) and even put in place: health insurers in Germany pay a small percentage per year per individual insured to support the self-help, information, and lobbying of health consumer groups

(Geissler 2011), a model that might be adapted elsewhere. All concerned actors have a stake in finding solutions to the present impasse but patients have the most to lose: it is time the organizations that represent them demanded a funding model that works.

Notes

1 This chapter was based on dissertation research funded through Dalhousie University from the CIHR training program in Ethics of Health Research and policy, from Dr. Janice Graham's CIHR grant MOP 74473 (Risks and Regulation of Novel and Therapeutic Products) and from a Norah Stephen Oncology Summer Studentship. Many, many thanks are due to my supervisory committee at Dalhousie: Janice Graham, Wendy McKeen, Paul Pross, Susan Sherwin and Ingrid Sketris, for ongoing scholarly advice and support, and to my external examiner, David Hess. The current version has benefited greatly from critical comments on earlier drafts from Ted Schrecker, from members of Françoise Baylis' Impact Ethics discussion group at Dalhousie, and from the volume editors Willy Viehoever, Peter Wehling and Sophia Koenen.
2 Abortion and the dissemination of birth control information had been illegal in Canada since 1869, subject to a maximum penalty of life imprisonment.
3 I use italics to indicate pseudonyms of activists I interviewed.
4 The Sub-committee was part of the Standing Committee on Health and Welfare, Social Affairs, Seniors and the Status of Women.
5 Over 17 years, Canadian Dollars $131.4 million out of $197 million went to these two categories. The remaining awards were distributed across four categories: Early Detection; Prevention and Risk Factors; Quality of Life; and Health Services.
6 I was a founding member of this group.

References

Amesbury, Barbra (ed.) (1995) *Survivors: In search of a voice – the art of courage*, Toronto: Woodlawn Arts Foundation.

Armstrong, Pat; Armstrong, Hugh; Choiniere, Jacqueline; Feldberg, Gina and White, Jerry P. (1994) *Take care: warning signals for Canada's health system*, Toronto: Garamond.

Batt, Sharon (1989) Cancer victims can learn from AIDS sufferers, *The Gazette*, Montreal, 4 July.

___ (1994) *Patient No More: The politics of breast cancer*, Charlottetown, PEI: Gynergy.

Best Medicines Coalition (2013) Statement on funding sources, Best Medicines Coalition website. Available online at: <www.bestmedicines.ca/system/files/BMC_Funding_State_07.pdf> (accessed 11 July 2013).

Bramswell, Helen (2000) Survival rates higher for U.S. cancer patients, group says, *Kitchener-Waterloo Record*, Ontario, 26 September, A4.

Breast Cancer Action Montreal (2001) Policy on corporate contributions, Breast Cancer Action Montreal website. Available online at: <www.bcam.qc.ca/policy> (accessed 11 July 2013).

Breast Cancer Prevention Panel (1993) *Breast cancer prevention: best guesses*, transcript, Montreal: Breast Cancer Action Montreal, 24 March.

Brophy, James T.; Keith, Margaret M.; Watterson, Andrew; Park, Robert; Gilbertson, Michael; Maticka-Tyndale, Eleanor; Beck, Matthias; Abu-Zahra, Hakam;

Schneider, Kenneth; Reinhartz, Abraham; DeMatteo, Robert and Luginaah, Isaac (2012) Breast cancer risk in relation to occupations with exposure to carcinogens and endocrine disruptors: a Canadian case control study, *Environmental Health*, 11(87), 1–17.

Brown, Maychai (2012) The demise of the Canadian Breast Cancer Research Alliance, Breast Cancer Action Montreal website. Available online at: <http://bcam.qc.ca/content/demise-canadian-breast-cancer-research-alliance> (accessed 7 July 2013).

Buist, Steve (2000) Cancer care report card doesn't tell the whole truth, *The Hamilton Spectator*, 26 September 2000, A1.

Canadian Breast Cancer Research Alliance (CBCRA) (2007) About CBCRA: public involvement, Canadian Breast Cancer Research Alliance website. Available online at: <http://breast.cancer.ca/WebNET.aspx?u=WebNETGuest&p=user&v1=guest&a=2#2,11> (accessed 13 June 2013).

Carter, Patricia I. (1999) Federal regulation of pharmaceuticals in the United States and Canada, *Loyola of Los Angeles International and Comparative Law Journal*, 21(2), 215–258.

Cherniak, Donna and Feingold, Allan (eds) (1968) *Birth Control Handbook*, 1st edn, Montreal: Students' Society of McGill University.

—— (1970) *Birth Control Handbook*, 4th edn, Montreal: Students' Society of McGill University. Available online at: <https://openlibrary.org/books/OL25240461M/Birth_control_handbook> (accessed 25 July 2014).

Cohen, Jillian Clare (2003/4) Canada and Brazil: dealing with tension between ensuring access to medicines and complying with pharmaceutical patent standards – is the story the same? Comparative Program on Health and Society, *Working Paper Series*, Toronto: University of Toronto. Available online at: <http://munkschool.utoronto.ca/cphs/papers/year/2003-2004> (accessed 5 July 2013).

Cooperstock, Ruth and Lennard, Henry L. (1979) Some social meanings of tranquilizer use, *Sociology of Health and Illness*, 1(3), 331–347.

DelVecchio Good, MaryJo; Good, Byron J.; Schaffer, Cynthia and Lind, Stuart E. (1990) American oncology and the discourse on hope, *Culture, Medicine and Psychiatry*, 14(1), 59–79

DeMatteo, Robert; Keith, Margaret; Brophy, James T.; Wordsworth, Anne; Watterson, Andrew E.; Beck, Matthias; Rochon Ford, Anne; Gilbertson, Michael; Pharityal, Jyoti; Rootham, Magali and Scott, Dayna N. (2012) Chemical exposures of women workers in the plastics industry with particular reference to breast cancer and reproductive hazards, *New Solutions: A Journal of Environmental and Occupational Health Policy*, 22(4), 427–448.

Epp, Jake (1986) *Achieving health for all: a framework for health promotion.* Ottawa, ON: Health and Welfare Canada. Available online at: <www.hc-sc.gc.ca/hcs-sss/pubs/system-regime/1986-frame-plan-promotion/index-eng.php> (accessed 8 July 2013).

Experts in chronic myeloid leukemia (2013) The price of drugs for chronic myeloid leukemia (CML) is a reflection of the unsustainable prices of cancer drugs: from the perspective of a large group of CML experts, *Blood*, 121(22), 4439–4442.

FemmeToxique (2012) Safe cosmetics campaign, Breast Cancer Action Montreal website. Available online at: <www.femmetoxic.com> (accessed 11 July 2013).

Floyd, Gordon (1996) Viewpoint: the voluntary sector in Canada's new social contract – more responsibility but no voice? *The Philanthropist*, 13(2), 39–45.

Geissler, Jan (2011) Health policy in Germany: consumer groups in a corporatist polity, in H. Lofgren; E. de Leeuw and M. Leahy (eds) *Democratizing health: Consumer groups and the policy process*, Cheltenham, UK and Northampton, MA: Edward Elgar, 127–142.

Greene, Barbara (1992) *Breast Cancer: unanswered questions*, Ottawa: House of Commons.

Harding, Jim (1986) Mood modifiers and elderly women in Canada: the medicalization of poverty, in K. McDonnell (ed.) *Adverse effects: women and the pharmaceutical industry*, Penang: International Organization of Consumers' Unions, regional office for Asia and the Pacific, 51–86.

Hess, David J. (2009) The potentials and limitations of civil society research: getting undone science done, *Sociological Inquiry*, 79(3), 306–327.

Hoey, John (1998) The arrogance of science and the pitfalls of hope, *Canadian Medical Association Journal (CMAJ)*, 159(7), 803–804.

Jenson, Jane and Phillips, Susan D (1996) Regime shift: new citizenship practices in Canada, *International Journal of Canadian Studies*, 14(1), 113–135.

Johnson, Erica (2000) Promoting drugs through patient advocacy groups, *Marketplace*, Vancouver: CBC-TV, 14 November. Available online at: <www.cbc.ca/marketplace/pre-2007/files/health/drugmarketing/index.html> (accessed 11 July 2013).

Kaegi, Elizabeth (on behalf of the Task Force on Alternative Therapies of the Canadian Breast Cancer Research Initiative) (1998a) Unconventional therapies for cancer 1: Essiac, *CMAJ*, 158(7), 897–902.

___ (1998b) Unconventional therapies for cancer 2: green tea, *CMAJ*, 158(8), 1033–1035.

___ (1998c) Unconventional therapies for cancer 3: iscador, *CMAJ*, 158(9), 1157–1159.

___ (1998d) Unconventional therapies for cancer 4: hydrazine sulfate, *CMAJ*, 158(10), 1327–1330.

___ (1998e) Unconventional therapies for cancer 5: vitamins A, C and E, *CMAJ*, 158(11), 1483–1488.

___ (1998f) Unconventional therapies for cancer 6: 714-X, *CMAJ*, 158(12), 1621–1624.

Kaegi, Elizabeth, with the Ontario Division of the Canadian Cancer Society (1998g) A patient's guide to choosing unconventional therapies, *CMAJ*, 158(9), 1161–1165.

Kaufert, Patricia (1998) Women, resistance and the breast cancer movement, in M. Lock and P. Kaufert (eds) *Pragmatic Women and Body Politics*, Cambridge: Cambridge University Press, 287–309.

Kelly, Patricia (1991) Testimony, a study of breast cancer: The Subcommittee on the Status of Women of the Standing Committee on Health and Welfare, Social Affairs, Seniors and the Status of Women, 22 October, Ottawa: House of Commons, 1–35.

Kelly, Patricia; Condy, Charmaine and Harder, Sandra (1997) *Together to an end: the first Canada–U.S. breast cancer advocacy conference, final report*, Burlington: Pisces.

Lalonde, Marc (1974) *A new perspective on the health of Canadians: a working document*, Ottawa, ON: Health and Welfare Canada.

Lang, Ronald (1974) *The politics of drugs: a comparative pressure-group study of the Canadian Pharmaceutical Manufacturers' Association and the Association of the British Pharmaceutical Industry, 1930–1970*, London: Saxon House, Lexington Books.

Lerner, Barron H. (2001) *The breast cancer wars: hope, fear and the pursuit of a cure in twentieth-century America*, New York: Oxford.

Lexchin, Joel (1984) *The real pushers: a critical analysis of the Canadian drug industry*, Vancouver: New Star.

—— (2008) New directions in Canadian drug regulation: whose interests are being served? in Ó. O'Donovan and K. Glavanis-Grantham (eds) *Power, Politics and Pharmaceuticals*, Cork: Cork University Press, 153–170.

Ley, Barbara (2009) *From pink to green: disease prevention and the environmental breast cancer movement*, New Brunswick, NJ, and London: Rutgers University Press.

Löwy, Ilana (2000) Trustworthy knowledge and desperate patients: clinical tests for new drugs from cancer to AIDS, in M. Lock, Allan Young and A. Cambrosio (eds) *Living and working with the new medical technologies*, New York: Cambridge University Press, 49–81.

Mayer, Musa (2005) When clinical trials are compromised: a perspective from a consumer advocate, *PLoS Medicine*, 2(11), 1060–1063.

McDonnell, Kathleen (ed.) (1986) *Adverse effects: women and the pharmaceutical industry*, Penang: International Organization of Consumers' Unions, regional office for Asia and the Pacific.

McKenzie, Donald C. (1998) Abreast in a boat: a race against breast cancer, *CMAJ*, 159(4), 376–378.

MacLeod, Robert (1990) Cancer society aide attacks "sexist" policy, *The Globe and Mail*, 6 December, A1.

McMahon, Eileen (1996/7) NAFTA and the Biotechnology Industry, *California Western Law Review*, 33(31), 31–48.

MacPhee, Rosalind (1994) *Picasso's woman: a breast cancer story*, Vancouver: Douglas and McIntyre.

McPherson, Paula (1992) Testimony, a study of breast cancer: The Subcommittee on the Status of Women: Standing Committee on Health and Welfare, Social Affairs, Seniors and the Status of Women, 25 February, Ottawa: House of Commons, 1(11), 19.

Mickleburgh, Rod (1993) Forum on breast cancer hailed as watershed event in Canada: patients emerge as full partners in setting priorities, *The Globe and Mail*, 17 November 1993, A6.

Moore, Kelly; Kleinman, Daniel L.; Hess, David and Frickel, Scott (2011) Science and neoliberal globalization: a political sociological approach, *Theory and Society*, 40(5), 505–532.

Moreira, Tiago (2009) Truth and hope in drug development and evaluation in Alzheimer's disease, in J. F. Ballenger; P. J. Whitehouse; C. G. Lyketsos; P. Rabins and J. Karlawish (eds) *Treating dementia: do we have a pill for it?* Baltimore, MD: Johns Hopkins University Press.

Morrison, Sylvia (1991) Testimony: a study of breast cancer, The Subcommittee on the Status of Women: Standing Committee on Health and Welfare, Social Affairs, Seniors and the Status of Women, 22 October, Ottawa: House of Commons, 1(1), 43–52.

Morrow, Marina (2007) "Our bodies our selves" in context: reflections on the women's health movement in Canada, in M. Morrow, O. Hankivsky, and C. Varcoe (eds) *Women's Health in Canada: critical perspectives on theory and policy*, Toronto: University of Toronto Press.

Murray, Susan (2000) Cancer report card sparks dispute. *Winnipeg Free Press*, 26 September, A4.

National Breast Cancer Research Framework (NBCRF) (2009) What is the National Breast Cancer Research Framework? Available online at: <http://framework.cbcfontarioreport.ca> (accessed 11 July 2013).

Nebenzahl, Donna (2003) Do drug firms call the tune? *The Gazette* (Montreal), 9 April, D1, D4.

Patterson, James T. (1987) The dread disease: cancer and modern American culture, Cambridge, MA: Harvard University Press.

Payer, Lynn (1988) *Medicine and Culture: varieties of treatment in the United States, England, West Germany and France*, New York: Holt.

Picard, André (2001) Charities "thank God" for drug firms' money, *The Globe and Mail*, 4 January 2001, A8.

Pross, Paul A. (1992) *Group Politics and Public Policy*, 2nd edn, Toronto: Oxford University Press.

Public Health Agency of Canada (2013) Multi-sectoral partnerships to promote healthy living and prevent chronic disease. Available online at: <www.phac-aspc.gc.ca/fo-fc/mspphl-pppmvs-eng.php> (accessed 25 November 2013).

Radcliffe, Nancy (1999) Tamoxifen survey report: results and comments. Available online at: <http://web.archive.org/web/20041206170508/http://bca.ns.ca/surveys/index.htm> (accessed 3 July 2013).

Radin, Patricia (2006) "To me it's my life": medical communication, trust, and activism in cyberspace, *Social Science & Medicine*, 62(3), 591–601.

Regush, Nicholas M. (1993) *Safety last: the failure of the consumer health protection system in Canada*, Toronto: Key Porter Books.

Rochon Ford, Anne (1993) An overview of select social and economic forces influencing the development of in vitro fertilization and related assisted reproductive techniques: new reproductive technologies and the science, industry, education and social welfare systems in Canada, *Ottawa: Research Studies of the Royal Commission on Reproductive Technologies*, 5(1), 75–139.

—— (1998) A Different Prescription: considerations for women's health groups contemplating funding from the pharmaceutical industry, Toronto: Institute for Feminist Legal Studies, York University.

Rule, Erik G. and Chapman, Haley (1999) Strategic alliances between disease-specific non-profit organizations and private sector pharmaceutical companies, paper presented at the Canadian Institute, 7 April, Toronto: Pricewaterhouse Coopers.

Sethna, Christabelle (2006) The evolution of the *Birth Control Handbook*: from student peer-education manual to feminist self-empowerment text, 1968–1975, *Canadian Bulletin of Medical History*, 23(1), 89–118.

Sibbald, Barbara (1999) Breast cancer conference marred by questionable presentations, critics charge, *CMAJ*, 161(5), 584.

Simpson, Christy (2004) When hope makes us vulnerable: a discussion of patient-healthcare provider interactions in the context of hope, *Bioethics*, 18(5), 428–447.

Sinding, Christina; Barnoff, Lisa and Grassau, Pamela (2004) Homophobia and heterosexism in cancer care: the experience of lesbians, *Canadian Journal of Nursing Research*, 36(4), 170–188.

Smith, Joanna (2012) Federal budget 2012: Health Canada cuts funding to women's health research groups, *Toronto Star*, 25 April. Available online at: <www.thestar.com/news/canada/2012/04/25/federal_budget_2012_health_canada_cuts_funding_to_womens_health_research_groups.html> (accessed 5 July 2013).

Tannock, Ian F. and Warr, David G. (1998) Unconventional therapies for cancer: a refuge from the rules of evidence? *CMAJ*, 159(7), 801–802.

Tardif, Marcella (1992) Testimony, a study of breast cancer, The Subcommittee on the Status of Women: Standing Committee on Health and Welfare, Social Affairs, Seniors and the Status of Women, Ottawa: House of Commons, 1(9), 34–43.

Tudiver, Sari (1994) The strengths of links: building the Canadian Women's Health Network, *Report of the Winnipeg Consultation Organizing Committee*, Winnipeg, 1–17.

Waller, Margaret and Batt, Sharon (1995) Advocacy groups for breast cancer patients, *CMAJ*, 152(6), 819–822.

Waserman, Lori (1997) *Before pink ribbons: understanding the invisibility of breast cancer in the Canadian women's health movement during the 1970s and 1980s*, unpublished thesis, Ottawa: Carleton University.

Weiss, Raymond B.; Rifkin, Robert M.; Stewart, F. Marc; Theriault, Richard L.; Williams, Lori A.; Herman, Allen A. and Beveridge, Roy A. (2000) High-dose chemotherapy for high-risk primary breast cancer: an on-site review of the Bezwoda study, *The Lancet*, 355(9208), 999–1003.

World Health Organization (WHO) (1986) *The Ottawa Charter for Health Promotion*, Geneva: World Health Organization. Available online at: <www.who.int/health-promotion/conferences/previous/ottawa/en> (accessed 10 July 2013).

8 Beyond scientific controversies

Scientific counterpublics, countervailing industries, and undone science

David J. Hess

Introduction

The role of patient associations, health movements, and other actors outside the medical profession and associated research community has changed dramatically during recent decades. To some degree, the changes are broad ones that affect science in general: as the technological complexity and industrial diversity of societies has increased, the scientific field has become both more important politically and more politicized. Social movements and civil society organizations have been drawn into political conflicts about the regulation of both new and old technologies, and they have politicized issues of therapeutic choices and research agendas. At the same time, the relations between the scientific field and industry have also changed because new professional specialties and new industries also seek to influence research agendas. The growth of industrial funding and the allure of revenues from patents have also provided scientists with the incentives to respond to industrial needs; however, some medical researchers have become aligned with health reform movements and patient advocacy organizations, and their involvement tends to enhance and politicize divisions within the scientific field over research agendas.

This study adopts a perspective on patient advocacy movements and medical research that is based on the political sociology of science and technology (Moore et al. 2011). Central concepts from the sociology of scientific knowledge remain important, such as the proposition that the making of scientific knowledge is socially shaped or negotiated. However, the focus of attention in a political sociological perspective is on power differentials and the relations between the scientific field and other social fields (such as the medical profession, civil society, the pharmaceutical industry, and the state). In this project I focus particularly on the meso-level construction of scientific research fields rather than the micro-level of specific knowledge claims, on the unequal power relations between challengers and incumbents in the therapeutic and research fields, and on the relationship between the sociology of scientific knowledge and the sociology of scientific ignorance.

This chapter will outline a conceptual framework, present case study materials based on one health reform movement, and then discuss the broader theoretical implications.

Background concepts and framework

There are various ways to classify patient advocacy organizations (Epstein 2008); the focus here is on the relationship to health policy, corporate power, and social change. From this perspective, one can think of health advocacy organizations as forming a continuum from traditional interest groups, which attempt to increase research resources and therapeutic access, to reform movement organizations, which challenge mainstream approaches to disease and treatment and draw attention to the politics of research agendas and therapeutic choices.

Advocacy organizations close to the pole of traditional interest groups attempt to increase research resources and therapeutic access for a social segment, such as persons afflicted by a particular disease. The disease may be a common one, such as breast cancer or AIDS, or a rare one, for which resources and treatment options are limited because of the demographics. In either case, the primary goal with respect to research funding is the allocation of resources. Resources may come from the reallocation of existing health-related resources or from the reallocation of resources to health research and care from other social fields. In either case, medical specialists and pharmaceutical companies may advise and encourage advocates to lobby organizations that provide funding to free up resources. Conflicts tend to arise over treatment options as defined by the mainstream of the researchers and health-care providers.

At the other pole of health-related advocacy, health movements challenge the dominant frameworks of disease categorization, etiology, and/or treatment. For example, patients suffering from an unrecognized disease face not only an issue of funding allocation but also a controversy within the research community over the etiology and sometimes over the very existence of the disease. With respect to contested disease etiology, patient advocacy organizations that seek more research into alternative causes of a disease find themselves at odds with what Brown has called the "dominant epidemiological paradigm" (Brown 2007). Likewise, advocacy organizations may also contest treatment options and seek greater funding for research on (and greater access to) therapies that are outside the medical mainstream. The contestations over treatment options are often linked to those over etiologies, but the two types of contestations can be distinct. In other words, advocacy groups can share the dominant etiological paradigm while rejecting the mainstream approaches to treatment, or vice-versa. There can also be radically different theory-treatment packages, which in turn are associated with complementary and alternative medicine (CAM) professions.

Both the interest group pole and the movement pole of health advocacy draw attention to specified ignorance or non-knowledge, that is, areas of potentially fruitful future research that could be completed (Merton 1987; Gross 2009). At the interest group pole, the articulation of non-knowledge tends to define the future research agenda in ways that are consistent with mainstream researchers, and hence their view of non-knowledge is generally "positive" or desirable both for the advocacy group and for the mainstream research community. In contrast, reform movement organizations tend to draw attention to future research areas that mainstream researchers and associated industrial groups (the leaders of the medical profession and dominant corporations in the pharmaceutical industry) reject as negative non-knowledge. For example, advocates of CAM cancer therapies draw attention to the value of nutritional and nutraceutical therapies as alternatives to mainstream chemotherapy. Thus, a conflict emerges over the identification of systematic pockets of non-knowledge that are created by the shared assumptions of the dominant agents in the research and industrial fields. Elsewhere we have discussed this form of non-knowledge as "undone science" (Frickel et al. 2010; Hess 2007, 2011; Woodhouse et al. 2002). There is also an element of what Gross calls "nescience," that is, a form of scientific ignorance that is only knowable in retrospect, after a surprise. However, due to the impossibility of seeing nescience in advance, this form of scientific ignorance does not play the same role in the politics of agenda-setting as does the specified ignorance of positive and negative non-knowledge.

Whereas in the interest group type of advocacy organization, the partnership is among civil society organizations, mainstream researchers, and corporate funders, in the reform movement type of advocacy organization, the partnership is often with some combination of scientists outside the mainstream, alternative or CAM clinicians, and countervailing industrial firms such as nutraceutical organizations. When scientists "go public" with their claims about epistemic gaps and systematic non-investigation of research leads and hypotheses, they form a counterpublic, often in alliance with civil society organizations (Hess 2011). When the aspirations of the counterpublic receive acceptance by the mainstream of the research field, and the new research agendas receive funding and legitimacy, a process of epistemic modernization occurs (Hess 2007). In other words, the research field becomes open to reforms of its research priorities, methods, and conceptual frameworks based on the inclusion of the perspectives of previously excluded groups. The change can lead to a situation in which undone science, as identified by civil-society reform organizations, gets done. However, other possible outcomes include marginalization and intellectual suppression, which can lead into the dynamics of backfire (Delborne 2008; Martin 2007, 2010).

Networks of reform-oriented civil society organizations and dissenting researchers tend to lack the resources to mount a successful challenge to the dominant epidemiological and therapeutic paradigms. However, if the counterpublics form coalitions with countervailing industries, their political power and economic resources increase. In the case of the CAM cancer counterpublics discussed below, the countervailing industries provide resources such as research institutions and peer-reviewed publications from the CAM professions and funding from the nutraceutical industry. Although there is an element of grassroots organizing and democracy in the counterpublics, their political power is contingent on building alliances with countervailing professions and industries (on countervailing power in industrial transitions, see Hess 2013).

Although these conditions of counterpublics and countervailing powers are likely to be general across a wide range of technology-oriented reform movements in societies that have parliamentary institutions and high levels of influence by private capital on the political system, the case study that follows will focus on a specific health reform movement in the United States. The methodology focuses on the long-term, meso-level of the broad historical transition of the research and therapeutic fields. More generally, the concept of social fields as quasi-autonomous but inter-connected social spaces of contestation informs the methodology (Bourdieu 2005). The historical narrative is divided into two sections based on a periodization divide during the 1990s. The research is based on years of interviews, conference participation, and participation in patient advocacy events, and it also draws on extensive reading of both the popular and scientific literature. The long-term warrant of ethnographic research has enabled a picture to develop of the transition of the field that was not evident when the research first began during the 1990s.

The CAM cancer field in twentieth-century United States

During the period prior to World War II, the fields of cancer etiology and treatment in the United States were more open and pluralistic than today. Although the theory that cancer was an infectious disease with a bacterial etiology was widely accepted before World War I, slowly other etiologies emerged based on studies of cancer and environmental toxins, viruses, and genetic predisposition. During the first half of the twentieth century, there was little evidence of cancer-related patient advocacy organizations or other types of civil society advocacy work in either the United States or Europe. However, there were networks of scientists and clinicians who had developed theories of cancer etiology and treatment approaches that offered an alternative to surgery. Among the prominent networks were those who continued to support the theory of bacterial etiology by developing therapies that included antimicrobial interventions such as vaccines and dietary changes. This network of researchers included William Coley and Thomas Glover, and it survived in the US after World War II principally in the networks that developed in support of the work of Royal Raymond Rife and

Virginia Livingston (Hess 1997). Another prominent and influential early approach was the treatment of cancer advocated by John Beard, who believed that proteolytic enzymes produced by the pancreas held cancer cells in check (Moss 2008a, 2008b).

After World War II, chemical weapons became the basis for the new generation of cancer chemotherapy drugs, and the credibility for vaccine and enzyme therapies declined in the mainstream medical community. However, during this period the field of complementary and alternative medicine (CAM) approaches to cancer diversified, and there were more extensive networks of clinicians and patients. A prominent network in the US was support for the therapy Krebiozen, which was based on a substance isolated from the serum of horses that had been injected with the bacterium *Actinomyces bovis.* The therapeutic claims were highly controversial, but at its peak during the 1950s, the network included political and labor leaders as well as doctors. Emmanuel Revici and Max Gerson, two European émigrés to the US, attracted networks of clinicians and patients in support of their complex nutritional and biological therapies. Some prominent herbal therapies, notably the Hoxsey and Essiac formulas, also attracted networks of patient advocates (Hess 2004; Moss 1996).

In most cases, solid clinical evidence in the form of peer-reviewed studies was absent, and health authorities prosecuted practitioners. At the high end of scientific credibility, Livingston and her fellow researchers published in peer-reviewed journals, and Revici and Gerson were medical doctors who conducted scientific research and found linkages between nutrition and cancer that later became more widely accepted. In contrast, the herbal formulas came from folk medicine traditions, and although the therapies attracted a following of patients who claimed to have been successfully treated, they lacked the scientific research credibility of the Livingston, Revici, and Gerson networks. Even more controversial were the Krebiozen supporters, who were plagued by widespread claims of fraud. Some of the networks were able to establish clinics, generally in Mexico, which institutionalized some CAM approaches to the point that they could survive the death of the founder (Hess 2004; Moss 1996).

A patient-based health reform movement emerged in support of laetrile, a food-based pharmacological intervention for cancer that was claimed to be toxic only to cancer cells. The laetrile phenomenon was the source of formal advocacy organizations, some of which survive today. In 1963, the laetrile patient Cecile Hoffman founded the International Association for Cancer Victims and Friends (the word "Victors" was later switched for "Victims"), and she partnered with the Tijuana-based physician Ernesto Contreras to obtain therapy in Mexico when it was not available in the United States. The Contreras Oasis Hospital eventually grew into one of the largest of the Tijuana cancer treatment centers. Over time the patient organization and the Contreras Oasis Hospital diversified to support a wide range of CAM cancer therapies. In 1973 the Los Angeles chapter of the association formed the Cancer Control Society, which continues to host an annual meeting that brings together cancer patients with CAM practitioners. Beginning in 1984, the conference also provided tours of the Tijuana cancer clinics, including those associated with the Gerson, Hoxsey, Rife, laetrile, and other CAM approaches (Hess 1999).

A galvanizing moment in the development of the CAM cancer therapy movement was the prosecution of the physician John Richardson. Because he was a member of the John Birch Society, his prosecution triggered the mobilization of an estimated 500 chapters and 30,000 supporters in favor of the legalization of laetrile (Culbert 1974; Markle and Petersen 1980). Michael Culbert, another patient advocate leader and cofounder of the International Council for Health Freedom, noted in an interview with me that the laetrile movement was not monolithically right-wing, because it also included hippies and countercultural supporters (Hess 1999). Despite the diversity of political viewpoints of the laetrile movement during the 1970s, there was a strong libertarian stream in the CAM cancer therapy movement in the United States. That stream continues today in expressions of concern with government control of medicine and electronic record keeping (e.g., Citizens Council for Health Freedom 2013). Another source of support for laetrile and CAM cancer therapies in general was the National Health Federation, an organization founded in 1955 to promote more open markets for vitamin supplements and unconventional medical therapies (Markle and Petersen 1980). Furthermore, in 1977 the firing of Ralph Moss, the assistant public affairs director of Memorial Sloan Kettering Cancer Center who exposed the cover-up of successful laetrile experiments, added another dimension to the laetrile movement. He went on to found a patient support and educational organization, Cancer Decisions, and he became a leader in calls for scientific support of research into CAM cancer therapies. His book *The Cancer Industry*, originally published in 1980, chronicles the problems in clinical trials for laetrile and other CAM cancer therapies, and it discusses the suppression that clinician-researchers faced during the 1970s and 1980s (Moss 1996). He also became a student of German cancer clinics and the leading American expert on the options available for patients who have the resources to travel to Germany.

Laetrile was not the only CAM cancer therapy that was emerging during the 1970s. There were also networks of clinicians, researchers, and patients in support of the work of Linus Pauling and Ewan Cameron on vitamin C and cancer, Michio Kushi on macrobiotics, Joseph Gold on hydrazine sulfate, Stanislaw Burzynski on antineoplastons, and Lawrence Burton on immuno-augmentative therapy. During the early 1980s the cancer research community responded to the laetrile and vitamin C claims by conducting clinical trials that had negative results, but CAM cancer therapy advocates claimed that the studies suffered from fatal design flaws (Hess 1999; Moss 1996; Richards 1981). Because the CAM community was not included in the design and execution of the clinical trials, the resulting experimenters' regress only increased the gap between the two communities.

In 1986 Congressman Guy Molinari joined with patient advocates and 40 other Congressional representatives to ask the Office of Technology Assessment of the US Congress to call for an investigation into bias against CAM cancer therapies, partly in response to the repression of immuno-augmentative therapy (Office of Technology Assessment 1990). Patient advocate Frank Wiewel, whose father was a Burton patient, led a march on Washington against the suppression of CAM cancer therapies and was the original requestor of the Office of Technology Assessment study (Hess 1999). A group of CAM advocates led by journalist Robert Houston tracked the errors in the subsequent report and called for corrections (Hess 1999). The report evaluated existing research on a wide range of CAM cancer therapies and became a battleground for conventional and CAM cancer researchers. The publication of the report is sometimes mentioned as one of the reasons why the Office of Technology Assessment was closed, but it also served as a trigger for Congressional reforms that led to the establishment in 1991 of the Office of Alternative Medicine of the National Institutes of Health. In 1998, amid charges that the office was too soft on alternative medicine, it was restructured as the National Center for Complementary and Alternative Medicine (NCCAM).

Epistemic modernization and liberalization

During the 1990s two significant changes occurred in the development of the field of research and therapies for CAM and cancer. The founding of the Office of Alternative Medicine (later NCCAM) marked a regime change in which the integration of CAM therapies was to proceed, based on evidence. Thus, a new era of epistemic modernization was supposed to occur, in which the integration of CAM and mainstream therapies would become possible based on scientific research. The change coincided with the professionalization of CAM providers, especially the growth of degree programs and licensing arrangements for naturopaths and acupuncturists. Researchers representing CAM professions were added to the NCCAM advisory board, including a naturopath, an acupuncturist, and a chiropractor in 2011. Cancer patient advocates, including one whom we interviewed for *Women Confront Cancer*, also were allowed to join the advisory panel of NCCAM, at least during the initial period (Wooddell and Hess 1998).

In general, the integration of CAM research coincided with a complementarization process, that is, the focus of research on complementary rather than alternative uses of CAM cancer therapies. Furthermore, in a process akin to bioprospecting among indigenous herbal medicines, the dominant networks of the research and therapeutic fields colonized the CAM field by taking ideas and subjecting them to a filtration process that translated them into patentable pharmaceutical products. There are numerous examples, including the ideas of William Coley (who is now recognized as the father of cancer immunology even if his therapies have long been rejected) and the idea of anti-angiogenesis. In the translation from, for example, shark cartilage to an anti-angiogenesis drug, the biological product was simplified and patented (Hess 2006).

The complementarization process also included the integration of CAM researchers, especially those associated with research and education institutions, including schools of naturopathic and chiropractic medicine. On the surface, there was a significant change from the era of the Mayo Clinic trials for vitamin C and laetrile, which excluded CAM researchers and physicians from participation in the design and execution of the trials. However, the new conditions for research also put the therapy through a filter that has a dual bias: against alternative modalities in favor of complementary modalities and against the total, individualized protocol in favor of a standardized therapeutic unit such as a drug or food supplement. Advocates of alternative approaches were told to prove their therapeutic mettle with clinical trials, but the funding was very restricted for the research, and NCCAM did not fund direct, head-to-head research on alternative cancer therapies versus conventional therapies. Guidelines of equipoise (projected equivalent benefit for patients) made it ethically difficult to offer, for example, the herbal formula Essiac and standard chemotherapy as competing arms in a clinical trial. The exception was patients with a very poor prognosis for whom conventional therapies have little efficacy, such as pancreatic cancer patients, but with that population it is possible that nothing will work well.

The research agenda at NCCAM can be tracked via its funding record and the results of funded studies. The analysis in Table 8.1 provides one example of how to analyze undone science in a systematic and quantitative way. The analysis is focused on results from NCCAM-funded studies over a

Table 8.1 Summary of Cancer-Related Research Results, 2001–2011

Year	*N*	*Cancer Prevention*	*Cancer Treatment*	*Cancer Population*
2011	18	–Vitamin E, clinical	0	CAM provider use
2010	30	–Gingko Baloba, clinical	+White tea, subclinical; –Shark cartilage, clinical; +Green tea, subclinical	0
2009	30	0	+Acupuncture and cancer pain in rats, subclinical	0
2008	44	+Probiotics, clinical	+Massage and patient mood, clinical	CAM provider use
2007	8	0	0	0
2006	12	–Vitamins C & E, meta	–Vitamins C & E, meta	0
2005	2	0	–Shark cartilage, clinical	0
2004	2	0	0	0
2003	0	0	0	0
2001	1	0	0	0
Total	147	4	7	2

+ or - indicates positive or negative results.
National Center for Complementary and Alternative Medicine (2012).

ten-year period that were included in its "spotlight" pages as they were archived in December 2011. The ten-year time frame makes it possible to gain a better picture of the nature of the research and direction of results. One can see that cancer is only a relatively small percentage of the data set of research results. Even though cancer affects more than one-third of the population and was a central disease in the political process that led to the establishment of the original Office of Alternative Medicine within the National Institutes of Health, cancer is the topic of only about 9 percent of the 147 completed studies in this data set. Furthermore, within the group of 13 cancer studies, most of the research is on prevention, subclinical efficacy, or behavior. Shark cartilage is the only CAM cancer therapy for which clinical results were available. Both studies tested shark cartilage in a complementary modality, and both had negative results (the first was stopped early due to low patient adherence and no apparent benefit). Although shark cartilage was widely hyped and was the basis of both positive subclinical results and conversion into anti-angiogenesis drugs, it was hardly one of the main lines of CAM cancer therapy. With respect to the main lines of CAM cancer therapy (e.g., proteolytic enzymes, autogenous vaccines, the Gerson diet, the Revici lipids, immuno-augmentative therapy, antineoplastons, vitamin C, laetrile, hydrazine sulfate, and the herbal formulas such as Essiac), little more was known about clinical efficacy in 2011 than in 1991, when the Office of Alternative Medicine was founded. Even vitamin C, for which the Mayo Clinic trials substituted an oral dose for intravenous injections (a crucial design flaw according to CAM advocates because high plasma levels could not be attained), remained unfunded. In other words, although there was a blossoming of research on a wide range of diseases and some research on cancer, the fundamental questions raised by the history of conflict remained undone science.

The one exception to the pattern of undone science for alternative modalities of CAM cancer therapies was the head-to-head clinical trial of an enzyme-and-supplements therapy in the lineage of John Beard, which was originally funded by the National Cancer Institute at the request of Nicholas Gonzalez, a physician who had trained at the Memorial Sloan Kettering Cancer Center. The case of Nicholas Gonzalez is especially important because it was originally heralded as representing a new era of cooperation and integration, and it allowed a direct comparison of his therapy with chemotherapy for inoperable pancreatic cancer patients (that is, the Gonzalez therapy was not tested as additional to chemotherapy). The equipoise limitation, which generally restricted direct comparisons of a conventional chemotherapeutic cocktail with a CAM cocktail, could be met because the life expectancy was low, and the survival benefit from the conventional therapy was also very low. However, ten years later, Gonzalez found to his surprise that the study had been published in the *Journal of Clinical Oncology* without any correspondence with him or the other lead investigator (Chabot et al. 2009). He initiated an investigation and alleged that the recruited patients for the nutrition arm were not comparable to the control arm of the clinical trial, that the claim that the chemotherapy patients did better than the Gonzalez patients was unfounded, and that the lead investigator had financial ties to the chemotherapy drug used in the trial. The NIH office responsible for investigating the trial concurred that the arms were not comparable, and the details are chronicled in his book *What Went Wrong* (Gonzalez 2012). As Gonzalez wrote:

> My colleague Dr. Linda Isaacs and I initially approached this project with some enthusiasm, believing it to be a wonderful opportunity to bring the conventional academic world and "alternative" researchers, so often at odds, together for the benefit of science and for patients suffering terrible illness. But as the years passed we came to realize with some disappointment that there was no new dawn breaking, no new age of cooperation between the academic and alternative universes, that the same biases against treatment methods developed outside of the mainstream still reigned supreme, and that scientists and physicians at the highest levels of academia would do anything, even change the truth to prove an unconventional therapy has no value.
>
> (Gonzalez 2009)

In short, the one, high-profile, NIH-funded direct comparison of a major alternative cancer therapy against a standard chemotherapeutic agent in the control arm ended in the same kind of accusations that had characterized the clinical trials for other alternative cancer therapies, such as vitamin C and laetrile. In this sense little had changed since the 1980s, even with a highly respected and well-credentialed researcher and clinician such as Gonzalez. His experience shows quite clearly the limitations of the epistemic modernization of CAM research. The outcome became well known in the CAM communities, and it confirmed the general belief that cancer therapy was the most firmly guarded area of biomedical orthodoxy and the perception that NCCAM was not willing to wade into those waters. The results of the Gonzalez trial and the data on the funding patterns suggest that although the research field has changed significantly since 1991, there are also fundamental continuities that have not addressed the issues of undone science.

The second historical change during the 1990s involved the liberalization of therapeutic access. With respect to cancer treatment, some medical doctors began to include CAM therapies in their oncology practices under the new term "integrative medicine," and hospitals also began to offer integrative cancer care. CAM therapies available in the hospital settings were generally limited to mind-body therapies such as yoga and to nutritional counseling, and people with whom I spoke in those centers indicated that their physical location and social position were very marginal. In the late 1990s, the Center for Mind-Body Medicine at George Washington University and the National Cancer Institute began sponsoring conferences on "comprehensive cancer care," where the new approach to integrative cancer treatment provided a different vision of CAM cancer therapies from those of the Cancer Control Society, which was connected with the alternative cancer therapies of the Tijuana clinics. The conferences included patient advocates and did not exclude the "alternative" side of CAM cancer therapies, but the sessions also clearly showcased the evidence-based medicine paradigm and the practices of integrative oncology. In these practices, patients generally received conventional chemotherapeutic and/or immunological treatment along with access to mind-body therapies and counseling on diet, supplements, and lifestyle changes. They gained access to complementary therapies as long as they followed the conventional drug regimen, but in most cases patients were not given a choice between conventional treatment and alternative cancer therapies.

The limited liberalization of the therapeutic field occurred at roughly the same time as the liberalization of the dietary supplements industry. Prior to the passage of the Dietary Supplements and Health Education Act (DSHEA) of 1994, food supplements existed in a liminal regulatory state between food and drugs. The Food and Drug Administration adopted the view that vitamins and dietary supplements were drugs if they exceeded a potency of greater than 150 percent of the Recommended Daily Allowance, but those regulations were reversed by the Proxmire Amendment of 1976. In response, the Food and Drug Administration used its regulatory authority over food additives to limit the availability of food supplements. DSHEA responded to the situation by clearly classifying food supplements as food, and it allowed manufacturers to make limited health claims (such as structure and function support), but it did not allow them to make disease claims (Bass 2011). For practical purposes, DSHEA placed supplements outside regulatory oversight from the Food and Drug Administration unless they could be proven to be unsafe, but manufacturers of supplements could only make claims about structure and function, not about the efficacy of supplements for the treatment of diseases. In effect, the existence of a disease claim associated with a supplement, rather than a material or design boundary, determined its classification as either food or drug. The law had been widely supported by the nutritional supplements industry as well as CAM advocates. However, some consumer advocacy organizations and the pharmaceutical industry criticized the act for exposing consumers to worthless expenditures on supplements, and periodic battles flared up in the United States Congress between opposing coalitions.

Similar conflicts emerged at the global trade level in Codex Alimentarius regulations for food supplements. Although the Codex guidelines are technically voluntary, the World Trade Organization recognizes them in resolving trade disputes, and Codex guidelines are likely to have increasing influence in global trade policy (Halfon 2010). An enduring concern is that the US may harmonize its supplements law with Codex, which has tended to follow the stricter, European approach. CAM advocates and the nutritional supplements industry in the US and some other countries worry that the change would render illegal the over-the-counter sale of high-dose supplements by converting them into prescription drugs that would either be extremely costly or simply unavailable because of the lack of regulatory approval. Nutritional advocacy organizations and the dietary supplements industry have been especially vigilant over attempts to harmonize US regulations to Codex. The US government's Food and Drug Modernization Act of 1997 contains anti-harmonization language, and at the urging of advocacy organizations, language that would have facilitated harmonization was deleted from the 2010 Food and Drug Modernization Act (Alliance for Natural Health 2010).

The concern among CAM and "health freedom" advocates with harmonization has some empirical support in the experience with the North American Free Trade Act. Patients have been going to Mexico for CAM cancer treatment since the 1960s, and it is in Mexico that they can gain access to the alternative end of the spectrum of CAM cancer therapies. Access to this end of the spectrum contains both the risks of lack of efficacy and the potential, albeit often small, for a positive response when conventional options are ineffective; however, it is interesting that on the bus tour of these clinics I learned that many of the prospective patients were family members of US doctors who were fairly knowledgeable about the field. The number of clinics in Tijuana grew during the 1980s and 1990s, but the North American Free Trade Agreement also made possible the Mexico-United States-Canada Health Fraud Work Group, or MUCH, which closed some of the Tijuana clinics. Although some clinics closed permanently, in general they proved resilient, and in 2011 at least 20 clinics were still functioning in Tijuana. However, business had slowed due to the recession and the rise of kidnappings and other forms of violence, which have nearly ended the city's tourism industry (Moss 2005, 2011). Furthermore, the liberalization of the therapeutic field in the United States also meant that for some patients the integrated therapies offered in the United States were adequate. Patients generally lack the knowledge to distinguish among the different forms of CAM cancer therapies, so unless they are very well read, they are not able to distinguish the complementary therapies available in US integrative practices from the alternative therapies available in the Mexican clinics, not to mention the considerable overlap between the two based on the legal status of food supplements in the US and the different levels of doses used for supplements.

Due to liberalization of the therapeutic field, the locus of health advocacy has also shifted. The patient advocacy organizations that were so active at the height of the laetrile, vitamin C, and immuno-augmentative therapy controversies have not disappeared but have shifted their attention toward more routinized activity such as holding conferences and providing patient support services. Likewise, the alternative practitioners have not disappeared but increasingly have been displaced by a continuum of health-care practitioners who offer a range of CAM therapies, but mostly on the complementary side of integrative care. With the rise of evidence-based integration and the liberalization of the supplements market, advocacy work has shifted to the preservation of the relatively deregulated nutraceutical market against attempts by coalitions of pharmaceutical companies, consumer advocates, and some medical professionals to reduce availability by putting over-the-counter supplements behind a costly prescription barrier.

Although scientifi c controversies continue and the problem of undone science for alternative cancer therapies remains unresolved, the liberalization of access to therapies and supplements has been accompanied by a new type of engagement with science and the public. The Alliance for Natural Health USA has sponsored campaigns to limit the regulatory authority of the Food and Drug Administration with respect to health claims for food supplements. For example, the organization worked with Congressman Ron Paul, who was also a presidential candidate for the Republican Party nomination in 2012, to support various amendments that would enable the manufacturers of food supplements to make a broader scope of disease claims. The "Stop Censoring Medical Science" campaign includes the proposed Free Speech about Science Act, which would allow manufacturers of nutritional supplements to reference peer-reviewed scientifi c studies about the health effects of the supplements and would prevent the Food and Drug Administration from using those health claims to trigger a change of status of the supplement from food to drug (Alliance for Natural Health USA 2012). For example, growers of cherries or manufacturers of supplements based on cherries currently cannot make reference to peer-reviewed studies that suggest that the consumption of cherries may reduce heart-attack risk. The law would enable manufacturers to publicize peer-reviewed studies, but it would preserve the right of government agencies to intervene to stop false and misleading claims. Here, the historical question of science and the public good, the right of patients to have the undone science done so that they know what works and what does not, is amplified by a second question: the right of the supplements industry to make public the results of evidence-based medicine to nutraceutical consumers. It also raises the question of what constitutes a peer-reviewed publication from a regulatory perspective.

Discussion

A signifi cant strand of work on science, technology, and health has utilized the concept of biological citizenship to analyze historical changes such as the ones described here. From this perspective, advocacy for CAM during the period before the 1990s involved the change from a rights-based citizen, who demanded freedom of access to medical therapies, to a more choice-based citizen, who is faced with a bewildering combination of CAM and conventional therapies under the tent of integrative medicine and a liberalized market of nutraceuticals. The contrasting modalities of citizenship might be compared with a rights-based form of biological citizenship, in which patients or victims use their biological condition to legitimate demands for rights of access to health care, and a form of biological citizenship based on biomedical potential, consumer hope, and individual health (Petryna 2002; Rose 2007; Wehling 2011). Similar changes have been noted elsewhere in studies of neoliberalism, such as the growth of the entrepreneurial self and the emergence of health practices as a field of consumer choice (Moore and Hoffmann 2014; Ong 1999).

Although the concept of changes in health-related citizenship can help to identify underlying cultural shifts in the forms of health advocacy, it needs to be articulated with a broader institutional analysis of changes in relations between patient advocacy and industry. The field of patient advocacy has undergone dramatic changes in which industrial sponsorship has elevated some organizations to a dominant position in the advocacy field while also changing the forms and goals of advocacy (Baggott and Forster 2008; Batt 2012; Jones 2008; O'Donovan and Glavanis-Grantham 2005). As a result, organizations that retain a more critical perspective on the dominant epidemiological and therapeutic paradigms tend to occupy a subordinate position in the advocacy field, a pattern that has occurred in various types of social movement fields, from health advocacy (Batt 2012) to hunger advocacy (Poppendieck 1998) to environmental advocacy (Dowie 1995). It is among the subordinate positions in the civil society fields of advocacy organizations that one finds articulations of general political citizenship founded on action based on the public interest rather than rights anchored in a biological condition. In this situation, the mode of operation is less an interest group that seeks to have more resources (for a particular disease, or greater access to a particular drug) and more that of a reform movement in which there is a broader goal of social change.

Furthermore, the enactment of citizenship in this circumstance is not reducible to the ideal of the *moi commune* or rational-critical discourse in the traditional of utopian, Western, democratic theory because the counterpublic that emerges in the case of CAM politics is not innocent of sectional interests. The patient advocates and CAM-oriented researchers articulate a general social reform goal – a more democratic politics of therapeutic evaluation and access – that goes beyond the interest group politics of advocating for greater resources for one social segment over another, but the CAM counterpublic is also aligned with countervailing professional groups and industries, which have their own sectional interests. Just as elites articulate a public interest that is in alignment with those of the dominant political and industrial organizations, so the counterpublic articulates an alternative public interest that has its own sectional alignments. In other words, alliances among mainstream advocacy organizations, mainstream researchers, the medical profession, and the pharmaceutical industry enter into conflict with alliances among CAM advocacy organizations, researchers, professions, and countervailing industries such as the nutraceutical industry.

Thus, I am not arguing that those in the dominant position in the fields of health research, care, and policy cannot articulate a public interest; they do with clarity. Elites from the industrial field tend to form alliances with political, scientific, and civil society elites to ensure that an articulation of official public interest is aligned with the sectional interests of the industrial elites. In the case of cancer there is an alignment of the leading medical associations, mainstream cancer charity and advocacy organizations, leading scientific researchers, and the pharmaceutical industry in favor of an approach to treatment that is based on patented drugs that are tested in clinical trials. The dominant networks constitute an official public that articulates the grounds and limitations of narratives of cancer treatment and disease, based on a spectrum of choices that have been certified as scientifically valid and medically safe and efficacious. They work well with the interest group pole of patient advocacy organizations, which accept the dominant etiological and therapeutic paradigms (and often receive large donations from the pharmaceutical industry), and they tend to limit political conflict to the allocation of resources within that field or over increases of resources to that field. The official view of the cancer research agenda has strong merits, because on the surface it is grounded in evidence-based medicine, and the scientific field is charged with providing a source of neutral arbitration of disputes within the confines of a field of biomedical research and therapy that is oriented toward patented drug interventions.

In a pluralistic state, competing coalitions present their arguments for policy changes in a relatively neutral setting (a legislative committee and an executive agency), and the public representatives evaluate competing claims and make decisions. Thus, conditions of competition and neutral decision-making by government units charged with acting in the general public interest make it possible for sectional interests and articulations of public interest to coincide, because the sectional interests provide information that a neutral arbiter can evaluate. However, as political sociologists have documented, governments do not generally operate according to a classical, pluralist model. Likewise, as this study has shown, in the case of CAM research that is sponsored by the US government, there are layers of prioritization: away from CAM-related cancer research in general, within CAM research away from cancer research and away from clinical trials of treatment, and within clinical trials away from the head-to-head study of alternative therapies.

Counterpublics emerge from the subordinate positions of social fields (government, industry, civil society, and science) to contest the epistemic claims, political ideologies, and policy directions of official publics. Although counterpublics are often linked to historically excluded groups in society (e.g., hourly labor, women, and ethnic minority groups), the connection is historically contingent and can include networks of people who occupy relatively privileged social addresses but are in the subordinate position of the social fields that they inhabit (Fraser 1997; Harding 1998, 2008; Hess 2011). A scientific counterpublic emerges when scientists and clinician-researchers located in a subordinate position in the scientific field step out of their roles as researchers and enter other social fields (such as the media, government, civil society, and industry) to advance an alternative arrangement of knowledge agendas in the scientific field as better serving a broad public interest. In the case of advocacy for CAM cancer therapies in the US, there is full counterpublic of researchers, clinicians, patient advocacy leaders, nutritional companies, political officials, and health freedom organizations. The clinical field has seen the growth and professionalization of CAM providers, and the therapeutic field has seen the growth of the nutritional supplements industry. Both pose a challenge to the medical profession and the pharmaceutical industry, and the skirmishes over professional and industrial position take place over a long time horizon in multiple fields, including regulatory policy, legislation, patient recruitment, research agendas, funding priorities, and the interpretation of research design and results. Although not innocent of sectional interest, the counterpublic also advances an agenda for research and policy based on its opposition to the vision of public interest articulated by the official public. Thus, one does not conclude that patient advocacy organizations represent the public interest in opposition to the sectional interest of the mainstream of research and clinical practice. Instead, both the counterpublic and official public construct contrasting visions of public interest that are aligned with their sectional interests. Indeed, battles also occur within civil society between mainstream organizations such as the American Cancer Society and CAM-oriented clinicians and advocacy organizations.

The counterpublic also draws attention to undone science, that is, science that is systematically blocked because it is in conflict with the research agendas of the dominant agents in a scientific research field and associated industrial fields (e.g., the pharmacological orientation of the cancer therapy research field, oncology profession, and pharmaceutical industry). For the counterpublic, research into CAM cancer therapies is a form of positive non-knowledge, whereas during the early period of the CAM-mainstream relationship, the official public viewed the CAM challenge as negative non-knowledge, a worthless and unproven approach based on dubious science. Not only were alternative cancer therapies not worth the investment of public research resources, but the practice of CAM cancer therapies also represented a threat to the public interest, because some of the therapies were potentially dangerous. Even if the therapies were generally recognized as safe, they represented an opportunity cost because innocent cancer patients could be bilked of their money and miss the opportunity for potentially life-extending conventional therapies. The fact that the history of the CAM cancer field does have its share of hucksters and unproven folk remedies, even as it has brilliant scientists such as Revici, suggests that the construction of a threat to the public interest has some basis. In other words, with respect to CAM cancer therapies, there is a risk of both Type 1 and Type 2 errors, that is, rejecting an effective CAM therapy and accepting an ineffective one.

Conclusion

The historical changes described above as the epistemic modernization of the CAM cancer research field and the liberalization of policy governing therapeutic and nutraceutical markets include reconstructions of notions of citizenship but go beyond them. The relationships between the official publics and counterpublics and between their articulations of the conditions of public good also changed. During the post-liberalization period, the older "hard line" approach of the official public's stance of opposition to alternative medicine has not disappeared, but it has become moderated by the limited acceptance of CAM based on the filtration criterion of evidence-based medicine, which enables some complementary modalities of CAM cancer therapies to enter into conventional practice under the rubric of integrated medicine. Funding appears for research on CAM therapies, and the repressive strategy appears to give way to a more rationalized, integrative strategy. Leaders of CAM professions are brought into the funding process, such as the Advisory Council of the NCCAM, and papers are published in peer-reviewed literature. Patients are allowed to have their vitamins and yoga as long as they take their drugs, too.

However, the liberalization of the therapeutic field occurs on the terms of the dominant agents in the field. Biomedical integration proceeds slowly and in a limited way, much as other forms of integration occur (such as the slow process whereby men of the dominant ethnic groups have admitted some ethnic minorities and women into management positions). The funding priorities of the official public continue to marginalize and even discredit alternative modalities for cancer treatment. The result of medical integration is "A" deletion in the CAM, so that it tends to become "COM" (complementary only medicine). Just as radical feminist and minority activists had to leave their radical politics on the doorstep of entry into the corporate world that embraced "integration" as a social policy of liberalization, so CAM advocates must leave their alternative aspirations on the doorstep of entry into the biomedical mainstream. There is little funding available to test the prospect of alternative cancer therapies, and the blockage is legitimated by an ethics system that limits clinical trials to situations of equipoise of benefits to patients. In short, there is a process of incorporation (of CAM into the integrated mainstream) and also of transformation (of CAM into COM). As I have shown elsewhere, these dynamics of complementarization apply to other alternative industrial movements, specifically to a subtype of those movements that I have studied as "technology- and product-oriented movements" such as organic foods, open-source programming, and solar energy (Hess 2005, 2007, 2013).

Although both epistemic modernization and therapeutic liberalization have been limited, the historical change has been accompanied by a decline in the high levels of popular mobilization that occurred during the laetrile period. To some degree the historical change is a product of the success of the reform movement. The liberalization of the therapeutic field means that it is both more diverse and less polarized than it was during the 1960s and 1970s. Patients have access to a wider range of both conventional and CAM therapies, and patients who wish to gain access to a more complete range of alternative therapies can go to Mexico, Germany, or other countries. Clinician-based patient advocacy organizations sometimes mobilize to support a particular doctor when faced with prosecution, but the general patient advocacy organizations play a broader role in holding conferences and educating patients about options. If a significant regime change were to occur, with multiple crack-downs on multiple practitioners, it is possible that the patient organizations would become quickly mobilized. Thus, a general conclusion is that the change of epistemic modernization and therapeutic liberalization has been accompanied by a relative quiescence of patient advocacy organizations in this field. They have not disappeared, but they are not mobilized in the more directly political ways that were evident before the 1980s.

The CAM cancer case is also of general interest to the study of social movements, civil society, and science. The social movements literature includes studies of the effects of social movements, and one of the conclusions is that it is not always easy to determine a causal relationship between mobilizations and policy outcomes (Giugni 1998; Amenta et al. 2010). In some cases, governments have responded to advocacy by establishing post-market monitoring or holding consultation exercises, but it remains to be seen how much change such programs will effect (Böschen et al. 2011). In the case of CAM cancer therapies in the US, on one level there has been a substantial change since the 1980s, but on another level nothing has changed. One of the important lessons from the study of the CAM cancer therapy movement in the US is the need to pay more attention to the role of countervailing industries in relationship to the issue of the effects of social movements. The history described here disturbs the idea of industrial cooptation of social movements by suggesting that attention could be focused more on the coalitions of civil society organizations, scientists, and different industries. Without the constant surveillance of the nutraceutical industry, it is likely that the relatively open access that US consumers enjoy for food supplements and that CAM clinicians and patients have to high-dose supplements for therapeutic purposes would quickly evaporate. These are the conditions of democracy in a society in which political power is heavily influenced by the visions of public interest that are formulated by large industrial corporations. Democratic contestation in a corporatocracy implies that counterpublics may achieve limited political success, but they are more likely to do so when they can take advantage of countervailing industrial power.

References

Alliance for Natural Health USA (2010) ANH-USA victory! Supplements are exempted from Codex language in food safety bill, April 13. Available online at:

<www.anh-usa.org/anh-usa-victory-supplements-are-exempted-from-codex-language-in-food-safety-bill> (accessed 30 March 2013).

___ (2012) Free Speech about Natural Health Science: it's time to fight back! Available online at: <www.anh-usa.org/free-speech-about-natural-health-science> (accessed 30 March 2013).

Amenta, Edwin; Caren, Neal; Chiarello, Elizabeth; and Su, Yang (2010) The political consequences of social movements, Annual Review of Sociology, 36, 287–307.

Baggott, Rob and Forster, Rudolf (2008) Health consumer and patients' organizations in Europe: towards a comparative analysis, Health Expectations, 11(1), 85–94.

Bass, Scott (ed.) (2011) Dietary Supplement Regulation: a comprehensive guide, Washington, DC: Food and Drug Law Institute.

Batt, Sharon (2012) *From grassroots to pharma partnerships: breast cancer advocacy in Canada*, unpublished Ph.D. dissertation, Dalhousie University.

Böschen, Stefan; Kastenhofer, Karen; Rust, Ina; Soentgen, Jens; and Wehling, Peter (2011) Scientifi c non-knowledge and its political dynamics: the cases of agribiotechnology and mobile phoning, *Science, Technology, & Human Values*, 35(6), 783–811.

Bourdieu, Pierre (2005) *The Social Structures of the Economy*, Malden, MA: Polity Press.

Brown, Phil (2007) *Toxic Exposures: contested illnesses and the environmental health movement.* New York: Columbia University Press.

Chabot, John; Tsai, Wei-Yang; Fine, Robert; Chen, Chunxia; Kumah, Carol; Antman, Karen and Grann, Victor (2009) Pancreatic proteolytic enzyme therapy compared with gemcitabine-based chemotherapy for the treatment of pancreatic cancer, *Journal of Clinical Oncology*, 28(12), 2058–2063.

Citizens Council for Health Freedom (2013) *Our Goals.* Available online at: <www.cchfreedom.org/about.php> (accessed 30 March 2013).

Culbert, Michael (1974) *Freedom from Cancer*, New York: Pocket Books, Simon and Schuster.

Delborne, Jason (2008) Transgenes and transgressions: scientific dissent as heterogeneous practice, *Social Studies of Science*, 38(4), 509–541.

Dowie, Mark (1995) *Losing Ground: American environmentalism at the close of the twentieth century.* Cambridge, MA: MIT Press.

Epstein, Steven (2008) Patient groups and health movements, in E. Hackett, O. Amsterdamska, M. Lynch and J. Wajcman (eds) *The Handbook of Science and Technology Studies*, 3rd edition, Cambridge, MA: MIT Press, 499–539.

Fraser, Nancy (1997) *Justice Interruptus: critical reflections on the "postsocialist" condition.* New York: Routledge.

Frickel, Scott; Gibbon, Sahra; Howard, Jeff; Kempner, Joanna; Ottinger, Gwen and Hess, David (2010) Undone science: charting social movement and civil society challenges to research agenda setting, *Science, Technology, & Human Values*, 35(4), 444–473.

Giugni, Marco (1998) Was it worth the effort? The outcomes and consequences of social movements, *Annual Review of Sociology*, 24, 371–93.

Gonzalez, Nicholas (2009) The Truth about the NIC-NCCAM Clinical Study, Available online at: <www.dr-gonzalez.com/jco rebuttal.htm> (accessed 30 March 2013).

___ (2012) *What Went Wrong: the truth behind the clinical trial of the enzyme treatment of cancer*, New York: New Spring Press.

Gross, Matthias (2009) *Ignorance and Surprise: science, society and ecological design*, Cambridge, MA: MIT Press.

Halfon, Saul (2010) Confronting the WTO: intervention strategies in GMO adjudication, *Science, Technology, & Human Values*, 35(3), 307–329.

Harding, Sandra (1998) *Is Science Multicultural? Postcolonialisms, feminisms, and epistemologies*, Bloomington, IN: Indiana University Press.

—— (2008) *Sciences from Below: feminisms, postcolonialities, and modernities*, Durham, NC: Duke University Press.

Hess, David (1997) *Can Bacteria Cause Cancer?* New York: New York University Press.

—— (1999) *Evaluating Alternative Cancer Therapies*, New Brunswick, NJ: Rutgers University Press.

—— (2004) CAM cancer therapies in twentieth-century North America: examining continuities and change, in R. Johnston (ed.) *The Politics of Healing*, New York: Routledge, 218–230.

—— (2005) Technology- and product-oriented movements: approximating social movement studies and STS, *Science, Technology, & Human Values*, 30(4), 515–535.

—— (2006) Antiangiogenesis research and the dynamics of scientific research fields: historical and institutional perspectives in the sociology of science, in S. Frickel and K. Moore (eds) *The New Political Sociology of Science*, Madison, WI: University of Wisconsin Press, 122–147.

—— (2007) *Alternative Pathways in Science and Industry: activism, innovation, and the environment in an era of globalization*, Cambridge, MA: MIT Press.

—— (2011) To tell the truth: on scientific counterpublics, *Public Understanding of Science*, 20(5), 627–641.

—— (2013) Industrial fields and countervailing power: the transformation of distributed solar energy in the United States, *Global Environmental Change*, 23(5), 847–855.

Jones, Kathryn (2008) In whose interest? Relationships between health consumer groups and the pharmaceutical industry in the UK, *Sociology of Health and Illness*, 30(6), 929–943.

Markle, Gerald and Petersen, James (1980) *Politics, Science, and Cancer: the laetrile phenomenon*, Washington, DC: American Association for the Advancement of Science.

Martin, Brian (2007) *Justice Ignited: the dynamics of backfire*, Lanham, MD: Rowman & Littlefield.

—— (2010) How to attack a scientific theory and get away with it (usually), *Science as Culture*, 19(2), 215–239.

Merton, Robert (1987) Three fragments from a sociologist's notebooks: establishing the phenomenon, specifi ed ignorance, and strategic research materials, *Annual Review of Sociology*, 13, 1–28.

Moore, Kelly and Hoffmann, Matthew (2014) "The tip of the day": field theory and alternative nutrition in the US, in S. Frickel and D.J. Hess (eds.) Fields of knowledge: Science, politics and publics in the neoliberal age (*Political Power and Social Theory, Volume 27*), Bingley, West Yorkshire: Emerald Group Publishing Limited, 223–258.

Moore, Kelly; Hess, David; Kleinman, Daniel and Frickel, Scott; (2011) Science and neoliberal globalization: a political sociological approach, *Theory and Society*, 40(5), 505–532.

Moss, Ralph (1996) *The Cancer Industry*, Brooklyn, NY: Equinox Press.

—— (2005) Patient perspectives: Tijuana cancer clinics in the post-NAFTA era, *Integrative Cancer Therapies*, 4(1), 65–86.

—— (2008a) The life and times of John Beard, DSc. (1828–1924), *Integrative Cancer Therapies*, 7(4), 229–251.

___ (2008b) Enzymes, trophoblasts, and cancer: the afterlife of an idea (1924–2008), *Integrative Cancer Therapies*, 7(4), 262–265.

___ (2011) A visit to the Tijuana cancer clinics, *Townsend Letter for Doctors and Patients*, April. Available online at : <www.townsendletter.com/April2011/warcancer0411.html> (accessed 30 March 2013).

National Center for Complementary and Alternative Medicine (2012) Research Results by Date. Available online at: <http://nccam.nih.gov/research/results/spotlight> (accessed 30 March 2013).

O'Donovan, Órla and Glavanis-Granthan, Kathy (2005) Patients' organizations in Ireland: challenging capitalist biomedicine? Final Report to the Royal Irish Academy. Available online at: <www.ria.ie/getmedia/87b7f804-c1ba-4c66-8a46-00c57300b491/ODonovan.pdf.aspx> (accessed 30 March 2013).

Office of Technology Assessment (1990) *Unconventional Cancer Treatments*, Washington, DC: Government Printing Office.

Ong, Aihwa (1999) *Flexible Citizenship: the cultural logics of transnationality*, Durham, NC: Duke University Press.

Petryna, Adriana (2002) *Life Exposed: biological citizens after Chernobyl*, Princeton, NJ: Princeton University Press.

Poppendieck, Janet (1998) *Sweet Charity? Emergency food and the end of entitlement*, New York: Viking.

Richards, Evelleen (1981) *Vitamin C and Cancer: medicine or politics?* New York: St. Martin's Press.

Rose, Nikolas (2007) *The Politics of Life Itself: biomedicine, power, and subjectivity in the twenty-first century*, Princeton, NJ: Princeton University Press.

Wehling, Peter (2011) Biology, citizenship, and the government of biomedicine: exploring the concept of biological citizenship, in U. Bröckling, S. Krasmann and T. Lemke (eds) *Governmentality: Current Issues and Future Challenges*, London: Routledge, 225–246.

Wooddell, Margaret and Hess, David (1998) *Women Confront Cancer*, New York: New York University Press.

Woodhouse, Edward; Hess, David; Breyman, Steve and Martin, Brian (2002) Science studies and activism: possibilities and problems for reconstructivist agendas, *Social Studies of Science*, 32(2), 297–319.

9 Interpellating patients as future users of biomedical technologies

The case of patient associations and stem cell research[1]

Henriette Langstrup

Introduction

Over the last 30 years, patients and patient associations have become more legitimate, visible and influential actors in health care (Hogg 1999; Landzelius 2006). While many patient associations were initiated as institutions that could offer supplementary support to patients and raise the awareness of the general public, today they often play a more influential role in both the politics and the practicalities of health care (Brown et al. 2004; Wehling 2011). Activities aimed at directly influencing political decision-making (Wood 2000) and at supporting (Novas 2006) or challenging (Epstein 1996) research have become more widespread. Not least in relation to biomedical research and in particular within genomics, patient associations have been shown to be more involved (Stockdale 1999; Rabeharisoa and Callon 2002; Novas 2006). In these contexts they fund research, engage in public controversies over ethical and juridical issues related to genomics (e.g. cloning, use of embryonic, fetal or animal tissues, patenting of genes; see e.g. Horst 2003, 2007), and form partnerships with researchers to define and carry out research in cooperation (Epstein 1996; Rabeharisoa 2003; Rabeharisoa and Callon 2004; Wehling 2011).

In this chapter, I trace the ways in which various patients and their associations came to regard themselves as the users of future stem cell technologies and subsequently became involved in activities related to this strand of research at the advent of stem cell research in the early 2000s. How did patient associations come to jump on the bandwagons of not just clinical research with therapeutic benefits that are within reach but also a field like stem cell research, which at that time was almost exclusively a basic and experimental strand of research? I will use the notion of interpellation from Althusser (2005 [1971]) to analyze the ways in which patient associations' involvement with basic research is related to contemporary research policy and the way it enacts science as a series of entrepreneurial projects. Enacting scientific research as a project is obviously a mundane activity, but none the less one with certain consequences: it entails, among other things, that the activity described in these terms is directed toward certain more or less specific goals. I shall argue that this 'projectness' interpellates patients and their associations in specific ways. Through the lists circulating in the mass media of illnesses that, it was hoped, would become treatable or curable with the help of stem cell therapies, patients came to recognize themselves as – in Althusser's terms – the subjects of this logic, or more specifically as the projected users of stem cell technologies.

First I will present my analytical approach, arguing that the concept of interpellation is helpful in specifying the embodied and subjectively experienced moment of becoming attached to the network of technoscience. I then introduce the concept of projectness to describe a contemporarily privileged logic within science. Following this, the main part of the chapter aims at providing an empirical description of what Callon (2003, 2005) and Callon and Rabeharisoa (2008) have termed 'the emergence of concerned groups'. Based on interviews with Danish stem cell researchers and representatives from patient associations and on written material, I will flesh out three different responses (recognition, misrecognition and counter-interpellation) given by patient associations when interpellated by the projectness of stem cell research. Finally, I discuss how my results may add subtlety to the previously too sharply drawn distinction between the engagement of patients in research as either oriented toward exploitation for their own, urgent needs or towards exploration as an open-ended search for knowledge in a more traditional version of basic research.

Analytical approach

There is always an issue of identity at stake in the production of scientific projects (Callon 1986). Entrepreneurs must ensure that the actual interests and identity of the actors involved in the emergent networks of innovation are shaped as far as possible in accordance with the initial problematization, locking actors into the network (ibid.). The specificity of how the effect of identity comes about, however, often remains rather opaque. What are the more-specific points at which actors acknowledge the centrality of a project? What are the devices applied in order to create such an effect? Here I suggest that the concept of interpellation may be used to describe the way in which becoming attached to certain entrepreneurial projects entails becoming a specific kind of subject. Techno-scientific projects seem to hold a 'promise of identity' to the actors who accept their centrality. Interpellation as conceptualized by Althusser is the process through which the specific subject arises by being hailed by the larger Subject, or what he terms the 'ideological state apparatus'[2] (Althusser 2005 [1971]). In the specific instance of being hailed or interpellated (the example is that of a policeman calling out to a man on the street: 'You there!'), the individual comes to recognize him or herself as the specific subject to whom ideology speaks. The scene in the street continues with the individual being hailed turning toward the policeman. The specific subject arises as an effect of this scene, which connects the individual to the ideological (ibid.). It is the individual's instant and embodied recognition (s/he turns when hailed) that reproduces the ideology, hence the state. As Butler has argued, the scene should be seen as an allegory of 'a strange sort of middle ground' where neither the agency of the subject nor the authority of ideology is yet given, but only accomplished in the act of turning (Butler 1997: 107)[3]. However, 'ideology' has a singular ring to it and may be replaced by more plural and heterogeneous concepts when we want to understand scientific research projects. Haraway has particularly pointed to technoscience as 'more, less, and other than what Althusser meant by ideology; technoscience is a form of life, a practice, a culture, a generative matrix' (Haraway 1997: 50). Although technoscience does entail potential authority, this authority is not singular but rather may be thought of as coming in the form of various 'logics'. Where ideology suggests an overarching and ubiquitous force, a logic here denotes the way in which at certain times words, practices, and materialities make things hang together in an obvious and unquestioned manner (Mol 2008). As Mol argues, the term logic points to particular rationalities; it may not be verbalized or explicit but may be implicit, inscribed in practices, habits or technologies (ibid.). The reproduction of a logic through the turning of the interpellated individual should not be seen as unambiguous – the individual might turn in more ways than one, for example, the turn might entail doubt ('Who? Me?') or misrecognition ('Me? I don't think so'). It is through these various ways of turning toward the interpellator that a logic is constituted and transformed – whether the turn produces recognition, misrecognition or another response.

What remains of Althusser's concept, and the aspect I deploy in the analysis below, concerns the ways in which the concept of interpellation points toward a specific, bodily and materially practiced operation through which individuals come to regard themselves or those they represent as subjects of a certain logic and its practices, in my case as future users of stem cell technologies. Interpellation not only makes the subject recognize him or herself in certain ways but also sets in motion new actions related to and transformative of the logic.

The privileged logic of 'projectness'

The public funding of biomedical research worldwide is undergoing a transformation, whereby governments increasingly see their role in the allocation of public research funding to be the advancement of technological innovations associated with specific agendas such as economic growth and public health protection (The Danish Government 2003; Bouchard and Lemmens 2008). In this context of promotion of commercial research within public universities (see also Mirowski and Van Horn 2005) the activities of researchers have also changed, toward creating external alliances and presenting their activities in terms of projects oriented toward more or less unambiguous goals[4]. With projects set in specific time frames and with stated goals and objectives, it becomes possible to monitor research as it unfolds and to evaluate its process and results on the basis of its initial plans and objectives. Within this project form of organizing action, actors are to produce what the project aims at. John Law has suggested the term 'projectness' (Law 2002; Law and Singleton 2000) to identify a favored, singular version of the story of technological innovation, where technologies are developed as the result of a delimited time frame, clear goals and clever management (see Strauss 1988). I will use the term projectness to point to a certain contemporary and privileged logic which has shaped the way stem-cell science and potentially other strands of basic research interpellate patients. Specifying the potentiality of science in technological terms intensifies the production – through interpellation – of identities that are cast as potential users of such technologies (Oudshoorn and Pinch 2003). Future users, who in the present are possessors of heightened expectations and often of urgent needs, become highly manifest representations of future bedsides and future markets.

The work of forging durable relations to external parties as well as projected users is to be seen as an implicit part of the work that constitutes 'technoscience' (Latour 1987). Researchers have always had to operate as entrepreneurs (Latour 1988) or heterogeneous engineers (Law 2002). What can be argued to have changed is the increased visibility of and strategic attention to science as being in the business of forging relationships with society (Nowotny et al. 2001) and in the business of producing new technologies. In the area of the biosciences, this orientation promotes a new and more active role with regard to patients. Work done in 'the sociology of expectations' (Brown and Michael 2003) has already shown how hope and fear among the general public and patients are both products and drivers of research and innovation (e.g. Brown 2003; Moreira and Palladino 2005). Expectations constitute the projected future as it operates in the present (Brown and Michael 2003) and become central in forging the links that constitute technoscience – often independently of the actual fulfillment of these expectations and promises. When I use of the concept of 'projectness', it is to suggest that performing science in terms of a technology development project has a particular impact on the way in which promises are given and thus on the way in which 'communities of promise' (Brown 2003) are shaped. The promises given within a logic of projectness are already directed specifically at particular future users, who in turn come to feel obliged to respond not just to the promises of cures and therapies but also to the identities that they are promised. Promises taking the material form of lists of future users interpellate patients and their associations in very specific ways, as the following analysis will show.

The waiting list for a cure: performing stem cell research in project terms

Human embryonic stem cells (hESC) are cells that, given the right conditions (in a human uterus or in the laboratory), have the potentiality to become any cell in the human body. However, the research on hESC is concerned with the channeling of this potentiality into specific, stable cell lines of differentiated human tissues, which can be clinically applied to a number of illnesses and damages within the emergent field of regenerative medicine. The multipotency of stem cells is thus both the resource and the challenge for researchers within this field. However, the challenge of making specific the cells in the petri dish extends to the work of acquiring funding, mirroring the overall challenge for science in turning potentiality into marketable utility. Becoming every or any cell is not seen as a legitimate result within the frame of science as entrepreneurial projects: being *useful* in project terms means being useful for something or someone *specific*.

One central device in performing the potentiality of hESC research as leading to specific and useful end products is *the listing* of illnesses which, it is suggested, are or will become curable or treatable by stem cell technologies. Such lists can be found in scientific articles on stem cell research, in funding applications for stem cell research, and in mainstream media outlets. In the article often referred to as the one that heralded the arrival of a new medical paradigm with hESC research (Thomson et al. 1998), it was suggested that hESC would become useful for drug discovery and transplantation medicine; infertility treatment, juvenile diabetes and Parkinson's disease were more specifically listed as areas of application. The listing of illnesses has since been gradually extended. Looking at a Wikipedia entry on stem cell treatment, a list of no fewer than 15 potential treatments can be found (including cancer and baldness) (Wikipedia 2013). In some of these areas, therapeutic application is still some way off and the main association between a certain illness and a specific cell type is still located in the laboratory. In other areas, clinical studies are currently underway on human subjects (e.g. heart failure and osteoporosis; for patients' experiences with the former, see Huniche 2007). Listing potential areas of application can thus refer to very different levels of accomplishment with regard to the projected goal of regenerative medicine. How do such lists come into being within the research environment? In what follows, I move from a general description of stem cell research to the empirical field of Danish stem cell research as it unfolded in the early 2000s.

A number of basic researchers working with stem cells were interviewed about how they referred to particular areas of clinical application when applying for funds, writing articles or addressing various publics. One researcher working with dopamine-producing nerve cells reflected:

> I really think it is good to provide the clinical aim, but you shouldn't overlook the fact that if you have 2% dopamine producing cells [the cells that a person with Parkinson's disease lacks] out of the total cell population then it will not be wise to write an article that says a lot about Parkinson's and therapy (...). There is also politics to it, however, in that you want to sell the product that you are making. Especially in relation

> to the charities, of course, here we are pragmatists. They have an interest in reading something about therapies.
>
> (Interview with stem cell researcher)

For this researcher, the reference to clinical aims related to Parkinson's disease is a way of encompassing the interests of possible donors into publications and research proposals, even if the legitimacy of such claims might be open to criticism. He suggests that the reference to therapies – 'the products' – make the charities more likely to fund the research than a mere reference to the basic mechanisms currently studied in the laboratory. Other researchers interviewed had similar considerations:

> Funding from private charities is absolutely necessary to be able to do research ... It is easiest to get money if you are doing something which concerns disease in some way or another. You always write something in your research proposal about how you hope that this will lead to a cure for the disease. That is how it is, even if you know that it might not actually be within the timeframe of the three years you have drawn up ... This is the perspective which will get a patient association to fund your research. But it might actually be a much more fundamental thing [you wish to study].
>
> (Interview with stem cell researcher)

These researchers suggest that they have strategic considerations in relation to the naming of specific illnesses and the possibility that they may find a therapy or cure for these through their (often very basic) research. The research in this sense becomes a project of reaching certain therapeutic outcomes or even products for specific patient groups. Whether being asked by funding parties to describe outcomes of research or merely considering the possible publics who might read and act on their documents, the reference to diseases and therapeutic possibilities seems productive to these researchers in giving the research a more tangible sense of aim and legitimacy. The immense potentiality of stem cells is seen – both in the laboratory and discursively – as directed toward specific cell types. Thereby they are linked to specific diseases and patients, who thus come to be the ones for whom the research is useful – the prospective users of hypothetical technology. The research proposals and research articles not only identify certain patient groups but also aim at encouraging them to fund research. It is not solely the stem cell/researcher-nexus that defines this potential user – this is determined also by the existence of a *demand* for certain cell types:

> Everyone who works with stem cells throws themselves into the work of making the cell types which are on demand. [...] Often experts working on neural stem cells see that it would be wise if they could produce beta cells [for diabetes], which will gain them more publicity.
>
> (Interview with stem cell researcher)

Therefore the potentiality of stem cells is directed toward particular ends, partly through the calculations of researchers about meeting certain demands or market expectations. The experience that there are groups of patients who are waiting for cells, who are already prospective users of these cells, thus contributes to directing the multipotency of stem cells towards more specific ends. But who were these prospective users, how did they become defined as such, and in what ways did they relate to the potentiality of stem cell research?

Patient associations' engagement with stem cell research

The researchers quoted above suggested that the reference to specific illnesses and thus to patients provided a clear and legitimate aim by which their research could be presented and monitored as projects. I suggest that patients became interpellated by this logic as it was materialized in the listing of diseases, and that in their response to this hailing by the stem cell researchers they became the embodiment of an unfulfilled and persistent demand. Their responses to the listing of diseases were central for stem cell research to emerge as projects. However, they did not merely reproduce the logic of projectness, they also translated it in various ways. In the following I will look at specific ways in which Danish patient associations related to stem cell projects and how they came to regard themselves as prospective users of stem cell technologies. Furthermore, I shall explore how patient associations themselves intervened in the projects of research and how they sought to be incorporated into such lists.

Being on the list

A look at patient associations' web pages and other written sources produced by the associations demonstrated that the issue of stem cell research figured widely, but in very diverse ways[5]. In some associations, as in the Danish Multiple Sclerosis Society, most references to stem cell research were found in the 'questions and answers' section on the website, where patients and their relatives had posed questions to professionals about whether stem cell research might help cure multiple sclerosis now or in the future[6]. Being 'on the list' as a possible recipient of future stem cell therapies mobilized patients and relatives to pose questions. The patient association both responded to such mobilization by answering questions and participated in it by mediating and producing the texts that examined the current research projects and their projected goals. Websites of patient associations provided news articles referring to or reprinting national and international mainstream and scientific articles on the therapeutic potential of stem cell research, or more specific and self-produced material on the issue. Interviews with representatives from seven[7] of the identified associations revealed more nuances to the experience of being 'hailed' as a potential beneficiary through the listing of particular diseases. In particular, the media's presentation of the potentiality of stem cell research was in many interviews highlighted as particular points in time when both patients and the associations came to recognize themselves as connected to stem cell research. These media representations specified how and for whom the projects were or might be useful. The Parkinson's Association was one of the few associations found to be strongly engaged with stem cell research at the time, and in explaining this engagement the head of the secretariat said:

> We hear about it [stem cell research] through the press, television, and read in the newspapers, and then we become interested. Not least because initially three diseases are being mentioned: diabetes, Alzheimer's and Parkinson.
>
> (Interview, head of secretariat, Parkinson's Association)

Rather than being mobilized through direct relations with, for example, Danish stem cell researchers, it was the popular media that initially engaged the association with stem cell research.

For Finn Kristensen, President of the Juvenile Diabetes Research Foundation (JDRF) in Denmark, it was likewise the encounter with such lists of curative prospects for diabetes through stem cell research that prompted his engagement. When Kristensen learned that his son had juvenile diabetes, he started searching the Internet to learn more about the disease. He found material there suggesting that juvenile diabetes might in the near future be curable through stem cell therapies. Much of this material came from or referred to JDRF – the largest charity supporting research into diabetes and internationally involved in lobbying for legislation allowing and benefiting stem cell research.

> I did my research on the Internet and the articles and material found here [on the web-site of JDRF] compared to that from Diabetesforeningen [the Danish Association for Diabetes] was much more appealing in my view. Much more forward-looking and innovative.
>
> (Interview with Finn Kristensen, JDRF-dk)

For Kristensen, the online encounter with JDRF and its slogan, 'Dedicated to Finding a Cure', was an instant recognition of what *he* should be and how *he* should act as a father of a child with diabetes. This recognition was instrumental in prompting him to contact JDRF. Supported by Danish diabetes researchers already in receipt of research funding from the foundation, he started a Danish branch of JDRF, arranging charity events and promoting stem cell research through an active engagement in political debates.

How should we understand this instant recognition when someone is addressed through the mediation of stem cell projects? In her study of

American oncology research, Good (2001) has suggested that it is through 'the daily and global circulation of popular, business and medical knowledge' that the public, clinicians, and most notably, patients, are taken into what she terms 'the biotechnical embrace' – an affective and enthusiastic response to the projected possibilities of medical research (Good 2001). Patients and relatives do not just feel embraced by the media stories and so become enthusiastic and hopeful; the stories of stem cells 'call out to' them in such a way that they come to feel obligated to act to confirm that they are in fact the users of these projected technologies.

Interpellation is not about consciously deciding to confirm than one is the subject who has been summoned, but rather an instant recognition that one is related to and thus defined by specific entities in the world, for example stem cell research (Althusser 2005 [1971]; see also Law 2000, 2002). As I have already stressed, this does not mean that Science with a capital S is a coherent institution engaged in defining patients as future users. Science has as much at stake here as the subjects being interpellated. Without subjects responding affirmatively to the interpellation of the listing of diseases, stem cell research as projects with specific goals will cease to exist: without funds, without legitimacy. Although the recognition of oneself as the subject being addressed in Althusser's version is a causal relation, the following empirical analysis shows that, at the level of the associations, there were different ways of turning toward the interpellator when called. In the following, I describe three different responses from Danish patient associations: recognition, misrecognition and counter-interpellation.

Recognition: a demand for cells

As already indicated above, some associations did at the time engage further with stem cell research – in particular JDRF and the Parkinson Association. They responded to the interpellation affirmatively, 'Yes, we are in fact the ones who need such cures' and took organizational action in order to participate in making real such projected goals and by extension their identities as users of the technology. For the Parkinson's Association these activities included earmarked funding for stem cell research and lobbying for less restrictive legislation on the use of hESCs (e.g. for therapeutic cloning). JDRF.dk grew, as a new national charity, out of Finn Kristensen's experiences of being interpellated – and thus continued JDRF's international work of promoting stem cell research through both financial and political means. In understanding these affirmative responses, it is important to acknowledge that these two associations had in common the specific feature of knowing their patients as people lacking one specific type of cells and the bodily location of these absent cells. Being in possession of this knowledge and being already engaged in research activities related to cell therapy meant these associations were woven at the onset into an existing network of expectations. They were already interpellated[8] as prospective users of some kind of regenerative treatment. Rather than the interpellation by stem cell research being the first time that these patients and their associations were made the subjects of a regenerative cure for their disease, the listing of Parkinson's and diabetes by stem cell researchers confirmed an existing self-conception relating to past relations forged with research on neuro-transplantation. The Parkinson's Association had already been connected to these research projects. However, this line of research and the surrounding network of expectation faced major challenges. Results of clinical trials providing Parkinson's patients with dopamine-producing nerve cells from aborted fetuses provided the so-called proof-of-concept for cell-based replacement therapy, but did not provide either satisfactory clinical effects or solutions to the ethical and logistical problems entailed in making a steady supply of fetuses manageable (Lindvall and Björklund 2004). As the head of the secretariat said, neuro-transplantation of fetal tissue 'isn't a realistic approach, because it simply isn't possible to procure all these fetuses' (Interview 2006). Stem cell research could provide dopamine-producing cells for transplantation, which need not have to come from aborted fetuses but rather from cell lines produced from embryos or even adult tissue. Stem cell research was thus conceived as a possible restoration of the Parkinson's patients' relation to cell research and thus of the self-conception of Parkinson's patients as prospective users of curative, regenerative treatment. What could in theory be seen as shattering hopes or as the unveiling of an unrealistic hype becomes in practice a resource for the creation of a new hope (Brown and Michael 2003). The Parkinson's Association both confirmed the identity ascribed to them through the media presentation of them as being on the list and took on activities devoted to making this prediction realizable.

Misrecognition: diffuse demands, illegitimate projects

The media's influence on interpellation and the responses given at organizational level is thus related to bodily or material aspects that go beyond the mere experience of identification of the individual subject. This also counted in relation to the association that at this point in time misrecognized or was reluctant to respond affirmatively to the interpellation[9]. Although many patients – most notably those on the list of possible recipients – seemed to have recognized themselves as subjects of this research, other associations in fact saw their obligation as being to stand guard against such identification. They feared that hopes would be unrealistically raised among patients by putting too much faith in popularized and hyped accounts of something as intrinsically unpredictable as basic research (Brown 2003). Among these were the Alzheimer's Association and the Multiple Sclerosis Association, which, despite some interest from the patient and relatives' representatives, were reluctant to initiate any particular activities in this area. This organizational reluctance and the fear of hyping expectations were related to the lack of a demand for specific cells. Although both illnesses – Multiple Sclerosis and Alzheimer's – are neurodegenerative illnesses, the damages causing the diseases do not originate from one specific type of cell located in a specific area of the nervous system but rather from many different mechanisms located in different areas of the neural system. As expressed by the head of the research committee in the Alzheimer's Association:

> there is still a good distance to go before stem cells will be applicable to daily clinical practice in neurology. And even longer in relation to Alzheimer's disease because it is such a diffuse degenerative disease. If you take Parkinson's disease, it is one particular area that degenerates. It will be easier to intervene here. But with Alzheimer's much more knowledge is needed.
>
> (Interview 2006)

A patient representative from the Multiple Sclerosis Association recounted her own initial interpellation when hearing of stem cell research in the media and the subsequent rejection of her questions when talking to the medical professionals in the association:

> There was this television program where they talked about it [stem cell therapies]. Then I tried to do a bit of research into the area and I found that there was some research in progress in Sweden. […] But when I talked to some of the doctors and researchers I know their response was, no, it was way too diffuse, because no one knew where things happened when a person had Sclerosis. But it was doable for people with Parkinson's, because there you'd know where it [the degeneration] happened.
>
> (Multiple Sclerosis Association, interview 2006)

This patient representative kept reading about stem cell research, going to meetings, and presenting her insights to patient and professional representatives in the association. However, as organizations, neither of the two ventured to promote or engage further in stem cell research at this point in time.

For the associations the reason to engage was, therefore, related to the degree that they could legitimately argue that they needed a specific cell type located at a specific site in the body. Without the knowledge of which specific cells their patients needed, the associations found it illegitimate to raise the hopes of their patients and relatives by talking in terms of cures. The project of engaging in stem cell research became as diffuse as the illness itself. So while the media presentations of stem cell research did interpellate these patients and their associations, the patient associations misrecognized the legitimacy of the call. By this, I do not mean to suggest that the success or failure of interpellation depends on biology. Rather, biology – the issue of specifying certain cells – was at that time mobilized also by those being interpellated to forecast the possible stability or frailty of the identity they were being offered. By misrecognizing the call, they also performed another version of science, another logic, in which they designated research as a venture for more knowledge, distinguishable from its application in developing cures and technologies. Highlighting and raising user demand among patients was seen in this logic as potentially obstructive to scientific progress.

Counter-interpellation: getting on the list

The engagement of one of the other associations found to be active in relation to stem cell research, the Danish Spinal Cord Injuries Association (Foreningen af Rygmarvsskadede, RYK), had taken a slightly different path. This association had not initially participated in expectations of neuro-transplantation of fetal tissue, these technologies being concerned mainly with Parkinson's disease and diabetes. More importantly, the association had not regarded its task as being to represent any interest in curative treatments for spinal cord injuries. If an injured person had earlier asked the association about the possibility of curing the injury, this would have been promptly dismissed as illegitimate. However, this attitude and practice changed as a consequence of interaction with one researcher in particular, eventually leading to engagement with neuro-transplantation.

In the late 1980s, spinal cord injuries were not on the list of those possibly treatable by these future therapies. Nevertheless, some of the active members of the association discussed among themselves whether this transplantation approach could be applied to their type of neural injury. For each individual injury, they too suffered a loss of particular cells located at a particular site in the nervous system. This led them to approach a neurological researcher who was studying Parkinson's and neural regeneration. Their own account of this meeting, presented in the association's own journal, marks a turning point in their relation to science and for their collective identity:

> Once upon a time there was a researcher and four wheelchair users meeting up in an empty parking lot at Aarhus University campus. It was midsummer, 1988, and spirits were high. The researcher explained about new trials being carried out abroad transplanting immature nerve cells as a step on the way towards the cure of damages to the central nervous system. The trials dealt with Parkinson's disease. But why not a cure for persons with paraplegia and tetra? When would it be our turn? (Rasmussen 2001).

Although the researcher told them that injuries to the spinal cord always included damage to more than one type of tissue and that the relations between the location of the damage and the brain is complex, the researcher also agreed to take the question seriously even though his area of expertise was Parkinson's disease. As a direct consequence of this meeting, in 1990 and 1998 two scientific conferences on spinal cord repair were held in Denmark.

The results of the conferences were communicated to the members of the association as an article entitled, 'Will we ever walk?' and 'We will walk'. The change from a question to an assertive claim marked a change in the association's involvement in the research and a change in its identity. With the latter claim, 'We will walk', the association began a more direct engagement with regenerative research through active funding. Where they had initially been the interpellators of the researcher as the person who should get spinal cord injuries onto the list for neurological repair, they were now 'called in' by the same researcher to participate as partners in funding a PhD study on stem cells as a way to repair spinal cord injuries.

> We had to loosen up a bit on the demand for an achievable goal within a set timeframe. With stem cells this is not realistic. But we told ourselves, no one does any research on spinal cord injuries in Denmark at present, so we might make a difference.
>
> (RYK representative, interview 2006)

The association had initially maintained a policy of only supporting research projects that they were certain would result in something usable for people afflicted with a spinal cord injury, thus mirroring the political preference for scientific research as innovative projects. However, becoming involved with basic researchers meant that the uncertainties related to this kind of research began to be part of the considerations of the association, just as the hopes and expectations of the injured had found their way into the laboratories of the researchers. This transformation of the association from actively distancing itself from the hopeful assemblies of the injured forming around genetic and other biomedical research agendas to actively engaging in the establishment of research projects aimed at finding a cure did not happen in the Danish context without opposition, in particular from clinicians with relations to RYK. Much like the professional representatives of the Alzheimer's Association and the Multiple Sclerosis Association, the clinicians suggested that the hopes for a cure for spinal cord injuries generated by the hype of stem cells were unfounded and that such research would generate disappointment and use the resources for care in the wrong way. However, RYK, which is run only by people who themselves have a spinal cord injury, found no such conflict. In response to the 'false hopes' argument, they argued that the possibilities and hopes were not necessarily related to themselves. 'I am going to stay in this chair. It won't be us [being cured] [...] Our legs wouldn't cope, our psyche wouldn't cope – those that will benefit from this are not even injured yet!'. With this statement, they highlighted that becoming a prospective user of stem cell technology is not necessarily a personal identity. Rather, it is a collective identity, which includes future subjects and implies an obligation to work for them in the present. Interestingly, by becoming involved with research into neuro-transplantation and stem cell research, the very conception of what and whom the association represented seemed to change, as did the time frame of their engagement. Although initially engaging with science to get on the list and in practice also engaging with the format of projects, the members of this association nevertheless willingly accepted that they were involved in uncertain projects that might not directly benefit their own health. The very act of engagement thus interacts with and changes both what is seen to be useful and for whom it will be useful. The effects of interpellation and counter-interpellation are, therefore, not the mere reproduction of a logic of projectness through obedient subjection to the role of advocating users; interpellation, as I have used the term, also entails a reconfiguration or translation of both the subjects and the logic in question.

Discussion

In their extensive work on the French patient association AFM (Association française contre les myopathies), Rabeharisoa and Callon have highlighted several developments in the ways in which patient associations engage with research (Rabeharisoa 2003; Rabeharisoa and Callon 2004; Callon and Rabeharisoa 2008). One central change suggested has been the addition within these organizations of a logic of exploration, meaning engaging in more open-ended basic research, to the existing logics of exploitation, i.e. engaging in activities (research and other) with more immediate benefits for their patients (Rabeharisoa and Callon 2004). Likewise, Barbot has described how the notion of being 'an active patient' has changed in relation to the engagement of AIDS associations in France; from one in which the patient should engage to become knowledgeable about his or her own illness toward one where a patient should be active as an experimenter and knowledge producer (Barbot 2006). On the one hand, these observations correspond to the findings presented here; on the other hand, my results suggest that there are more nuances to the relationship between exploration and exploitation when we look at the dynamics between interpellator (science) and interpellated (patient associations). Science policy has become more oriented toward exploitation, thus promoting the view that scientists in the first instance direct their research toward specific, useful ends to attune research with public interests, legitimacy, and market opportunities. Currently, the logic of projectness and the preference for being able to identify prospective users is privileged within the larger assembly of biomedical research, not only within patient associations. This acute need for 'usefulness' has thus confirmed patient associations' call for a science that takes their needs into consideration rather than science for its own sake. On the other hand, it seems increasingly to have also become the task of patient associations to critically consider the legitimacy of the new and long sought-after identity as 'users' that they are promised. In my study this happens in the case of misrecognition, where the call was at the time seen as illegitimate, because no active use of stem cell technology is foreseeable for this patient group. The lists of future cures and therapies were in this case actually seen as obstructive to explorative research. In the case of RYK and counter-interpellation, the perceived obstacles to exploitation and usefulness for their patient group were what mobilized the association. To get 'on the list' and become engaged in research, the associations had to accept uncertainties, unclear time frames, and the fact that they as individual subjects might not be the ones who would benefit from the research. The case of RYK thus shows how engagement starting out within a logic of projectness can lead to a translation of what a project might be and how and for whom usefulness should be assessed.

My research thus suggests that when looking not just at the patient associations in isolation, but also at the nexus between science and patients, there is a privileged logic of projectness at play, and that this logic quite forcefully interpellates patients and their associations. My study also shows that this does not mean that patient associations are subject to this logic as a deterministic ideology, as their responses in various ways confirm, question or translate this logic. It is also clear that the responses may change over time, as new knowledge and techniques come into being: patients and their associations may move along the continuum, finding their hopes unanswered or new interpellations more legitimate. However, the initial, instant, and embodied attraction – the promise of identity – of these calls should not be overlooked. Although they raise hopes and expectations which often remain unfulfilled for the individual patient, they also mobilize patients to engage and, quite counter-intuitively, to become new advocates for more explorative and less project-like research.

In this chapter, I have used the concept of interpellation to analyze the engagement of patient associations with stem cell research. A more nuanced and less singular version of interpellation can help to demonstrate the variety in the relations forged between specific strands of basic research and specific patients and patient associations. It brings to our attention the ways in which certain privileged logics found within the emergent networks of biomedical research have subject effects, in the sense that such logics and their sociomaterial enactments hail individuals and demand that they respond by turning toward specific strands of research with the question 'Who? Me?' However, as I have sought to show, more than one response can be given to interpellation and patients themselves may very well act as the interpellators and not just those being subjectified by institutionalized powers. Although interpellation requires us to ask questions of ideology or logics and to acknowledge their involvement in creating subjects, it is the specificities of the responses we should focus our attention on if we wish to trace contemporary reconfigurations of the assemblages of biomedical science and technology.

Notes

1 This chapter is a slightly rewritten version of Langstrup 2011. Many thanks to the journal *Science, Technology & Human Values* for the permission to reprint this paper.

2 Althusser provides a list of such ideological state apparatuses including the church, the educational system, and the family (Althusser 2005 [1971]: 92).

3 The concept of interpellation has been deployed and discussed widely in post-structuralism (e.g. Zizek 1989) and elsewhere (e.g. Lévinas 1979). It is beyond the scope of this chapter to do justice to all the conceptual nuances suggested by these discussions.
4 In the Danish context the transformation of public science policy was stated with the catch-phrase 'from thought to invoice', underscoring the government's aim of furthering a more commercial and goal-directed orientation within publicly funded research (The Danish Government 2003).
5 Based on a search on the web pages of Danish patient associations in the winter of 2005–2006, I found nine associations that referred directly to stem cell research and the therapeutic possibilities this research might have for the disease in question: Danish Alzheimers Association, Danish Parkinson Association, Danish Cystic Fibrosis Association, Danish Heart Foundation, Danish Multiple Sclerosis Society, Danish Haemophilia Society, Danish Diabetes Assocation, Juvenile Diabetes Research Foundation in Denmark, and Danish Spinal Cord Injuries Association.
6 Looking at the answers given, the most frequent reply from specialist to patients and relatives was one explaining the basic science of stem cells, calling for patience from anyone waiting for a cure and underscoring the uncertainty and unpredictability of basic research.
7 Two associations were not included in the interview study. One, the Danish Diabetes Association, was in the process of shaping its policy in this area and found it premature to share these ongoing reflections and negotiations with outsiders, and the other, the Danish Haemophilia Society, did not respond to numerous invitations to join the study.
8 Althusser points out that subjects are always already interpellated (Althusser 2006 [1971]), but fails to discuss in what ways this interacts in practice with the specificities of the interpellation to be explained.
9 At the time of writing (2013), the Sclerosis Association – as the association is now called – is engaged more directly in both informing its members on ongoing research on stem cell therapy and sclerosis, funding basic and clinical stem cell studies, and recruiting members for an ongoing clinical study at Copenhagen University Hospital. More recent developments in the understanding of stem cells and sclerosis have thus moved the response of the Sclerosis Association in a more affirmative direction. The Alzheimer's Association is still less explicitly engaged with the subject, but has awarded a prominent stem cell researcher an honorary grant for his research on neurodegeneration and stem cells.

References

Althusser, Louis (2005 [1971]) Ideology and Ideological State Apparatuses (Notes toward an Investigation), in A. Sharma and A. Gupta (eds) *The Anthropology of the State: A Reader*, Malden, MA, Oxford and Carlton: Wiley-Blackwell, 86–111.

Barbot, Janine (2006) How to Build an 'Active' Patient? The Work of AIDS Associations in France, *Social Science and Medicine*, 62(3), 538–551.

Bouchard, Ron A. and Lemmens, Trudo (2008) Privatizing Biomedical Research: A 'Third Way', *Nature Biotechnology*, 26(1), 31–36.

Brown, Nik (2003) Hope against Hype: Accountability in Biopasts, Presents and Futures, *Science Studies*, 16(2), 3–21.

Brown, Nik and Michael, Mike (2003) A Sociology of Expectations: Retrospecting Prospects and Prospecting Retrospects, *Technology Analysis & Strategic Management*, 15(1), 3–18.

Brown, Phil; Zavestoski, Stephen; McCormick, Sabina; Mayer, Brian; Morello-Frosch, Rachel and Altman, Rebecca G. (2004) Embodied Health Movements: New Approaches to Social Movements in Health, *Sociology of Health & Illness*, 26(1), 50–80.

Butler, Judith (1997) *The Psychic Life of Power: Theories in Subjection*, Stanford: Stanford University Press.

Callon, Michel (1986) Some Elements of a Sociology of Translation: Domestication of the Scallops and the Fishermen of St Brieuc Bay, in J. Law (ed.) *Power, Action, and Belief: A New Sociology of Knowledge?* London: Routledge and Kegan Paul, 196–233.

—— (2003) The Increasing Involvement of concerned groups in R&D Policies: What Lessons for Public Powers?, in A. Guena, A.J. Salter and W.E. Steinmueller (eds) *Science and Innovation: Rethinking the Rationales for Funding and Governance*, Cheltenham: Edward Elgar, 30–68.

—— (2005) Disabled Persons of All Countries, Unite! in B. Latour and P. Weibel (eds) *Making Things Public: Atmospheres of Democracy*, Cambridge: MIT Press, 308–313.

Callon, Michel and Rabeharisoa, Vololona (2008) The Growing Engagement of Emergent Concerned Groups in Political and Economic Life: Lessons from the French Association of Neuromuscular Disease Patients, *Science, Technology, & Human Values*, 33(2), 230–261.

Epstein, Steven (1996) *Impure Science: AIDS, Activism, and the Politics of Knowledge*, Berkeley: University of California Press.

Good, Mary-Jo D. (2001) The Biotechnical Embrace, *Culture, Medicine and Psychiatry*, 25(4), 395–410.

Haraway, Donna (1997) *Modest_Witness@Second_Millennium.FemaleMan©_Meets_OncoMouse™*, New York: Routledge.

Hogg, Christine (1999) *Patients, Power & Politics: From Patients to Citizens*, London: Sage.

Hogg, Christine and Williams, Charlotte (2001) Whose Interests do Lay People Represent? Towards an Understanding of the Role of Lay People as Members of Committees, *Health Expectations*, 4(1), 2–9.

Horst, Maja (2003) *Controversy and Collectivity: Articulations of Social and Natural Order in Mass-mediated Representations of Biotechnology*, PhD Thesis, Doctoral School on Knowledge and Management, Copenhagen Business School.

—— (2007) Public Expectations of Gene Therapy: Scientifi c Futures and Their Performative Effects on Scientific Citizenship, *Science, Technology, & Human Values*, 32(2), 150–171.

Huniche, Lotte (2007) Med livet i hænderne: Kroniske hjertepatienters perspektiver på eksperimentel stamcellebehandling, in L. Koch and K. Høyer (eds) *Håbets teknologi: Samfundsvidenskabelige perspektiver på stamcelleforskning i Danmark*, København: Munksgaard, 225–250.

Landzelius, Kyra (2006) Introduction: Patient Organization Movements and New Metamorphoses in Patienthood, *Social Science & Medicine*, 62(3), 529–537.

Langstrup, Henriette (2011) Interpellating Patients as Users: Patient Associations and the Projectness of Stem Cell Research, *Science, Technology, & Human Values*, 36(4), 573–594.

Latour, Bruno (1987) *Science in Action*, Cambridge, MA: Harvard University Press.

—— (1988) *The Pasteurization of France*, Cambridge, MA: Harvard University Press.

Law, John (2000) On the Subject of the Object: Narrative, Technology, and Interpellation, *Configurations*, 8(1), 1–29.

___ (2002) *Aircraft Stories: Decentering the Object in Technoscience*, Durham, NC and London: Duke University Press.

Law, John and Singleton, Vicky (2000) Performing Technology's Stories: On Social Constructivism, Performance, and Performativity, *Technology and Culture*, 41(4), 765–775.

Lévinas, Emmanuel (1979) *Totality and Infinity: An Essay on Exteriority*, Boston, MA and Dordrecht: Kluwer Academic Publishers.

Lindvall, Olle and Björklund, Anders (2004) Cell Therapy in Parkinson's Disease, *NeuroRx*, 1(3), 382–393.

Mirowski, Philip and Van Horn, Robert (2005) The Contract Research Organization and the Commercialization of Scientific Research, *Social Studies of Science*, 35(4), 503–548.

Mol, Annemarie (2008) *The Logic of Care: Health and the Problem of Patient Choice*, London: Routledge.

Moreira, Tiago and Palladino, Paolo (2005) Between Truth and Hope: On Parkinson's Disease, Neurotransplantation and the Production of the 'Self', *History of the Human Sciences*, 18(3), 55–82.

Novas, Carlos (2006) The Political Economy of Hope: Patients' Organizations, Science and Biovalue, *BioSocieties*, 1(3), 289–305.

Nowotny, Helga; Scott, Peter and Gibbons, Michael (2001) *Re-Thinking Science: Knowledge and the Public in the Age of Uncertainty*, Cambridge: Polity Press.

Oudshoorn, Nelly and Pinch, Trevor (eds) (2003) *How Users Matter: The Co-Construction of Users and Technology*, Cambridge, MA: MIT Press.

Rabeharisoa, Vololona (2003) The Struggle Against Neuromuscular Disease in France and the Emergence of the 'Partnership Model' of Patient Organisation, *Social Science and Medicine*, 57(11), 2127–2136.

Rabeharisoa, Vololona and Callon, Michel (2002) The Involvement of Patients' Associations in Research, *International Social Science Journal*, 54(171), 57–63.

___ (2004) Patients and Scientists in French Muscular Dystrophy Research, in S. Jasanoff (ed.) *States of Knowledge: The Co-Production of Science and Social Order*, London: Sage, 142–160.

Rasmussen, Viggo (2001) *Gå Johnny*. Available online at: <http://ryk.dk/artikel/20/282> (accessed 15 August 2008).

Stockdale, Alan (1999) Waiting for the Cure: Mapping the Social Relations of Human Gene Therapy Research, *Sociology of Health & Illness*, 21(5), 579–596.

Strauss, Anselm (1988) The Articulation of Project Work: An Organizational Process, *The Sociological Quarterly*, 29(2), 163–178.

The Danish Government (2003) *Nye veje mellem forskning og erhverv: fra tanke til faktura – Regeringens handlingsplan*, Ministeriet for Videnskab, Teknologi og Udvikling.

Thomson, James A.; Itskovitz-Eldor, Joseph; Shapiro, Sander S.; Waknitz, Michelle A.; Swiergiel, Jennifer J.; Marshall, Vivienne S. and Jones, Jeffrey M. (1998) Embryonic Stem Cell Lines Derived from Human Blastocysts, *Science*, 282(5391), 1145–1147.

Wehling, Peter (2011) The 'Technoscientization' of Medicine and its Limits: Technoscientific Identities, Biosocialities, and Rare Disease Patient Organizations, *Poiesis & Praxis*, 8(2–3), 67–82.

Wikipedia *Stem cell therapy* (2013) Available online at: <http://en.wikipedia.org/wiki/Stem_cell_treatments> (accessed 30 May 2013).

Wood, Brian (2000) *Patient Power? The Politics of Patients' Associations in Britain and America*, Buckingham: Open University Press.

Zizek, Slavoj (1989) *The Sublime Object of Ideology*, London and New York: Verso Press.

10 Patient organizations as biosocial communities?

Conceptual clarifications and critical remarks[1]

Thomas Lemke

Introduction

After the start of the human genome project in 1990, media and public interest in molecular biology and genetics increased in the following years. Scientists working in the context of the project hoped to decipher the "book of life," but they also envisioned new medical options for the diagnosis and treatment of diseases. The press regularly reported new discoveries in the area of genetics (Gerhards and Schäfer 2006), and genetic modes of explanation gained more and more credibility in everyday culture (Nelkin and Lindee 1995; van Dijck 1998; Duden and Samerski 2007). One of the consequences of this "gene hype" (Fleising 2001) or "gene fetishism" (Haraway 1997: 141–148) was that not only specific and rather rare diseases but also forms of behavior and capacities like intelligence, aggressiveness, and sexual preference were conceived of as caused or at least significantly influenced by genetic factors (Wasserman and Wachbroit 2001; Pieri and Levitt 2008; Kim 2009).

In this historical constellation, the anthropologist Paul Rabinow coined the notion of biosociality in the early 1990s. He claimed that the human genome project and genetic research would give rise to a new social order in which the strict division between nature and culture would be overcome. According to Rabinow, biosociality denotes social identities and practices which refer to human nature as being culturally understandable and technologically re-formable. Rabinow's thesis has significantly shaped the scientific debate on the social, political, and ethical implications of bioscientific knowledge. It has been incorporated by many sociologists and anthropologists in empirical investigations examining developments in contemporary life sciences and assessing the social transformations brought about by increasing genetic knowledge (Hacking 2006; Atkinson et al. 2007; Gibbon and Novas 2008). In addition, in close connection with the related concepts of "biological" or "genetic citizenship", this concept has been widely used in order to understand and analyze the identities and activities of patient associations, and in particular their engagement with biomedical research (Petryna 2002; Heath et al. 2004; Rose and Novas 2005).

This chapter begins by highlighting the basic arguments and the central aspects of the biosociality thesis. I then explore notable receptions of this concept and the focus on self-help groups and patients' associations in the literature on biosociality. The third section points to some analytical problems and empirical shortcomings in the debate on biosociality. I concentrate on three apparent deficits: the narrowing of the biosocial problematic that is the result of the focus on patients' associations; the questionable idea of a stable and univocal biology as the basis for processes of identity formation; and finally, the lack of interest in power relations, which up until now have not been adequately addressed. The final part sums up the history of the concept of biosociality and evaluates its future perspectives.

Biosociality: two central arguments

Paul Rabinow's essay "Artificiality and Enlightenment: From Socio-Biology to Biosociality" (1996a) is one of the most influential contributions in science and technology studies to have been published in the past 20 years.[2] The notion of biosociality that Rabinow outlines in this essay joins together two central motifs that are repeatedly taken up and varied in the text. First, the neologism denotes conceptually the interaction and entanglement of life processes and social practices. "Biosociality" marks an epochal break, a new arrangement of the relation between nature and culture that is no longer characterized by a clear and univocal borderline between the two realms. Second, the notion refers to new forms of identity and the emergence of groups on the basis of biological knowledge. "Biosociality" attempts to account for novel alliances between patients, scientists, politicians, medical doctors, and biotech companies that give rise to new kinds of socialities formed around particular biological conditions. The two meanings are linked with one another, but the second one gained much more currency in the reception of Rabinow's contribution.

Rabinow's argument draws from the concept of biopower the French philosopher Michel Foucault developed in his work.[3] Foucault distinguished historically and analytically between different mechanisms of power opposing sovereign power to biopower. He uses this term to identify a form of power that has characterized Western modernity since the seventeenth century and which consists of two main dimensions: the disciplining of the individual body and regulation of the population (see Foucault 1980). Rabinow's thesis is that the two poles of "body" and "population" identified by Foucault are currently being "rearticulated," and that the human genome project and genome research play a decisive role in this process. According to Rabinow, a "post-disciplinary order" is developing that supersedes the strict division between nature and culture and is characterized by a new relationship towards processes of life. Rabinow argues that "our social and ethical practices change as this project [the Human Genome Project] advances" (1996a: 93). His ethnographic curiosity focuses on the question of how this happens (see also 1999: 12–13).

According to Rabinow's account, contemporary genetics revolutionize and transform social practices and life processes. Genetics operates – and this is a central difference between it and other natural sciences – on the micro-level of molecular intervention, and will therefore "be embedded throughout the social fabric" (Rabinow 1996a: 98). According to Rabinow, in the face of this epochal and comprehensive transformation, "new genetics" cannot be understood in the terms used in the past. As he sees it, we are no longer witnessing a biologization of the social, the translation of social projects into biological categories (as in the well-known models of socio-biology or social Darwinism), but a profound re-configuration of social relations by means of biology:

> In the future, the new genetics will cease to be a biological metaphor for modern society and will become instead a circulation network of identity terms and restriction loci, around which and through which a truly new type of autoproduction will emerge, which I call "biosociality". If socio-biology is culture constructed on the basis of a metaphor of nature, then in biosociality nature will be modeled on culture understood as practice. Nature will be known and remade through technique and will finally become artificial, just as culture becomes natural.
>
> (ibid.: 99)

Rabinow's diagnosis of a "dissolution of the category of 'the social'" (ibid.) and his call for a readjustment of the notion of society as "the whole way of life of a people" (ibid.: 99; see also Rabinow 1989) draws on several intuitions from the field of science and technology studies. Many authors working in this tradition treat nature and society not as two separated and isolated realms but as a continuum of hybrids and networks (Latour 1983; Callon 1986; Law 1987; Haraway 1991). In this perspective, the notion of society is seen as something to be avoided or abandoned, given the multiple and diverse processes of cooperation and translation between social and natural actors and networks. This also holds true for the concept of nature, if nature is understood as an autonomous ontological sphere. Science and technology studies stress the complex interactions between nature and society that render impossible any neat assignment or fundamental categorization.

Rabinow's notion of biosociality does not only refer to the idea of a new relation between nature and culture. The concept also points to "the likely formation of new group and individual identities and practices arising out of these new truths" (1996a: 102) in the context of genome research. Rabinow expects more and more precise genetic tests to be available in the future, which will make it possible to detect disease risks and will finally help to prevent the emergence of disease or make early treatment of symptoms possible. Technological innovations and increasing scientific knowledge will, in Rabinow's view, provide the material conditions for new forms of sociality, identity politics, and modes of representation that are based on knowledge about bodily attributes and genetic characteristics and will shape the relationships of individuals to themselves and others:

> [I]t is not hard to imagine groups formed around the chromosome 17, locus 16, 256, site 654, 376 allele variant with a guanine substitution. Such groups will have medical specialists, laboratories, narratives, traditions, and a heavy panoply of pastoral keepers to help them experience, share, intervene, and "understand" their fate.
>
> (ibid.: 102)

Thus, the biosociality thesis in Rabinow's account is closely linked to a two-pronged historical discontinuity. The re-articulation of nature and society is complemented by the idea of the emergence of new social identities based on of biological knowledge. These two developments are intimately related. The increasing artificiality of nature makes new forms of sociality possible, constituted by shared biological features. However, in spite of the strong accent he put on discontinuities and disruptions, Rabinow was cautious enough not to overemphasize the historical break. Quite on the contrary, he stressed that "older cultural classifications will be joined by a vast array of new ones, which will cross-cut, partially supersede, and eventually redefine the older categories" (ibid.: 105). In the same vein, Rabinow partly took back the strong thesis of a departure from disciplinary society by stating that "older forms of cultural classification of bio-identity such as race, gender, and age have not any more disappeared than medicalization and normalization have" (ibid.: 103).[4] Rabinow does not assume a process of succession or dissolution but rather a reciprocal interaction in which "post disciplinary practices will co-exist with disciplinary technologies" (ibid.).

Reception: patients' associations as biosocial communities

Many authors have picked up and further developed Rabinow's notion of biosociality, using it for empirical research. While its reception has been quite diverse and heterogeneous, it is nevertheless possible to discern a specific focus. Most of these works have not concentrated on the constitution of individual and collective identities through expert discourse and medical authorities. Instead, research on biosociality has put an emphasis on processes of subjectivation "from the bottom up". Sociologists and anthropologists working on biosocialities have been primarily interested in new forms of solidarity and sociality arising from shared knowledge of genetic properties and risks, communication of medical options for treating diseases, and engagement with ethical conflicts arising for decision making (see Gibbon and Novas 2008; Hacking 2006).[5]

The result was that research on biosociality focused on the practices of self-help groups and patient advocacy. These works stressed the increasing importance of these groups for the production, legitimization, and appropriation of genetic knowledge or biomedical knowledge in general. Rabinow himself had suggested this focus in the essay, in which he mentions as "examples" of biosocial communities "neurofibromatosis groups whose members meet to share their experiences, lobby for their disease, educate their children, redo their home environment" (Rabinow 1996a: 102).

It is possible to discern three aspects or arenas of the work of self-help groups and patients' associations that were taken up by empirical studies on biosociality.[6] First, self-help groups and patients' associations lobby to increase public interest in their concerns and to attract state funding for research projects related to their respective causes. Their goal is to sensitize the public to the concerns of the ill and their suffering, and to influence policymakers.

A good example of this form of political engagement is an initiative in the USA that was founded by parents whose children were suffering from epidermolysis bullosa (EB), a debilitating genetic condition that leads to wounded, blistered skin. The parents' group formed the core of an activist group known as DEBRA (the Dystrophic Epidermolysis Bullosa Research Association). In the late 1970s, a group of parents brought their children into the Senate Office Building on Capitol Hill to demonstrate to members of Congress the consequences of the disease and the suffering of their children. The encounter had a significant impact. Senators secured funding for biomedical research on EB. The engagement of DEBRA went beyond lobbying for resources to treat a so-called orphan disease:

> Members of DEBRA were subsequently instrumental in creating a registry of EB patients' tissue samples, which have been crucial to laboratory research on the disease. In forging alliances with legislators … and with biomedical researchers, members of DEBRA and other genetic advocacy groups are making citizenship claims on behalf of their genetically vulnerable offspring.
>
> (Heath et al. 2004: 155)

A second arena of activism concerns the struggle against material or ideological restrictions on access to medical technologies and bio-scientific knowledge. Self-help groups and patient organizations fight restrictive or exclusive concepts of intellectual property in the domain of biomedical and genetic research. Their concern is also directed against the use of genetic knowledge solely for commercial purposes, which can lead to limitations on further research and to increases in the cost of the development and dissemination of diagnostic and therapeutic devices.

To avoid these disadvantages, the advocacy group PXE International, which brings together parents with children suffering from pseudodoxanthoma elasticum (PXE), a rare genetic condition that affects elastic connective tissue, proposed a model of patenting that has been adopted by other advocacy organizations seeking treatment for rare genetic conditions. The agreement ensures open access to the gene for researchers who wish to work in this area, and it prevents royalty fees that might increase the costs of genetic testing. PXE International was founded by Pat and Sharon Terry, whose children are affected by the disease. The organization built up a tissue registry and documented family pedigrees. The Terrys were also active in research on the PXE gene, and did voluntary work in a laboratory in Boston. Their efforts were finally successful:

> In June 2000 Sharon Terry was a co-author on two of the three scientific journal articles announcing the discovery of a gene for PXE. PXE International and the University of Hawaii have agreed to file their application for the PXE gene as co-inventors.
>
> (Heath et al. 2004: 164; see also Novas 2006)

A third field of engagement on the part of self-help groups and patient organizations is their participation in ethics committees and parliamentary deliberation, as well as the drafting of guidelines for the regulation of technological procedures such as genetic testing (Rabeharisoa and Callon 1999; Rabinow 1999; Heath et al. 2004; Rose and Novas 2005). Advocacy groups on Huntington's disease, a genetic disorder that leads to physical and mental deterioration, play a paradigmatic role in this context. The "international guidelines," which consist of recommendations for human genetics counseling and the technical implementation of the genetic test, were drawn up by a committee made up of members of the international Huntington disease community and research groups (International Huntington Association and the World Federation of Neurology Research Group on Huntington's Chorea 1994). In the mid-1980s an indirect genetic test became available, and the two organizations set up a commission to regulate the use of the test. The recommendations of that commission were passed in 1989 and published by important medical journals. This body of rules was revised after the discovery of the "Huntington gene" in 1993. Its regulations are still valid today. This regulatory framing, and the recommendation that genetic counseling and psychosocial support should be combined, became a model for other diseases and it has been adopted by a number of self-help groups (Engel and Lohkamp 2003; see also Lemke 2004).

To sum up, we can conclude that studies working with the notion of biosociality have focused on the increasing significance of patient organizations and self-help groups for the fi nacing, coordination, and regulation of genetic research. These studies have examined how these direct alliances and networks between medical researchers and scientists on the one hand and patients and their families on the other were created, how forms of individual and collective identity were shaped by them, and how new practices of political and social engagement emerged (see Rabeharisoa and Callon 1999, 2002).

Blind spots: the limits of biosociality

Research on biosociality has focused on collective forms of action, group identities, and the political activism or social engagement of patients' associations and self-help groups. Studies in this area have explored the motifs that guide their work, the alliances they form, and the channels and networks they mobilize in articulating their interests.

However, these studies are also characterized by some empirical shortcomings and analytical deficits. As mentioned above, I will concentrate on three of these weaknesses: the narrowing issue of biosociality that is the result of the focus on patient associations; the questionable idea of a stable and univocal biology that is taken to be the basis of processes of identity formation; and finally the failure to examine power relations, which up until now have not been adequately addressed in the discourse on biosociality.

Biosociality narrowed down

Reception of the biosociality thesis is marked by a double limitation. First, it has to be noted that the research often takes into account only a fragment of the biosocial problem. Biosociality tends to be equated with forms of patient advocacy. The discussion so far has focused on collectives characterized by membership rules and organizational borders. The privileged status of patient advocacy has a downside: many other relevant empirical fields and questions are not or not sufficiently addressed. Scott Vrecko rightly notes that studies following Rabinow

> overlook the many other social (trans)formations that Rabinow suggests may arise in relation to the new biosciences. The cultural practices and forms Rabinow mentions as subject to biosocial reorganization are not only patient groups, but also educational programmes, the design and planning of homes, tastes and practices of consumption, the structure of industry … as well as linguistic and labour practices.
>
> (Vrecko 2008: 53)

It must be stressed that the research focus on patient organizations only makes it possible to account for a limited spectrum of ways in which identities are shaped by genetics; in addition, the critique extends to the often one-sided and selective way in which these organizations are analyzed.

The growing literature on genetic or biological citizenship, in particular, presents an astonishingly one-sided account of the role of self-help groups and patient associations. It promotes a political optimism that associates biological citizenship with the emergence of new forms of participation and democratic action subverting the dividing line between lay and expert knowledge (Lemke and Wehling 2009; Wehling 2011).

However, significant conflicts and tensions can arise between biomedical research and commercial motives on the one hand and the interests of the patients and their families on the other. Self-help groups and patients' associations have undergone a significant change in recent years. By addressing research interests and commercial imperatives, they risk losing their independence and freedom of action. Medical experts often influence the agenda of patient support groups and dominate important committees, especially where research funding and public education are concerned (Kerr 2003). Their chronic shortage of funds and the search for social recognition make patients' associations susceptible to a dynamic that leads them away from the initial idea of self-representation and championing themselves. While the notion of self-help in the medical realm was once fueled by the objective of bringing patients together so that they could fight for their needs, rights, and interests, many self-help groups today have become part of a biomedical network that is shaped by the career interests of researchers and the profit motives of the pharmaceutical industry (Health Action International 1999; Grüber and Wagenmann 2002; Breast Cancer Action Germany 2006).

Furthermore, it has to be noted that the studies concentrate on some patient organizations while neglecting others. The literature on biosociality focuses on groups and movements fighting for medical solutions to health problems, while oppositional groups and those critical of medical expertise and solutions do not resonate in the literature. Phil Brown and his colleagues have distinguished between three types of health social movements: first, "Health Access Movements" which seek equitable access to health care; second, "Embodied Health Movements" which address disease, disability, or illness experience by challenging established science on etiology, diagnosis, treatment, and prevention; and third, "Constituency-Based Health Movements" addressing health inequality and inequity based on categories such as race, ethnicity, gender, class, or sexuality differences (Brown et al. 2008). The three types of health movements are characterized by rather different relations to science and biomedicine; some of them actively oppose the definitions of disease promoted by mainstream science and the modes of explanation offered to them by genetics (Wehling 2011).

In a similar vein, Bill Hughes contrasts work in the wake of biosociality with approaches that derive from the field of disability studies. This direction of research rejects the biomedical paradigm and understands disability primarily as a social phenomenon. While disability studies stress the historical contingency and social construction of disability, referring to processes of oppression, normalization and exclusion, research on biosociality is mostly linked to the biomedical model that takes disability to be a physical or mental defect originating in an individual body:

> Biological citizens and biosocial groups begin with a clearly articulated and medicalised concept of self-identity. Such individuals and groups admit to and embrace a "vital deficit". Proponents of the DPM [Disabled Peoples's Movement] work hard to abrogate the negative ontology that has haunted disability throughout modernity. They do so because this negativity has its historical roots in the value-laden and socially tyrannical medical distinction between the normal and the pathological.
>
> (Hughes 2009: 686; see also Palladino 2002: 158, n. 23)

The nature of society

The search for a basis for identity building and strategies of political debate refers back to the more fundamental question of the ideas of biology and nature that inform the concept of biosociality and how they shape its reception. Reading the literature on biosociality, one sometimes gets the impression that biological criteria are regarded as a fixed and univocal material foundation for moral problematizations, political activism, and social mobilization. The research often assumes that the building of identities and the processes of political articulation rely on objective and given biological features that are shared by certain individuals and groups. This assumption is quite debatable. To start with, biology is itself marked by processes of development and is open for strategies of intervention and optimization. Also, the distinction between biological and non-biological factors and features is certainly not trivial and self-evident, but depends on predominant modes of interpretation and explanation. The "new truths" Rabinow refers to (1996a: 102) are neither simply given nor uncontested. Quite the contrary: the definition of diseases, the explanation of causal mechanisms, and the suggestion of strategies of intervention are scientifically and medically highly controversial fields (Lemke and Wehling 2009: 95; Wehling 2011).

Ironically, the idea of a univocal and stable biology contradicts central intuitions of the biosociality thesis, which stresses the tendency to dissolve the separation between nature and culture. As Vrecko rightly notes, Rabinow's essay "not only suggests that biological knowledge has an effect on social processes, but also that knowledges of and practices relating to the biological are affected by social concerns and forms" (Vrecko 2008: 53). The reception puts the accent again on the side of nature, by presenting biology as the basis for identity and collective action. It systematically disregards the complex associations between nature and culture that no longer allow for any hierarchical order or structural differences.

This theoretical regression is also visible in the fact that practices of biosocialization are understood as social practices only. Works that make use of the notion of biosociality focus on the emergence or transformation of patient groups, their self-image, and forms of action as a consequence of genetic knowledge and clinical research. However, the collective in question is mostly conceived of as an exclusively human collective. In this perspective, activity is thought to be a privilege of humans while technological artifacts or non-human beings like genes or animals are taken to be passive. Here again, we can note a limitation that has arisen from a failure to consider insights from science and technology studies (Barad 2007; Latour and Weibel 2005; Bennett 2010). As Michel Callon and Vololona Rabeharisoa rightly stress, non-human actors do have an important role in these biosocial processes:

> [T]his socialization ... is mainly effected by nonhumans. They are the ones that by circulating and linking heterogeneous entities produce and determine the shape of networks of alliances and solidarity. For example, the gene, whose deletions are responsible for the spinal muscular atrophy (SMA) disease, links patients and their families to various actors, including the researchers at the Necker Hospital who took samples of their DNA and ended up locating and identifying the gene, the clinicians who performed prenatal tests, the researchers who published articles on the activity of proteins produced by the gene or worked on models of transgenic mice, and so forth.
>
> (Callon and Rabeharisoa 2008: 240)

Stefan Beck (2011: 99–101) has made a similar point. He argues that users of the concept of biosociality might well be in danger of falling victim to the widespread ontological individualism of mainstream Western social science. What might be overlooked are relations and modalities of the social that owe their existence to alternative socialities not grounded in "society" but in heterogeneous material-discursive assemblages.

The power of identity

The point of departure of the debate on biosociality was an update and reformulation of the Foucauldian analysis of biopower. However, there is hardly any interest in the literature in investigating how contemporary power relations are transformed by the generation and circulation of genetic knowledge (see Rommetveit 2009: 180–181). Moral problematizations and ethical conflicts take the place of the analysis of forms of exclusion, discrimination and domination.

The fact that power relations have not been adequately addressed in the analysis of biosocial communities is the result of a series of blind spots. Kaushik Sunder Rajan has pointed to the specific conditions and limits of the notion of biosociality. He shows on the basis of ethnographic studies in India and the United States how, in the global capitalist economy, the improvement of the living conditions or the reduction of the suffering of some is intimately connected to the systematic exploitation of the bodies and the impairment of the health of others. Those who participate as "volunteers" in clinical studies in India and expose their bodies as fields of experimentation for biomedical trials are unlikely to profit from new therapies that might come out of this research: "The experimental subject ... is a condition of possibility for biosociality and the neo-liberal therapeutic consumer" (Sunder Rajan 2008: 178). There are two forms of risks involved here. While according to Sunder Rajan the biosocial subject uses risk information to modify itself and to build up new collective subjects, the experimental subject-position is "merely risked" (ibid.: 161) and there is, he argues, a structural impossibility of "such a figure being a *political* subject" (ibid.: 178–179).

In a similar vein anthropologist Nancy Scheper-Hughes, writing on the mechanisms of the organ trade and the global organ market, notes that life-saving measures for one person demand a bodily sacrifice of self-mutilation by another. While many individuals have benefitted enormously from the possibility of getting the organs they need, she demands that we should reflect on the violence associated with many of these new transactions which establish new relations of exploitation and inequality. As she puts it, "one man's biosociality is another woman's biopiracy" (Scheper-Hughes 2005: 150; see also 164).

Furthermore, we have to be aware that the re-articulation of identities on the basis of biological knowledge is not the exclusive domain of the self-organized practices of patient organizations. The new or transformed forms of identity or modes of action are to a significant degree determined by expert discourses. Media reports, internet publications, health education, medical guides, and popular science books contribute to the ways in which individuals take up genetic explanations and interpretations and integrate them in their everyday life (Oudshoorn and Somers 2007). One example is the growing market in direct-to-consumer genetic tests. While most of the genetic tests available today target certain rare diseases, the diagnostic industry is also addressing more widespread diseases that are often influenced by lifestyle or environmental factors. They offer predictive testing for breast cancer, thrombosis or osteoporosis and many other diseases. In this context, the promotion of biosocial identities becomes part of an explicit marketing strategy that is presented as a democratization of genetics. Anne Wojcicki, one of the founders of the globally operating genetic diagnostic enterprise 23andMe, sees a bright future ahead: "We envision a new type of community where people will come together around specific genotypes, and these artificial barriers of country and race will start to break down" (quoted by Weiss 2008).[7]

"Afterword"

In the epilogue ("Afterword: Concept work") of a volume edited by Sahra Gibbon and Carlos Novas on the notion of biosociality (Gibbon and Novas 2008), Rabinow has reviewed the reception of his concept. He points to the historical context in which the notion was coined and to its implicit limits. The thesis of "biosociality" was, Rabinow suggests, intimately linked to the scientific dynamic of the human genome project and the medical expectations and hopes that went along with it: "It may be that the 1990s will be seen as the Golden Age of Molecular Biosociality. There was hope, there was progress, there was a reason to be urgent even strident – there were reasons to want to be biosocial" (Rabinow 2008: 190).

In retrospect, Rabinow now argues, this scenario was far too optimistic. The sequencing of the human genome showed that genotype and phenotype are only in very few cases linked in a straightforward and unidirectional way. The results of genomic research challenged the so-called "central dogma" of molecular genetics that had determined the research agenda since the beginnings of genetic technology in the 1970s. According to this dogma, every gene carries information for the building of a protein. It became clear that such a reductionist understanding of gene function and gene regulation had to be replaced by more differentiated concepts. Genes are not usually determining factors; rather, their activity is influenced to a considerable degree by other genetic and cellular, but also by developmental processes and environmental factors (Oyama 2000; Neumann-Held and Rehmann-Sutter 2006). The increasing insight into the complexity of biological regulation supports a more cautious assessment of the future diagnostic and therapeutic options of molecular medicine (Lock 2005; Wynne 2005). Rabinow's recent conclusion sounds rather sober: "the hopes and hype of the genomic decade have failed to provide adequate diagnostic or risk assessment tools or treatments based on them" (2008: 192).

In spite of these displacements and developments, the notion of biosociality remains in Rabinow's reading an important tool for the analysis of the social implications of genomic research and the assessment of its scientific importance. Rabinow stresses that the concept was not intended to represent an epochal or universal notion, but was put forward as a heuristic instrument to assist understanding of the specific relations between genetic knowledge and genetic technologies on the one hand and the emergence of new individual and collective identities on the other. According to Rabinow, the obvious limits of the notion are at the same time a conclusive proof of its enduring analytic fertility: "These limitations were a confirmation of the approach not its refutation. Inquiry reveals specificities and limits, an excellent definition of critical thinking" (ibid.: 191).

We may easily subscribe to this assessment. However, it is more a programmatic claim than an empirical statement. As we have seen, the concept of biosociality is often used in research in a one-sided and selective way so that important dimensions of the biosocial problematic cannot be grasped. To realize the analytical potential of the concept, we must first give up the privileged treatment of genetic factors and features in explanations provided of the development of diseases and the emergence of identities (see also Kliems 2008). Beyond this, it is necessary for research on biosocialities to break with the empirical fixation on patient advocacy groups, to question essentialist concepts of a stable and univocal biology, and to explicitly address relations of power and dominance in the analysis of how collective and individual identities are shaped. For the study of patient associations, the critical review of the concept of biosociality and its reception in social science means trying to understand the interrelations of such associations with biomedical knowledge in a more comprehensive and multi-faceted manner. Returning to the original intention of the concept as outlined above means accounting for the mutual co-constitution of the "social" and the "biological". Therefore, biomedical knowledge is not one-sidedly responsible for constituting and transforming the identities of patients and their organizations; simultaneously, the ways in which medical research is conducted, interpreted, and applied are themselves shaped by various contexts and social factors, such as the needs and hopes of patients or the visions and interests of scientific experts.

Notes

1 I would like to thank Michael Schedelik for helping to prepare the manuscript and Gerard Holden who copy-edited the text.
2 The essay was first published in 1992 in a collection of articles edited by Jonathan Crary and Samuel Kwinter under the title *Incorporations*.
3 Rabinow is not only an eminent social scientist working on biotechnological innovations (1996b; 1999; Rabinow and Dan-Cohen 2005) but also one of the most important interpreters and editors of Michel Foucault's work in the Anglophone world (see Rabinow 1984; Dreyfus and Rabinow 1982).
4 In *French DNA* Rabinow points to a decisive difference between "older" markers of identity and forms of "biosociality". Here, he uses the term to mean "a biologization of identity different from the older biological categories of the West (gender, age, race) in that it is understood as inherently manipulable and re-formable" (1999: 13).
5 See, for example, the formulations by Margaret Lock, Ian Hacking, Veena Das and Renu Addlakha: "possibilities for new forms of identity making on the basis of shared knowledge about genes" (Lock 2005: 50); "societies formed around a biological condition" (Hacking 2006: 91); "the emergence of associational communities around particular biological conditions" (Das and Addlakha 2001: 511).
6 See for the following Kollek and Lemke 2008: 187–191.
7 I am grateful to Barbara Prainsack for pointing me to the biosocial dimensions of the genetic diagnostic industry.

References

Atkinson, Paul; Glasner, Peter and Greenslade, Helen (eds) (2007) *New Genetics, New Identities*, London: Routledge.
Barad, Karen (2007) *Meeting the Universe Halfway: Quantum Physics and the Entanglement of Matter and Meaning*, Durham, NC, London: Duke University Press.
Beck, Stefan (2011) Staging Bone Marrow Donation as a Ballot: Reconfiguring the Social and the Political Using Biomedicine in Cyprus, *Body & Society*, 17(2–3), 93–119.
Bennett, Jane (2010) *Vibrant Matter: A Political Ecology of Things*, Durham, NC and London: Duke University Press.

Breast Cancer Action Germany (2006) Ein anderes Rezept: Fundraising und Ethik in Frauengesundheitsorganisationen. Berlin: Breast Cancer Action Germany. Available online at: <www.bcaction.de/pdf/alternativen1.pdf> (accessed 13 March 2013).

Brown, Phil; Zavestoski, Stephen; McCormick, Sabrina; Mayer, Brian; Morello-Frosch, Rachel and Altman, Rebecca (2008) Embodied Health Movements: New Approaches to Social Movements in Health, in P. Brown (ed.) *Perspectives in Medical Sociology*, 4th edition, Long Grove, IL: Waveland Press, 521–538.

Callon, Michel (1986) Some Elements of a Sociology of Translation: Domestication of the Scallops and the Fishermen of St. Brieuc Bay, in J. Law (ed.) *Power, Action and Belief: A New Sociology of Knowledge?* London: Routledge, 196–233.

Callon, Michel and Rabeharisoa, Vololona (2008) The Growing Engagement of Emergent Concerned Groups in Political and Economic Life: Lessons from the French Association of Neuromuscular Disease Patients, *Science, Technology & Human Values*, 33(2), 230–261.

Crary, Jonathan and Kwinter, Sanford (eds) (1992) *Incorporations (Zone 6)*, New York: MIT Press.

Das, Veena and Addlakha, Renu (2001) Disability and Domestic Citizenship: Voice, Gender, and the Making of the Subject, *Public Culture*, 13(3), 511–531.

Dreyfus, Hubert L. and Rabinow, Paul (1982) *Michel Foucault: Beyond Structuralism and Hermeneutics*, Chicago, IL: The University of Chicago Press.

Duden, Barbara and Samerski, Silja (2007) "Pop genes": An Investigation of "the Gene" in Popular Parlance, in R. V. Burri and J. Dumit (eds) *Biomedicine as Culture. Instrumental Practices, Technoscientific Knowledge, and New Modes of Life*, New York and London: Routledge, 167–189.

Engel, Stefan and Lohkamp, Christine (2003) Die Möglichkeiten von Selbsthilfegruppen bei der Erarbeitung von Richtlinien für die Genetische Diagnostik, *Medizinische Genetik*, 15, 72–76.

Fleising, Usher (2001) In Search of Genohype: A Content Analysis of Biotechnology Company Documents, *New Genetics and Society*, 20(3), 239–234.

Foucault, Michel (1980) *The History of Sexuality*, Vol. 1. *An Introduction*, New York: Pantheon.

Gerhards, Jürgen and Schäfer, Mike S. (2006) *Die Herstellung einer öffentlichen Hegemonie: Humangenomforschung in der deutschen und in der US-amerikanischen Presse*, Wiesbaden: VS Verlag.

Gibbon, Sahra and Novas, Carlos (eds) (2008) *Biosocialities, Genetics and the Social Sciences: Making Biologies and Identities*, London and New York: Routledge.

Grüber, Kathrin and Wagenmann, Uta (2002) *Zwischen Kompetenz und Instrumentalisierung. Selbsthilfegruppen und biomedizinische Forschung*, Berlin: Institut Mensch, Ethik und Wissenschaft/Gen-ethisches Netzwerk.

Hacking, Ian (2006) Genetics, Biosocial Groups, and the Future of Identity, *Daedalus*, 135(4), 81–95.

Haraway, Donna (1991) *Simians, Cyborgs, and Women: The Reinvention of Nature*, London and New York: Routledge.

—— (1997) *Modest_Witness@Second Millenium.FemaleMan©_Meets_Oncomouse™*, New York and London: Routledge.

Health Action International (1999) *The Ties that Bind? Weighing the Risks and Benefits of Pharmaceutical Industry Sponsorship*, Amsterdam: HAI.

Heath, Deborah; Rapp, Rayna and Taussig, Karen-Sue (2004) Genetic Citizenship, in D. Nugent and J. Vincent (eds) *A Companion to the Anthropology of Politics*, Malden, MA: Blackwell, 152–167.

Hughes, Bill (2009) Disability Activisms: Social Model Stalwarts and Biological Citizens, *Disability & Society*, 24(6), 677–688.

International Huntington Association and the World Federation of Neurology Research Group on Huntington's Chorea (1994) Guidelines for the Molecular Genetics Predictive Test in Huntington's Disease, *Neurology*, 44, 1533–1536.

Kerr, Anne (2003) Genetics and Citizenship, *Society*, 40(6), 44–50.

Kim, Yong-Kyu (2009) (ed.) *Handbook of Behavior Genetics*, 3rd edition, Luxemburg, MN and Berlin: Springer.

Kliems, Harald (2008) Vita Hyperactiva: ADHS als biosoziales Phänomen, in J. Niewöhner; C. Kehl and S. Beck (eds) *Wie geht Kultur unter die Haut? Emergente Praxen an der Schnittstelle von Medizin, Lebens- und Sozialwissenschaft*, Bielefeld: Transcript Verlag, 143–169.

Kollek, Regine and Lemke, Thomas (2008) *Der medizinische Blick in die Zukunft. Gesellschaftliche Implikationen prädiktiver genetischer Tests*, Frankfurt am Main and New York: Campus.

Latour, Bruno (1983) Give Me a Laboratory and I Will Raise the World, in K. D. Knorr-Cetina and M. J. Mulkay (eds) *Science Observed*, Beverly Hills, CA: Sage, 141–170.

Latour, Bruno and Weibel, Peter (eds) (2005) *Making Things Public: Atmospheres of Democracy*, Cambridge, MA: MIT Press.

Law, John (1987) Technology and Heterogeneous Engineering: The Case of the Portuguese Expansion, in W. E. Bijker; T. P. Hughes and T. Pinch (eds) *The Social Construction of Technological Systems: New Directions in the Sociology and History of Technology*, Cambridge, MA: MIT Press, 111–134.

Lemke, Thomas (2004) *Veranlagung und Verantwortung: Genetische Diagnostik zwischen Selbstbestimmung und Schicksal*, Bielefeld: Transcript Verlag.

Lemke, Thomas and Wehling, Peter (2009) Bürgerrechte durch Biologie? Kritische Anmerkungen zur Konjunktur des Begriffs "biologische Bürgerschaft", in M. Weiß (ed.) *Bios und Zoë: Die menschliche Natur im Zeitalter ihrer technischen Reproduzierbarkeit*, Frankfurt am Main: Suhrkamp, 72–107.

Lock, Margaret (2005) Eclipse of the Gene and the Return of Divination, *Current Anthropology*, 46(5), S47–S70.

Nelkin, Dorothy and Lindee, Susan M. (1995) *The DNA Mystique: The Gene as a Cultural Icon*, New York: W. H. Freeman.

Neumann-Held, Eva M. and Rehmann-Sutter, Christoph (eds) (2006) *Genes in Development: Re-reading the Molecular Paradigm*, Durham, NC and London: Duke University Press.

Novas, Carlos (2006) The Political Economy of Hope: Patients' Organizations, Science and Biovalue, *BioSocieties*, 1(3), 289–305.

Oudshoorn, Nelly and Somers, André (2007) Constructing the Digital Patient: Patient Organizations and the Development of Health Websites, in R. V. Burri and J. Dumit (eds) *Biomedicine as Culture: Instrumental Practices, Technoscientific Knowledge, and New Modes of Life*, New York and London: Routledge, 205–222.

Oyama, Susan (2000) *The Ontology of Information*, Durham, NC and London: Duke University Press.

Palladino, Paolo (2002) Between Knowledge and Practice: On Medical Professionals, Patients, and the Making of the Genetics of Cancer, *Social Studies of Science*, 32(1), 137–165.

Petryna, Adriana (2002) *Life Exposed: Biological Citizens after Chernobyl*, Princeton, NJ: Princeton University Press.

Pieri, Elisa and Levitt, Mairi (2008) Risky Individuals and the Politics of Genetic Research into Aggressiveness and Violence, *Bioethics*, 22(9), 509–518.

Rabeharisoa, Vololona and Callon, Michel (1999) *Le Pouvoir des Malades: l'Association Française contre les Myopathies et la Recherche*, Paris: Les Presses de l'École des Mines.

Rabeharisoa, Vololona and Callon, Michel (2002) The Involvement of Patients' Associations in Research, *International Social Science Journal*, 54(3), 57–65.

Rabinow, Paul (ed.) (1984) *The Foucault Reader*, New York: Pantheon.

—— (1989) *French Modern: Norms and Forms of the Social Environment*, Chicago, IL and London: University of Chicago Press.

—— (1996a) Artificiality and Enlightenment: From Sociobiology to Biosociality, in P. Rabinow, *Essays on the Anthropology of Reason*, Princeton, NJ: Princeton University Press, 91–111.

—— (1996b) *Making PCR: A Story of Biotechnology*, Chicago, IL: University of Chicago Press.

—— (1999) *French DNA: Trouble in Purgatory*, Chicago, IL and London: University of Chicago Press.

—— (2008) Afterword: Concept Work, in S. Gibbon and C. Novas (eds) *Biosocialities, Genetics and the Social Sciences: Making Biologies and Identities*, London and New York: Routledge, 188–192.

Rabinow, Paul and Dan-Cohen, Talia (2005) *A Machine to Make a Future: Biotech Chronicles*, Princeton, NJ: Princeton University Press.

Rommetveit, Kjetil (2009) Bioethics, Biopower and the Post-Genomic Challenge, in J. Gunning; S. Holm and I. Kenway (eds) *Ethics, Law and Society*, Vol. 4, Farnham and Burlington, VT: Ashgate, 165–181.

Rose, Nikolas and Novas, Carlos (2005) Biological Citizenship, in A. Ong and S. J. Collier (eds) *Global Assemblages: Technology, Politics, and Ethics as Anthropological Problems*, Oxford: Blackwell, 439–463.

Scheper-Hughes, Nancy (2005) The Last Commodity: Post-Human Ethics and the Global Traffi c in "Fresh" Organs, in A. Ong and S. J. Collier (eds) *Global Assemblages. Technology, Politics, and Ethics as Anthropological Problems*, Malden, MA and Oxford, UK: Blackwell, 145–167.

Sunder Rajan, Kaushik (2008) Biocapital as an Emergent Form of Life: Speculations on the Figure of the Experimental Subject, in S. Gibbon and C. Novas (eds) *Biosocialities, Genetics and the Social Sciences*, London and New York: Routledge, 157–187.

van Dijck, José (1998) *ImagEnation: Popular Images of Genetics*, New York: New York University Press.

Vrecko, Scott (2008) Capital Ventures into Biology: Biosocial Dynamics in the Industry and Science of Gambling, *Economy and Society*, 37(1), 50–67.

Wasserman, David and Wachbroit, Robert (2001) *Genetics and Criminal Behavior*, Cambridge: Cambridge University Press.

Wehling, Peter (2011) Biology, Citizenship and the Government of Biomedicine: Exploring the Concept of Biological Citizenship, in U. Bröckling; S. Krasmann and T. Lemke (eds) *Governmentality: Current Issues and Future Challenges*, London and New York: Routledge, 225–246.

Weiss, Rick (2008) Genetic Testing Gets Personal, *The Washington Post*, 25 March 2008, A01. Available online at: <www.washingtonpost.com/wp-dyn/content/story/2008/03/24/ST2008032402911.html> (accessed 18 March 2013).

Wynne, Brian (2005) Reflecting Complexity. Post-genomic Knowledge and Reductionist Returns in Public Science, *Theory, Culture and Society*, 22(5), 67–94.

Part III

Democratizing biomedicine?

The role of patient associations and health social movements

11 Changing contexts for science and society interaction

From deficit to dialogue, from dialogue to participation – and beyond?

Massimiano Bucchi

Introduction

During the past two decades, enduring public concern over certain science and technology issues, and growing citizens' demands for involvement in such issues, as well as multiplying examples of non-experts who actively contribute to shaping the agenda of research in fields like biomedicine have led to a rethinking of the very meaning of science and citizens' interactions in several arenas[1]. In many countries and at the European level, funding schemes and policy documents have now changed their keywords from "public awareness of science" to "citizen engagement", from "communication" to "dialogue", and from "science *and* society" to "science *in* society". Does the change of keywords actually reflect a change in the practice and understanding of these interactions? Or it is – as some scholars have suggested – in many cases a reappearance of the traditional, "deficit" approach in a new guise? Which theoretical model(s) can best help us interpret this changing scenario? What are the possible consequences for public engagement in biomedical research? This chapter focuses on trends and transformations of science/society interactions as the broader context for understanding civil society actors' and patient organization's role in the (bio)medical research processes.

The deficit model of public understanding of science and its discontents

Although the antecedents of such debates can be traced back to long-standing controversies about participatory democracy that have touched science and technology issues since the 1970s (see, e.g., Dickson 1984), the theme of public participation with regard to science has made itself felt with new force in conjunction with the crisis of the so-called defi cit model of public understanding of science[2] (Wynne 1991, 1995; Bucchi and Trench 2014). This model emphasizes the public's inability to understand and appreciate the achievements of science, owing to prejudicial public hostility as well as to misrepresentation by the mass media, and adopts a linear, pedagogical, and paternalistic view of communication to argue that the quantity and quality of the public communication of science should be improved. To make up for this deficit, public and private bodies have – especially since the mid-1980s – launched schemes aimed at promoting public interest in and awareness of science. These initiatives have ranged from "open house" days, which have become a routine feature at most laboratories and research institutions, to science festivals and training courses in science journalism.

Despite their variety, these activities, as well as the studies conceived within the framework of the deficit model, share certain assumptions and features, namely:

1 the assumption that public understanding of science largely coincides with scientific literacy, i.e., with the ability to understand science "correctly" as it is communicated by the experts, which is measured by the ability to answer appropriate questions on scientific methods and contents;
2 the assumption that this understanding, once achieved, guarantees favorable attitudes toward science and technological innovation;
3 the tendency to problematize the relationship between science and the public only as regards the latter term of the relationship, i.e., the public.

Especially since the early 1990s, however, these assumptions have been strongly criticized on several grounds. For example, it has been pointed out that the equation between public understanding and the ability to answer questions about science has long restricted the discussion to the somewhat redundant observation that members of the public do not reason in the same way as professional scientists. Also disputed is the assumed link between exposure to science in the media, level of knowledge, and a favorable attitude toward research and its applications. As regards biotechnologies, for example, research has shown a substantial degree of skepticism and suspicion even among the sections of the population most exposed to scientific communication and best informed about biotechnological topics (Bucchi and Neresini 2002). In general, therefore, it does not seem that the opposition of certain sectors of the general public to particular technical-scientific innovations is due solely to the presence of an information deficit. Rather, the phenomenon requires more systematic and detailed analysis.

More generally, the disjunction between expert and lay knowledge cannot be reduced to a mere information gap between experts and the general public as envisaged by the deficit model. Lay knowledge, and patient knowledge in particular, is not an impoverished or quantitatively inferior version of expert knowledge; it is qualitatively different. Factual information is only one ingredient of lay knowledge, in which it interweaves with other elements (value judgments, trust in scientific institutions, the person's perception of his or her ability to put scientific knowledge to practical use) to form a corpus no less sophisticated than specialist expertise (Wynne 1989, 1995).

Thus, despite significant communication efforts, persistent public concern over certain science and technology issues, and growing citizens' demands for involvement in such issues, as well as various instances of non-experts actively contributing towards shaping the research agenda have led to a rethinking of the very meaning of public communication of science in several arenas. For instance, in 2000 a report from the UK House of Lords acknowledged the limits of science communication based on a paternalistic, top-down science-public relationship, and detected a "new mood for dialogue". In 2002, the Copus (Committee on the Public Understanding of Science), set up in 1985 by the Royal Society and other institutions to support public awareness activities, was also brought to an end by its very founders after they had come to the conclusion that "the top-down approach which Copus currently exemplifies is no longer appropriate to the wider agenda that science communication is now addressing" (Copus 2002). As mentioned in the Introduction to this chapter, funding schemes and policy documents, in many countries and at the European level, have now changed their keywords from "public understanding of science" to "citizen engagement", from "communication" to "dialogue", and from "science *and* society" to "science *in* society". Initiatives aimed at eliciting public input on science and technology issues and decision-making about science and technology have flowered. In some countries, such as Switzerland or Denmark for example, specific agencies have been established to undertake "participatory technology assessment" of upcoming innovations on behalf of parliaments or governments (Joss and Bellucci 2002; Hennen 2012).

The concept of "knowledge co-production" has been introduced by scholars to describe intense forms of participation of non-experts in the definition and accreditation of scientific knowledge – as when patient organizations actively contribute to defining the priorities of medical research or when citizen groups gather epidemiological data that lead experts to rethink the cause of a certain pathology (Brown and Mikkelsen 1990; Moore 2006; Callon and Rabeharisoa 2008; Hess 2009). These forms have been interpreted as representing a major change not only with regard to the deficit model, but also with regard to its sociological critique. According to Callon (1999), for instance, the critical version of public understanding of science – as reflected in the dialogic option – shifts the priority from "the education of a scientifically illiterate public" to the need and right of the public to participate in the discussion, on the assumption that "lay people have knowledge and competencies which enhance and complete those of scientists and specialists". However, both models are seen as sharing "a common obsession: that of demarcation. [The first model], in a forceful way, and [the second model], in a gentler, more pragmatic way, deny lay people any competence for participating in the production of the only knowledge of any value: that which warrants the term 'scientific'" (ibid.: 89). On this basis, the need has been invoked for another, more substantial shift to a model of knowledge co-production in which non-experts and their local knowledge can be conceived as neither an obstacle to be overcome by virtue of appropriate education initiatives (as in the deficit model), nor as an additional element which simply enriches professionals' expertise (as in the critical-dialogical model), but rather as essential for the production of knowledge itself. Expert and lay knowledge are not produced independently in separate contexts, after which they encounter each other later; rather, they result from common processes carried forward in "hybrid forums" in which specialists and non-specialists can interact (Callon et al. 2001).

Science and public participation: a proposed interpretative framework

Public participation in science is an emerging phenomenon with uncertain boundaries, and the difficulties of defining it are compounded by the fact that it has simultaneously become a key focus of social mobilization, policy initiatives, and scholarly analysis. Moreover, a plurality of points of view and motives of interest for public participation can be identified within each of these areas. However, for my purposes here, public participation may be broadly defined as the diversified set of situations and activities, more or less spontaneous, organized, and structured, whereby non-experts become involved in, and provide their own input to, agenda setting, decision-making, policy forming, and knowledge production processes related to science (Callon et al. 2001; Rowe and Frewer 2005). Given such a broad definition, I propose here an interpretative framework able to account also for "spontaneous/uninvited" participatory forms, i.e., those not deliberately elicited by a sponsor in all their varieties: public mobilization and protests, patient associations shaping the research and care agenda, and community-based research (Brown 2007; Wynne 2007; Callon and Rabeharisoa 2008).

This framework is partly based on the one used by Callon and colleagues (2001) to classify hybrid forums, and adopts as horizontal axis one of its key dimensions: the intensity of cooperation among different actors in knowledge production processes (Callon et al. 2001: 175). While intensity should, of course, be understood as a continuum, some key gradations can be identified. Callon et al. (2001) speak of "access points" where non-experts can intervene. One such point is the moment when laboratory results are "translated" to real-life situations, which is a crucial stage in the stabilization of scientific knowledge (ibid.: 89ff.). At that point, contradictions and conflicts may emerge between specialist and lay knowledge, with non-experts questioning the extent to which laboratory data can be applied to their own specific situation. This was, for example, the case of people living close to the Sellafield nuclear reprocessing site, who used data they had collected themselves to contradict the reassuring statistics of experts on the number of leukemia cases in their area and eventually obtained an official enquiry (Wynne 1996), and the case of the Cumberland sheep farmers whose concrete experience of the peculiarity of Cumbrian soil disputed predictions based on expert models that the contamination would soon disappear (Wynne 1989). A second and more substantial degree of participation corresponds to the access point offered by what Callon and colleagues (2001) call "the definition of the research collective", for instance, when members of AIDS patient associations managed to gain involvement in the design of experiments and drug trial tests, thereby broadening the research collective to include non-researchers.

The public may even participate in the initial recognition of research problems, for example by bringing a particular event or series of events out of the limbo of happenstance and into the realm of problems warranting expert interest and attention. The public may also accumulate the initial stock of knowledge required to make professional research possible and worthwhile. For instance, in the 1980s it was the action by Woburn, Massachusetts, residents in gathering on their own initiative epidemiological data and information on a suspiciously high number of childhood leukemia cases in their area that eventually persuaded MIT to initiate a research program that uncovered genetic mutations caused by trichloroethylene (Brown and Mikkelsen 1990; see also Brown et al. 2006). Similarly, the mobilization of patient associations like the French *Association Française contre les Myopathies* (AFM) has been crucial in prompting fruitful research on genetic diseases.

The vertical axis of the diagram plots the extent to which public participation is elicited/invited by a sponsor, which could be defined, with a certain amount of simplification, as the degree of "spontaneity" of public participation. Here again, the variable should be viewed as a continuum, with the sponsored, structured participatory initiatives described by Rowe and Frewer (2005) at the upper end of the axis and protest movements and research activities of patient and resident organizations at the lower end (e.g., Brown 2007). Figure 11.1 gives a graphical representation of the space defined by these two dimensions, together with some illustrative examples.

A wide variety of forms and cases of public participation can be mapped in this space. The upper left quadrant comprises forms typically elicited by a sponsor and characterized by low-intensity participation by non-experts in knowledge production, e.g., a public opinion survey. The lower left quadrant contains spontaneous mobilizations that do not significantly impact the dynamics of research, e.g., residents' protests against the decision to locate a radioactive waste site in their area. The lower right quadrant includes "spontaneous" forms of knowledge co-production, such as those exemplified by the Woburn residents or by the AFM. Finally, a participatory initiative like a consensus conference on a science issue organized by a sponsoring institution can be placed in the upper right quadrant (high degree of elicitation, high degree of intensity).

Over time, public participation with regard to a certain issue may move along one or both dimensions: for instance, when a public protest induces an institutional sponsor to organize a consensus conference or a citizen

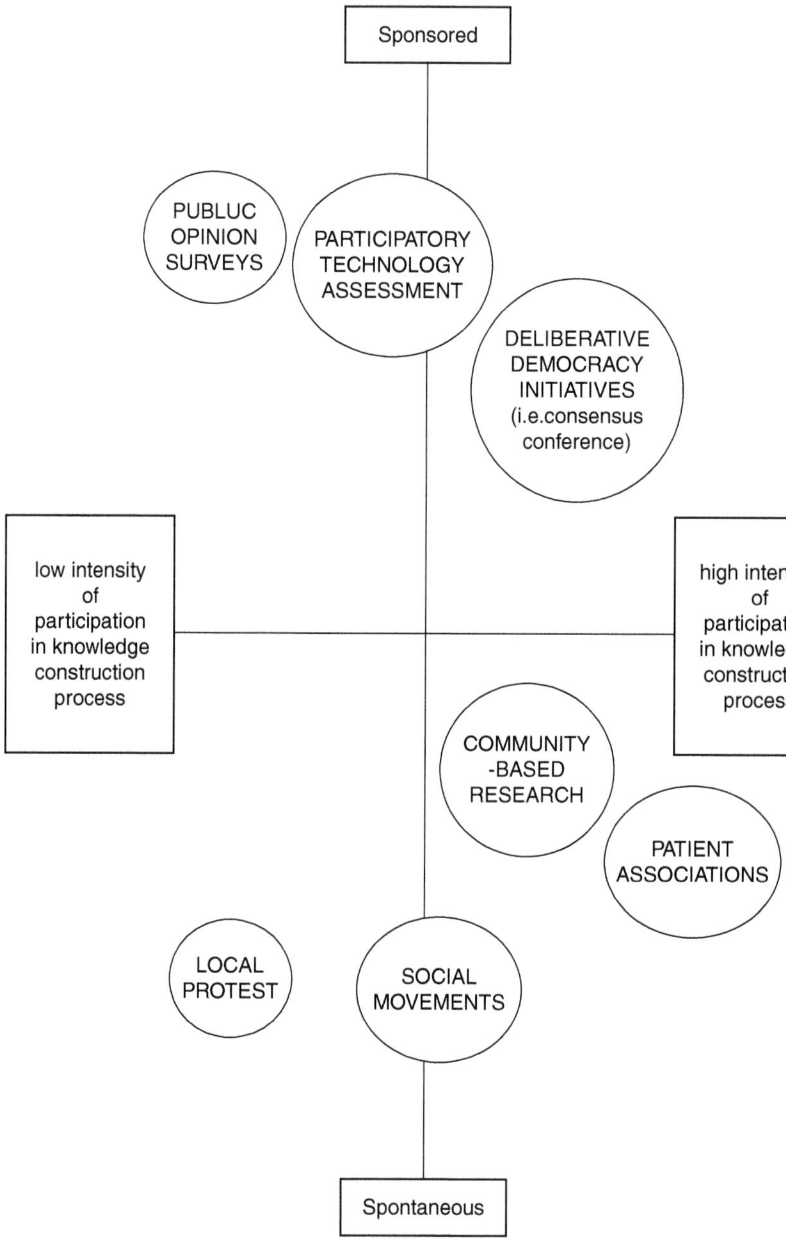

Figure 11.1 A map of public participation in science and technology.

panel, or when patient families or associations initially get together to lobby research institutions or drug companies and in the long run decide to establish their own research facilities.

The "open-endedness" of public participation is also emphasized in this interpretative framework. The idea of open-endedness means that the output of public participation is rarely entirely predictable on the basis of its structural features or on the basis of the sponsor's objectives; a public protest, for instance, may lead to renegotiation of a consensual decision, just as a participatory initiative originally designed to produce a consensus document may bring to light and radicalize conflicting positions, both among actual participants and – especially when the conflicts are reported by the media – in the broader public arena. Some degree of apprehension toward this open-endedness may be regarded as a key factor accounting for the sometimes resurgent temptation, on the part of research bodies and other institutions, to tame unruly public participation. This is often attempted by launching formal initiatives, and eventually performatively reinforcing traditional normative models, which selectively channel and circumscribe the public's role and contribution within pre-established agendas and formats (Wynne 2007).

The interpretative framework outlined above could be integrated by other relevant considerations. In particular, the use of inevitably broad labels such as "non-experts" or "lay public" should not lead us to flatten the intrinsic variety of citizens' involvement and their significantly differentiated capability and interest to shape knowledge production processes. Indeed, some of the most intense examples of participation actually involve highly motivated, very well informed groups – "quasi-experts" among non-experts, so to speak – that leave large parts of the public potentially disenfranchised. Sponsored and institutionalized forms of participation are by definition selective, and even those aimed at the widest possible involvement – such as the voting referendum – entail a substantial degree of self-selection. In other words, the question of "who participates" remains open for future research to the same degree as the question of "which forms of participation" represent citizens in which ways.

From deficit to dialogue, from dialogue to participation: changing contexts for science and society interaction?

Does the change of keywords – from deficit to dialogue, from dialogue to participation – actually reflect a change in the practice and understanding of science-society interactions? Or is it, as some scholars have suggested, in many cases a reappearance of the traditional deficit model in a new guise (Wilsdon et al. 2005; Trench 2006)? How are these changes redefining the forms of science and society interactions? Which theoretical model(s) can best help us interpret this changing scenario? Or, to quote another scholar, "how dead is the deficit model?" (Trench 2006).

To answer these questions, I would suggest that we first need to pay attention to the issue of context. One of the lessons from the "sociological turn" in science communication studies is that public communication of science cannot be understood in a *vacuum*. Rather, it should always be looked at not only within the context of experts/citizens interaction but also within the broader context of science in society.

This apparently simple recommendation has several significant implications. One is that we cannot straightforwardly apply models of science communication, such as a diffusionist, popularization notion of science communication, that were largely developed within the context of a science largely performed by relatively few state-based institutions to a science which is characterized, among other things, by pervasive relationships with the markets, a global outlook, and considerable emphasis on public relations, a configuration for whose communication prerogatives scholars have coined the label "PUS inc." – "the Public Understanding of Science, Incorporated" (Bauer and Gregory 2007). Moreover, contemporary science is increasingly challenging the very notion of a sharp distinction between producers and users of knowledge which rests on the basis of a diffusionist, deficit, transfer vision of science communication.[3] Companies, environmental organizations, and patient groups have established themselves as legitimate sources and providers of science communication.

Another feature of the contemporary science in society context is its intrinsic heterogeneity and fragmentation: communication is subject to the contradictory pressures of knowledge privatization and commodification, open access and sharing of research results, and citizen demands for greater involvement. All of this makes implausible the use of a single model to account for the varieties of contemporary expert/public configurations.

Table 11.1 sets out three key models of expert/public interaction – deficit, dialogue, and participation – together with their vision of science/society interaction and their broader ideological contexts. These models should be conceived as ideal types rather than as mutually exclusive categories. Most situations would have to be described as a combination of the three models. In this framework, the deficit model does not need to disappear: it becomes the default, "zero degree" of expert/public interaction processes.

This is why it is important to distinguish the many different facets of such models. While there are good reasons why we should abandon the expectation that public skepticism can be overcome by injecting knowledge, the deficit model's top-down, transfer vision of communication may be a reasonable proxy to describe situations characterized, for instance, by a low degree of public mobilization on science issues that have relatively low public resonance.[4] Over time, public/expert interaction with regard to a certain issue may move across models and their combinations: for instance, an emerging topic like nanotechnology may lend itself to deficit-like communication in its initial stages and later become the subject of public consultation/mobilization; vice versa, knowledge produced on a rare genetic pathology in situations of intense interaction between experts and non-experts may subsequently

Table 11.1 A multi-model framework of science-society interaction

Model of interaction	*Emphasis*	*Dominant versions*	*Aims*	*Ideological contexts*
Transfer Popularization One-way, one-time	Content	DEFICIT	Transferring knowledge	Scientism Technocracy Rhetoric of the knowledge economy
Consultation Negotiation Two-way, iterative	Context	DIALOGUE	Discussing the implications of research	Social responsibility Culture
Knowledge co-production, deviation Multi-directional, open-ended	Content & Context	PARTICIPATION	Setting the aims, shaping the agenda of research	Civic science Democracy

Adapted from Trench (2006) and Bucchi (2008).

become the focus of a deficit-like communication initiative. Studies highlighting the connection between an increase in the public salience of a certain science issue – or even in the level of knowledge – and mounting concern on the part of the public (Mazur 1981; Bucchi and Neresini 2002) might have actually identified the "tip of the iceberg" of these shifting configurations.

Coherence between communication patterns and the aims and ideological contexts deserves particular attention, as it may also help clarify why, for instance, institutions like the European Commission have encountered difficulties in relation to the consistency of the different claims they make about public participation in science and technology. It seems to be difficult to combine a participatory, co-production approach to science communication with an emphasis on technocracy and the rhetoric of the knowledge economy, which forms the basis of much EU policy strategy in the area of research and would rather lend itself to more traditional, deficit-transfer communication strategies (Trench 2006). Unlike deficit configurations, participation is also by definition multi-directional, open-ended, and potentially subject to conflict. Some degree of apprehension about this open-endedness may be regarded as a key factor accounting for the sometimes resurgent temptation, on the part of research bodies and other institutions, to "tame" unruly public participation through formal initiatives, or bluntly preaching dialogue and participation while practicing the deficit approach. More generally, there is always tension between opening up the black box of deficit communication for participation and putting participation back into the deficit box, with groups and institutions publicly struggling to impose their communicative definition of the situation – deficit, dialogue, or participatory-like. Indeed, a meta-level of science communication can be imagined at which actors are constantly engaged in defining (as participatory, dialogic, or deficit) the configuration of their interaction on a certain issue.

An interaction pattern should also not necessarily overlap with the aims and interests of a specific category of actors. Research and policy institutions may (in a deficit-like fashion) promote dialogic/participatory situations; citizens may contribute (in a dialogic/participatory fashion) to relegating to the deficit realm an issue in which they have little interest, or on which they feel comfortable reducing their role to quasi-passive spectators of knowledge as channeled by the experts for their own cultural benefit, aesthetic appreciation, or entertainment. In this light, rather than "which model accounts best" for expert-public interactions, one of the key sociological questions becomes "under what conditions do different forms of science-society interactions emerge?"

While a detailed analysis of such conditions would require a treatment of its own, a tentative list could in principle include:

- the degree of public salience of a certain science issue;
- the level of public mobilization on that and neighboring issues;
- the visibility and credibility of science institutions and actors involved;
- the degree of controversy/disagreement among science experts, as perceived by the public;
- the degree of institutionalization and the stability of professional boundaries in the science field of concern;
- the degree of social consensus on the overarching political and cultural context of science issues.

It may be expected, for instance, that an issue in the field of particle physics with low public impact and mobilization, little controversy among the experts, propelled by visible research institutions, in a context in which understanding of the fundamental laws of nature is a socially shared and undisputed aim, may lend itself to a deficit-like pattern in which the public is invited and willing to appreciate the spectacle of science's achievements. Likewise, it was unlikely that an issue like GMOs, touching many publicly relevant themes like food, safety, biodiversity and resource distribution, with a certain amount of experts' disagreement as publicly perceived, propelled by corporate actors in a context that is highly sensitive, alerted, and mobilized to questions of environment and globalization, would be containable in the deficit box. However, variations in the above-mentioned conditions and in other possible aspects of these questions may be reflected in a significant redefi niton of the interaction pattern. If a discovery in astrophysics is framed as "the Holy Grail of cosmology", as happened with the discovery in 1992 of radioactivity in the outer reaches of the known universe which was taken to represent the echo of the Big Bang at the origin of the universe, the situation may slide into a more dialogic, open interaction pattern in which the very boundaries between science and religion may be open to question (Miller 1994; Bucchi 2000).

It should be emphasized that the social, political, and cultural contexts have a bearing on more than the introduction of new knowledge by the experts. Emerging trends in popular discourse can give a completely different status and meaning to already existing scientifi c results, turning a transfer-deficit situation into an intense communicative short circuit. Despite a significant advance in human cloning announced by a team of scientists in 1993, cloning was not an issue in countries like Italy until the announcement of Dolly the sheep established a connection to a debate which had developed over issues such as embryos, in vitro fertilization, and abortion (Neresini 2000). The broader political context may also be decisive in setting the scene for interaction. Switzerland's or Scandinavia's tradition of civic participation is refl ected in the relevance given to that participation with regard to science, to the point of being incorporated into legislative prescription and dedicated institutional agencies (see e.g., Joss and Bellucci 2002).

Some general historical trends can be identified in the variations of these conditions. For instance, it is hard to deny that the increasing level of general education among citizens of many countries or the expanded potential access to science information through the internet has made participatory configurations more frequent and accessible today, particularly in areas like biomedicine and the environment (Nowotny et al. 2001; Trench 2007; Barker 2008; Akrich 2010). Other broad trends may include:

- the increasingly pervasive role of the media in questioning not only policy decisions on science but more specifically the connection between expertise and policy making;
- the rising demand for public participation as part of more general criticism of the capacity of traditional democracies to represent and include citizens' points of view when addressing global challenges, with crucial decisions increasingly being taken at levels not directly subject to citizens' influence – the so-called "democratic deficit" which is frequently a matter of concern with regard to, for instance, European or international institutions (Burns and Andersen 1996; Levidow and Marris 2001).

Other conditions, however, may be much less stable. Several studies written from sociological and historical perspectives suggest, for instance, that the inclination of scientists to open up their communicative boundaries to non-experts is neither a new nor a steadily growing phenomenon, but could rather be described in terms of alternating cycles of openness and closure (deviation and popularization) in a sort of pendulum movement (Hirschman 1982; Bucchi 2007).

Furthermore, the consequences of these conditions seem far from straightforward. For instance, when researchers mobilize in the public sphere to protest against budget cuts or against state regulation of certain research fields, or simply advocate greater public concern with science, they may contribute to a growing public perception of scientific expertise as interest-laden, thus damaging the credibility of traditional decision-making arrangements which involve only experts and policy makers (Bucchi and Neresini 2004). This in turn suggests an ironic and somewhat paradoxical generalization of the above-mentioned "open-endedness" principle: citizen pressures for more participation which have contributed to undermining the deficit approach may have been stimulated, among other things, by scientists' advocacy of that selfsame approach.

However, one should also resist the temptation to interpret the different analytical models of interactions among experts and the public as a chronological sequence of stages in which the emerging forms obscure the previous ones, with the dialogue version obliterating the deficit one or the participatory version substituting for the dialogue one. The interpretative framework proposed here seeks to account for the simultaneous coexistence of different patterns of interaction that may coalesce, depending on specific conditions and on the issues at stake.

Participation should not be reified as a circumscribed, static event or as a prerogative which can be switched on and off at will. Rather, it should be viewed as a process which fluidly assumes different contingent configurations. A certain notion of the relationship between professional experts and the public – for instance, as segregated categories in the deficit model, or as inextricably intertwined in the co-production model – is in itself a result of, and not a precondition for, the struggles, negotiations, and alliances taking place in those configurations.

Thus, on the one hand, changing styles and formats of science society interaction shape the opportunity structure for lay experts, patient organizations, and health social movements. On the other hand, their strategies for science mobilization may also contribute to redefine styles of science-society interaction and their formats[5]. Further research will be needed to better understand how different styles and formats of expert/non-expert interactions may configure different opportunities for such actors; and how different strategies may contribute to such redefinition. The role of civil society actors – such as patient organizations in the area of biomedicine – must be recognized as one of the key dynamics at the core of those co-evolutionary processes (Nowotny et al. 2001; Jasanoff 2004, 2005), redefining the meanings of science and the public, knowledge and citizenship, expertise and democracy.

Notes

1 Parts of this chapter draw on materials previously published by the author.

2 *Deficit* actually refers to a specific element of the model, namely the emphasis on the knowledge asymmetry between experts and the public as a basis and rationale for communicative interaction. It would actually be more accurate to refer to this model

as a *diffusionist* conception, which, in addition to the deficit element, incorporates a notion of communication as unproblematic one-way transfer, having no impact whatsoever on the processes of knowledge production (*popularization*). However, since *deficit* has become the standard label for the whole constellation among policy makers and scholars, I will use it here with that same general meaning. See Bucchi and Trench (2014).

3 "Post-academic science", "Mode-2 Science", are two of the labels used by scholars to indicate these emerging configurations of research in contemporary society (Gibbons et al. 1994; Ziman, 2000; Nowotny et al., 2001; see also Bucchi (in press).

4 Different reappraisals of the deficit model can be found in Sturgis and Allum (2004) and Dickson (2005).

5 On the concept of "style" with regard to science communication and science in society interactions, see Bucchi (2013).

References

Akrich, Madeleine (2010) From Communities of Practice to Epistemic Communities: Health Mobilizations on the Internet, *Sociological Research Online*, 15(2). Available online at: <www.socresonline.org.uk/15/2/10.html> (accessed 14 February 2014).

Andersen, Svein S. and Burns, Tom R. (1996) The European Union and the Erosion of Parliamentary Democracy: A Study of Post-Parliamentary Governance, in S. Andersen and K. A. Eliassen (eds) *The European Union: How Democratic is It?*, London: Sage, 227–251.

Barker, Kristin (2008) Electronic Support Groups, Patient-Consumers, and Medicalization: The Case of Contested Illness, *Journal of Health and Social Behavior*, 49(1), 20–36.

Bauer, Martin and Gregory, Jane (2007) From Journalism To Corporate Communication in Post-war Britain, in M. Bucchi and M. Bauer (eds) *Journalism, Science and Society: Science Communication between News and Public Relations*, London: Routledge, 33–52.

Brown, Phil (2007) *Toxic Exposures: Contested Illnesses and the Environmental Health Movement*, New York: Columbia University Press.

Brown, Phil; McCormick, Sabrina; Mayer, Brian; Zavestoski, Stephen; Morello-Frosch, Rachel; Gasior Altman, Rebecca and Senier, Laura (2006) "A Lab of Our Own": Environmental Causation of Breast Cancer and Challenges to the Dominant Epidemiological Paradigm, *Science, Technology & Human Values*, 31(5), 499–536.

Brown, Phil and Mikkelsen, Edwin J. (1990) *No Safe Place: Toxic Waste, Leukemia, and Community Action*, 1st edition, Berkeley: University of California Press.

Bucchi, Massimiano (2000) A Public Explosion: Big Bang in the UK Daily Press, in M. Dierkes and C. von Grote (eds) *Between Understanding and Trust: The Public, Science and Technology*, Harwood: Reading.

—— (2007) Scientists' Engagement in Society as Shifting Involvement, Presentation at the EUI Research Working Group, 24 May.

—— (2008) Of Deficits, Deviations and Dialogues: Theories of Public Communication of Science, in M. Bucchi and B. Trench (eds) *Handbook of Public Communication of Science and Technology*, London and New York: Routledge, 57–76.

—— (2013) Style in Science Communication, *Public Understanding of Science*, 22(8), 904–915.

—— (in press) Norms, Competition and Visibility in Contemporary Science: The Legacy of Robert K. Merton, *Journal of Classical Sociology*.

Bucchi, Massimiano and Neresini, Federico (2002) Biotech Remains Unloved by the More Informed, *Nature*, 416(3878), 261.

—— (2004) Why are People Hostile to Biotechnologies? *Science*, 304, 1749.

—— (2008) Science and public participation, in E. Hackett; O. Amsterdamska; M. Lynch and J. Wajcman (eds) *Science and Technology Studies Handbook*, Cambridge MA: MIT Press, 449–472.

Bucchi, Massimiano and Trench, Brian (2014) *Handbook of Public Communication of Science and Technology*, 2nd edition, London and New York: Routledge.

Callon, Michel (1999) The Role of Lay People in the Production and Dissemination of Scientific Knowledge, *Science, Technology & Society*, 4(1), 81–94.

Callon, Michel; Lascoumes, Pierre and Barthe, Yannick (2001) *Agir dans un monde incertain: Essai sur la démocratie technique*, Paris: Seuil.

Callon, Michel and Rabeharisoa, Vololona (2008) The Growing Engagement of Emergent Concerned Groups in Political and Economic Life: Lessons from the French Association of Neuromuscular Disease Patients, *Science, Technology & Human Values*, 33(2), 230–261.

Copus (2002) Statement on Copus by the British Association, the Royal Institution and the Royal Society, *www.copus.org.uk*, Available online at: <web.archive.org/web/20030202072854/http://www.copus.org.uk/news_detail_091202.html> (accessed 9 April 2014).

Dickson, David (2005) The Case for a "Deficit Model" of Science Communication, *SciDev.Net*, 27 June. Available online at: www.scidev.net/global/communication/editorials/the-case-for-a-deficit-model-of-science-communic.html (accessed 20 April 2014).

—— David (1984) *The New Politics of Science*, New York: Pantheon.

Epstein, Steven (1996) *Impure Science: AIDS, Activism and the Politics of Knowledge*, Berkeley CA: University of California Press.

Gibbons, Michael; Limoges, Camille; Nowotny, Helga; Schwartzman Simon; Scott Peter and Trow Martin (1994) *The New Production of Knowledge: Dynamics of Science and Research in Contemporary Societies*, London: Sage.

Hennen, Leonhard (2012) Why do We Still Need Participatory Technology Assessment? *Poiesis & Praxis*, 9, 27–41.

Hess, David J. (2009) The Potentials and Limitations of Civil Society Research: Getting Undone Science Done, *Sociological Inquiry*, 79(3), 306–327.

Hirschman, Albert (1982) *Shifting Involvements: Private Interest and Public Action*, Princeton, NJ: Princeton University Press.

Jasanoff, Sheila (2004) *States of Knowledge: The Co-production of Science and Social Order*, London: Routledge.

—— (2005) *Designs on Nature. Science and Democracy in Europe and the United States*, Princeton, NJ: Princeton University Press.

Joss, Simon and Bellucci, Sergio (eds) (2002) *Participatory Technology Assessment: European Perspectives*, London: Centre for the Study of Democracy.

Levidow, L. and Marris, C. (2001) Science and Governance in Europe: Lessons from the Case of Agbiotech, *Science and Public Policy*, 28(5), 345–360

Mazur, Allan (1981) Media Coverage and Public Opinion on Scientific Controversies, *Journal of Communication*, 31(2), 106–115.

Miller, Steven (1994) Wrinkles, Ripples and Fireballs: Cosmology on the Front Page, *Public Understanding of Science*, 3(4), 445–453.
Moore, Kelly (2006) Powered by the People: Scientifi c Authority in Participatory Science, in S. Frickel and K. Moore (eds) *The New Political Sociology of Science: Institutions, Networks, and Power*, Madison: University of Wisconsin Press, 299–325.
Neresini, Federico (2000) And Man Descended from the Sheep: The Public Debate on Cloning in the Italian Press, *Public Understanding of Science*, 9(4), 359–382.
Nowotny, Helga; Scott, Peter and Gibbons, Michael (2001) *Re-Thinking Science: Knowledge and the Public in an Age of Uncertainty*, Cambridge: Polity Press.
Rowe, Gene and Frewer, Lynn J. (2005) A Typology of Public Engagement Mechanisms, *Science, Technology & Human Values*, 30(2), 251–290.
Sturgis, Paul and Allum, Nick (2004) Science in Society: Re-evaluating the Deficit Model of Public Attitudes, *Public Understanding of Science*, 13(1), 55–74.
Trench, Brian (2006) Science Communication and Citizen Science: How Dead is the Deficit Model? Paper presented at PCST9, Seoul, 17–19 May.
___ (2007) How the Internet Changed Science Journalism, in M. Bucchi and M. Bauer (eds) *Journalism, Science and Society: Science Communication between News and Public Relations*, London: Routledge, 133–142.
Wilsdon James; Wynne Brian and Stilgoe, Jack (2005) *We need to infuse the culture and practice of Science with a new set of social possibilities: The Public Value of Science – Or how to ensure that science really matters*, London: Demos.
Wynne, Brian (1989) Sheepfarming after Chernobyl: A Case Study in Communicating Scientific Information, *Environment Magazine*, 31(2), 10–39.
___ (1991) Knowledges in Context, Science, *Technology & Human Values*, 16(1): 111–21.
___ (1995) Public Understanding of Science, in S. Jasanoff; Gerald E. Markle, James C. Petersen, and Trevor Pinch (eds) *Handbook of Science and Technology Studies*, Thousand Oaks, CA: Sage, 361–389.
___ (1996) May the Sheep Safely Graze? A Refl exive View of the Expert-Lay Knowledge Divide, in S. Lash, B. Szerszynski and B. Wynne (eds) *Risk, Environment and Modernity, Towards a New Ecology*, Thousand Oaks, California: Sage Publications, 44–83.
___ (2007) Public Participation in Science and Technology: Performing and Obscuring a Political–Conceptual Category Mistake, *East Asian Science, Technology and Society: An International Journal*, 1(1), 99–110.
Ziman, John (2000) *Real Science: What it Is, and What it Means*, Cambridge: Cambridge University Press.

12 The virtues (and some perils) of activist participation

The political and epistemic legitimacy of patient activism

Peter Wehling and Willy Viehöver

Introduction

In his reflections on the emergence of the figure of the "lay expert" in medical sociology, more than ten years ago, Lindsay Prior was quite skeptical about the reliability of patients' experiential knowledge when it comes to dealing with complex medical issues:

> Lay people ... often have detailed knowledge of other people as well as of themselves ..., and intimate knowledge about the circumstances in which they live .... And all in all, they are experts by virtue of "having experience". Yet, experience on its own is rarely sufficient to understand the technical complexities of disease causation, its consequences or its management. This is partly because experiential knowledge is invariably limited, and idiosyncratic. It generates knowledge about the one instance, the one case, the single "candidate" .... Above all, lay people can be wrong.
>
> (Prior 2003: 53; see also Prior et al. 2011)

More recently, and more cautiously, Steven Epstein has argued in a similar manner that social science work on patient activism "to date has been insufficiently critical of the tendency to valorize or romanticize lived experience as a basis for reliable knowledge, or to treat experience as a sort of bedrock resistant to critical interpretation" (Epstein 2011: 265).

As these quotations underscore, it continues to be unclear and controversial on what grounds patients and social movement activists are able to meaningfully contribute to and participate in the production of medical knowledge. However, what is in dispute here is not only the effectiveness or rationality but also the legitimacy of patients' and activists' engagement in research and research policy, since confusing medical knowledge production with idiosyncratic or erroneous lay assumptions can hardly be considered legitimate. Although there are several respects in which we do not share Prior's negative view of "experiential knowledge",[1] we would like to take such objections as an occasion to discuss and further clarify the questions of why and how the "public shaping" of medical research by patient associations, advocacy groups and health social movements can be justified and made sense of. One can roughly distinguish two types of justifications which are usually given for patient participation in research (see Martin 2008). The first of these is democracy-based, arguing that those who are affected by an illness should have a say in debates and decisions concerning medical research on this illness, and the second is knowledge- or expertise-based and suggests that patients, activists and advocates are able to make important and valuable cognitive and epistemic contributions to medical knowledge production. However, tentatively drawing this distinction immediately raises a number of questions. How do democracy-based and knowledge-based justifications relate to each other: are they complementary or mutually exclusive? How, in this context, should we conceive of "democracy" on the one hand and "knowledge" or "expertise" on the other?

In this chapter we will address these issues both from a democratic theory and from a sociology of science perspective, in order to contribute to specifying the political, normative and epistemic foundations of patient participation. Throughout the chapter, we will draw for purposes of illustration on examples of patient associations' engagement with medical research, mainly from the field of rare diseases. In the next section, we will argue that patient involvement is best understood in the framework of an "activist" model of democratic participation which differs from common conceptions of both representative and deliberative democracy.[2] In the third section we will use insights from the sociology of science and from science and technology studies (STS) in order to emphasize the importance, creativity, and legitimacy of patients' engagement in research and research politics. However, with regard to both democratic and epistemic legitimacy some ambiguities and potential perils have to be taken into consideration – fourth section. Therefore, in conclusion, we will outline some ideas for new political and institutional procedures which are intended to both foster patients' participation and increase its transparency and legitimacy.

Beyond "pure" deliberation: the activist model of participation

In recent decades a number of scientific and technological developments, above all nuclear energy and agri-biotechnology (genetically modified organisms, GMOs), have been intensively contested and ultimately rejected by large parts of society. Such rather unexpected political events have prompted calls for more participation of concerned citizens and civil society groups in scientific and technological matters or, more broadly, for the democratization of science and technology development. As is well known, in many countries one important reaction of political and scientific institutions to such demands consisted in initiating and organizing specific participatory exercises, resulting in the emergence of what has been termed "invited" (Wynne 2007) or "sponsored" (Bucchi and Neresini 2008) public participation. This is contrasted with "uninvited" or "spontaneous" engagement, which we will discuss later. Among the most widely used formats of invited public participation are the Danish consensus conferences, citizen's juries and similar exercises. In such formats, a group of unorganized "laypersons" are invited by governmental or scientifi c institutions to address a controversial topic of relevance for science and technology policy with the aim of declaring an independent stance on it at the end of the procedure. Recently, however, many scholars, but also representatives of civil society organizations (CSOs), have emphasized that these models of participation suffer from a number of limitations (see for instance Powell and Colin 2009; Braun and Schultz 2010; Hess 2011; Bogner 2012; Wynne 2014). Apart from the fact that they are often singular short-term events and in most cases fail to have any noteworthy political or scientific impact, they are also questionable with regard to their background assumptions about the effectiveness and democratic legitimacy of participation.

Regarding the *effectiveness* of participation, Maria Powell and Mathilde Colin (2009: 327) have convincingly argued that

> the recruitment of unorganized and nonopinionated citizens (usually volunteers) with little background on the scientific issue at hand is puzzling, given that these are the citizens who are least likely to have the energy, capacity, or collective power to engage with scientists and/or make their voices heard on the political level over the short or long term.

The results of such procedures, therefore, are not very likely to offer new insights and their impact on the development of science and technology or research policies will usually be quite limited. In addition, this approach appears to be equally questionable with regard to the *democratic legitimacy* of public participation. For on this understanding precisely those attributes appear to be hindrances to legitimate engagement in participatory processes which would enable civil society actors to make substantial contributions, namely independent knowledge (such as "experiential expertise") and normative values, articulated interests, argumentative skills and political or professional engagement. Underlying this view is a peculiar conception of "pure" or "purifi ed" deliberation that must not be "distorted" by prior knowledge, individual or group interest, or political involvement (see Braun and Schultz 2010). Corresponding to what might be termed the "classic ideal of deliberative democracy" (Mansbridge et al. 2010: 66), the source of legitimacy in this model lies in the assumption that participants who suspend their own interests (which are held to foster biased judgments) become both willing and able to acknowledge nothing but the Habermasian "force of the better argument". Thus, it is assumed, they will be in a position to define and promote the common or public good.

In addition, there also exist a wide range of procedures of "invited" participation in science and technology, such as "stakeholder dialogues", that expressly address and involve collective, organized actors instead of individual citizens. However, these forms of participation do not effectively modify the overall picture outlined above, since organizations are regularly addressed as advocates or lobbyists for a narrow and pre-defined interest without having a say in more fundamental debates on the direction and goals of research and technology development, which are usually exempted from discussion. In general, in such procedures there is little space for contestation, conflict and radical dissent (Hess 2011); instead, as Kathrin Braun and Susanne Schultz (2010: 415) have argued, "publics based on the idea of consensus and education are held in higher regard and ascribed a higher moral authority (and authenticity) than those based on the idea of conflict and struggle".

If we compare this model of participation with what patient associations, for instance in the field of rare diseases, actually do when they engage in medical research,[3] we become aware of a distinctive model of public participation which can be termed "activist" and differs from the deliberative one in several important respects. First, patients (or their relatives and carers) frequently do not wait for an "invitation" to participate but simply start to engage in medical research according to their own needs and priorities; moreover, they do so continuously, not only for a couple of weeks or months. Second, they purposefully organize themselves, based on their experience that only as a larger organized collective they will ever have the resources and the power to gain influence on medical research, research policies and decision-making on health care. Third, they strive to become as knowledgeable and well-informed as possible about the issues that appear relevant to them, in order to both cope with their illness and interact with scientists on an equal footing. However, this is not necessarily tantamount to acquiring biomedical knowledge but can also be achieved by collecting and systematizing patients' experiential knowledge. Fourth, patients and patient associations are far from suspending their specific interests, as is demanded by the deliberative model as an ostensibly necessary precondition for legitimate participation. Quite to the contrary, their primary aim is just to put the interests, experiences and views of a particular group of patients on the agenda of science and research policy. Fifth, patients do not always accept the given direction of biomedical research as an unquestionable fact and a result of superior scientific rationality. Instead, they occasionally radically challenge the "dominant epidemiological paradigm" (Brown et al. 2012), arguing for a completely different focus of research or even for stopping medical research on their condition in order to demedicalize it.

In our view, this activist model of engagement of interested collective actors promises not only greater effectiveness than the participation of unorganized, uninformed and presumably "unbiased" citizens but also an at least equivalent political and democratic legitimacy. In the activist model of public participation, the sources of democratic legitimacy are to be found in the fact that the specific needs, interests, and values of a particular group of persons, who are affected by illness and disease and often disadvantaged in society or the health care system, are collectively represented and strongly articulated both in the scientific and political sphere. In this view, it is essential for democratic societies that social actors, in particular marginalized and vulnerable groups, are both able and allowed to express their own interests, in order to make sure that they can speak for themselves and are not misrepresented by others: "Those who know their interests best, namely (in general) those whose interests they are, need to deliberate with others about those interests, come to understand them, express them, and stand up for them" (Mansbridge et al. 2010: 72). Thus, instead of suspending their interests as the starting point for "pure" deliberation, participants can even become more clearly aware of what their interests are in the process of deliberation. According to Jane Mansbridge and coauthors, "including self-interest in deliberative democracy reduces the possibility of exploitation and obfuscation, introduces information that facilitates reasonable solutions and the identification of integrative outcomes, and also motivates vigorous and creative deliberations" (ibid.: 72f.). It is therefore crucial to distinguish collectively articulated and reflected interests from mere short-term and surface preferences such as consumer choices on markets (ibid.: 68, n. 15). This is the reason why *organized* groups are so important for the expression of interests; patient associations often (though of course not always) offer a forum where immediate needs, individual preferences, or "idiosyncratic" views can be reflected and balanced, with the aim of articulating collective interests and values (see Fung 2003 and Tomes and Hoffman 2011 with regard to patient organizations). To put it differently, common group interests are neither a spontaneous preference nor an objective and static "given" determined by objective conditions of life, but are themselves the results of (more or less open and fair) processes of interaction, discussion and interpretation within social groups.[4] For this reason, interest-based, activist participation of organized groups goes far beyond the kind of "privatized consumer orientation" (Young 1996: 121) toward politics, or science and technology, which deliberative democrats rightly reject.

As these considerations underline, there are good reasons to accept that the expression and promotion of one's own interests should not generally be excluded from democratic deliberation. Insisting on these interests is not necessarily illegitimate and disruptive, nor will it "contaminate" deliberative discussions. To the contrary, the articulation of interests, such as the need for treatment of one's illness, can even provide a source of legitimacy for citizen or civil society participation. This applies in particular to those cases in which the interests of some social groups have been neglected by more powerful actors, or hegemonic definitions of the public good go unchallenged since these disadvantaged groups do not become aware of their opposing interests or fail to publicly articulate them. In addition, there are good reasons to doubt whether a statement issued at the end of a consensus conference by randomly selected citizens who were not previously familiar with the topic under discussion can claim higher representative or procedural legitimacy than uninvited activist participation. Indeed, both this kind of statement and the process of opinion-making within the group of citizens can easily be influenced by contingent factors such as group dynamics, time pressure, procedural routines or subtle directing by moderators or scientific experts (see Bogner 2012). Thus, under "real-world conditions" the democratic legitimacy of such procedures is frequently much weaker than theories of deliberative democracy suggest. Moreover, the advantages of the activist model become even more evident when we look at why and how interest-based collective participation proves to be beneficial for science and scientific pluralism.

Patients and activists in medical knowledge production

The sociology of science and STS have produced a good deal of evidence showing that science, contrary to idealized notions of scientific progress, does not proceed according to a universal logic of rational and value-free truth-seeking. By contrast, the issues of *what* gets studied and *how* it is studied are essentially shaped by a combination of "external" interests and influences such as the availability of funding, which mainly comes from the state and the economy, and specific "internal" criteria for selecting research topics and priorities.[5] In biomedicine, the following internal criteria can be identified:

- a research project promises to deliver (positive and statistically significant) results within a rather short period of time;
- the findings are likely to be publishable, and eventually published, in high-ranking, peer-reviewed journals;
- the research objects are (more or less) easily accessible, observable and possibly manipulable in controlled experimental settings – which, for instance, favors the search for genetic causes of disease over investigating environmental ones (Müller-Wille and Rheinberger 2012: 217);
- research allows deploying advanced technical equipment such as neuroimaging or genome sequencing.

It is quite obvious that these criteria for selecting research priorities and designing experimental settings are questionable and frequently will diverge from the criteria patients might have.

What Phil Brown and colleagues have termed the "dominant epidemiological paradigm" (DEP) of breast cancer research, with its focus on genetic and individual life-style factors instead of possible environmental causes of the disease, illustrates how such internal criteria and external influences interact and reinforce each other (see Brown et al. 2012: 24ff.). To the extent that such paradigms one-sidedly favor certain theoretical or methodological approaches over others, or even exclude important and pressing social or medical problems from scientific attention, biomedicine obviously is in need of challenges and inputs from other "external" sources. Among such important sources we can identify patient associations and health social movements, since they are able to mobilize independent knowledge and experiences and, therefore, in many instances act as a counterpart to the powerful influences exerted by governments, industry, the media and the institutions of mainstream science. To put it differently, patients and activists (or civil society organizations more generally) are important or even indispensable actors in what we have elsewhere termed the "polycentric governance" of scientific knowledge production (Wehling and Viehöver 2013; see also Brown et al. 2006).

By articulating and insisting on the experiences, interests and needs of particular social groups, patient organizations perform three important and closely related tasks which may help science to operate more comprehensively and socially responsibly: first, initiating and building networks among scientists as well as among researchers and patients: second, participating in research agenda setting: third, directly contributing to medical knowledge production, which not only includes providing scientists with useful and complementary expertise but also acting as a kind of epistemic "corrective" of (mainstream) biomedical research.

Building networks

Patient groups frequently provide important organizational and social resources for medical knowledge production. By regularly organizing national or international conferences on their diseases, by building personal relationships with individual scientists, by monitoring scientific journals for important new findings, by communicating such findings or by directly asking research teams from different institutions, disciplines or countries to collaborate with each other, patient associations initiate and create networks of researchers who might otherwise not even have taken notice of each other (see also Panofsky 2011). This often goes hand in hand with criticism of an excessive and dysfunctional orientation towards competition in contemporary science and research policies. Patients counter this neoliberal preference for competition with appeals to cooperation and the sharing of results, methods and ideas among those who conduct research on the same disease. In addition, in many cases patient associations' support is practically indispensable as a way of bringing together medical researchers and patients, thus enabling the former to observe patients, to collect blood samples or to organize clinical tests of new treatments. However, patient associations' contributions are not restricted to recruiting research participants; even more important is the fact that many of them issue guidelines for clinical trials and assess the clinical settings with a view to their prospects of scientific success and to ethical acceptability, and also to compatibility with the everyday lives of patients.

Participating in research agenda setting

Patient associations and health social movements engage in diverse and often conflicting ways in research agenda setting, that is to say in debates around the question of what should get studied in science. In this context, they frequently focus on what sociologists of science have termed "undone science" (Hess 2009, 2010; Frickel et al. 2010), that is, in other words, problems and issues that are important for patients or activists but are deemed uninteresting by mainstream science or have even escaped its attention. This has obviously been the case with rare or "orphan" diseases, many of which had been neglected by mainstream medical and pharmaceutical research. Yet in recent decades patient associations have succeeded in drawing medical, political and public attention to this class of diseases, culminating in the obligatory development and implementation of national action plans for rare diseases in all European Union member states by 2013. More generally speaking, medical or health care research is often not carried out because it is not economically profitable or generates excessive costs, because it is not politically opportune and not supported by powerful actors, or because it does not seem to be scientifically attractive, as for instance when it promises poor reputational rewards, research funds or media attention or presents few career opportunities. Thus, for patient associations their participation in research agenda setting often means more than just trying to push their concerns onto the agenda; it might also include contesting the underlying criteria for selecting research topics and determining research priorities. However, patient organizations themselves can and do also make use of such criteria in order to draw attention to their own issues, for instance by offering research grants or helping researchers to get media coverage. While challenging the biased mechanisms of agenda setting in mainstream science might in principle be the more adequate reaction, it is nevertheless an open question whether or not this is also more successful and instrumental than strategically using these mechanisms in order to achieve patient associations' goals.

Engaging in knowledge production

As numerous examples have demonstrated, patient associations and social movement activists are able to substantially contribute to medical knowledge production (see Caron-Flinterman et al. 2005 and Brown et al. 2012 for various examples). Generally speaking, it is not even surprising that patients, or their relatives and carers, often possess rather detailed experiential knowledge about the course of a disease, the efficacy of therapies or the everyday medical or social needs of patients, and in some cases even of possible causes of disease.[6] In addition, patient associations often collect, pool and systematize this knowledge – what Michel Callon and Vololona Rabeharisoa have termed "research in the wild" (Callon and Rabeharisoa 2003) and what comes close to the concept of "popular epidemiology" as developed by Brown (1992) and others. In many of these cases patients' knowledge and experience is more or less instrumental for and complementary to biomedical research; it adds to and refines the empirical data base of scientific knowledge production. By contrast, however, in a number of other cases patient groups, based on their local or experiential knowledge, act more radically as a kind of epistemic "opponent" or "corrective" of biomedical research, often with support from critical, non-mainstream scientists. One of the most prominent examples of such an epistemic challenge is the "Environmental Breast Cancer Movement" in North America, which has contested the "dominant epidemiological paradigm's" approach to breast cancer etiology and treatment and its priority on genetic and individual life-style factors (Brown et al. 2006; Brown 2007; Ley 2009; McCormick 2009a, 2009b). There are, however, many more instances which highlight patient associations' and health movements' role as epistemic opponents of (mainstream) biomedical science. This role is central in almost all cases of "contested illnesses" (Moss and Teghtsoonian 2008; Brown et al. 2012) as well as in many struggles and conflicts about the medicalization or demedicalization of certain conditions and disorders, among them ADHD, autism, shyness, obesity, fibromyalgia, transsexuality and deafness. From an STS and sociology of science perspective, these instances of epistemic opposition to biomedical knowledge claims are theoretically more interesting than those (nevertheless equally important!) cases where patient associations and health social movements are essentially supportive of "normal" and unchallenged scientific knowledge production. Such opposition sheds light on the limits and potential dangers of "pure" and self-sufficient scientific autonomy and, in addition, highlights the value and productivity of epistemic and cognitive diversity and dissent, both within and outside science. Scientific autonomy can become problematic when it results in the dominance or hegemony of a single paradigm, based on and accompanied by the successful marginalization or even exclusion of alternative theoretical and methodological approaches and the blocking of "external" influences. Diversity, by contrast, makes it possible to ask unfamiliar research questions and to investigate different research objects in different research sites, such as the household in cancer research (Brown et al. 2012), and to experiment with dissenting, non-mainstream theoretical concepts, research methods or therapeutic options. Thus cognitive diversity and epistemic plurality can reasonably be considered as valuable in themselves, and this is acknowledged (at least to a certain degree) even by philosophers of science like Philip Kitcher who otherwise hold a strong realist conception of the "one" scientific truth (see Kitcher 2011: 193ff.). The virtues of diversity remain unaffected even if patients' or activists' views ultimately turn out to be "idiosyncratic" or simply "wrong", as Prior suggests in the quotation at the head of this chapter. While patients' and activists' ideas are, without doubt, often erroneous, they will nevertheless in many cases be fruitful since they may prompt mainstream science to rethink, specify and possibly modify its background assumptions, research priorities or theoretical conclusions.

Against this backdrop, one can reasonably argue that patients' and activists' engagement in medical research can indeed claim epistemic legitimacy, and some authors have suggested that we should even understand the increasing involvement of civil society groups as part of an "epistemic modernization of science" (Moore et al. 2011), the roots of which can be seen as far back as the 1950s.[7] The concept of "emergent concerned groups", as developed by Callon and Rabeharisoa (2008), points in the same direction in stating that the dynamics of technoscience itself (as well as of economic markets) continuously produce social groups which are affected by and therefore concerned about the consequences of these dynamics, and so both *legitimately* and *productively* engage in shaping scientific and technological developments (see also Callon et al. 2009; Viehöver and Wehling 2011).

Challenges to the legitimacy of activist engagement

Given this strong endorsement from both "post-deliberative" democratic theory and the sociology of science and STS, are there any problems and pitfalls at all relating to activist civil society participation in science and technology? In the illuminating paper on the success (or failure) of patient groups and health movements quoted earlier, Epstein (2011: 263ff.) identifies three complications and obstacles: the problem of *representation* (that is, who legitimately speaks for the patients, by whom and how are their needs and experiences represented), the problem of *expertise* (that is, to what extent do divisions emerge between "lay experts" and "ordinary" group members), and the problem of *incorporation and co-optation* by political and scientific institutions or economic actors. Obviously, these are not only obstacles to "success" in a narrow, instrumental sense of effective goal-achievement, but also comprise major challenges to the democratic and epistemic legitimacy of patient and social movement activism. Since we cannot discuss these problems and their impact on political and epistemic legitimacy in detail here, we would like to draw attention to a specific threat to the legitimacy of patient activism which is closely linked to the "problem of representation" but simultaneously broadens the perspective, as it relates to the issue of legitimate representation both *within* patient associations and *among* them.

We will briefly illustrate this challenge by using two recent examples from patient and advocacy activism. The first example relates to advocacy for newborn screening (NBS) in the United States and has been described in detail by Rachel Grob in both a monograph (2011a) and a book chapter (2011b). While it seems uncontroversial that NBS enables early detection and timely prevention or treatment of disease and thus can help to avoid suffering and pain and can even save children's lives, one must nevertheless admit that this holds true only on the condition that appropriate prevention or treatment are actually available. Additional problems may arise as a consequence of the ambiguity of test results, unpredictable variations of diseases (including the possibility that some children who test positively will never develop any symptoms), and the fact that some diseases become manifest only in later life (see also Timmermans and Buchbinder 2013).

However, given the potential benefits of NBS individual parents as well as advocacy groups in the USA and elsewhere have increasingly urged the addition of "their" respective diseases to NBS programs.[8] Yet, as Grob observes,

> parents' advocacy efforts – both as individuals and as leaders in formal advocacy organizations – are not limited to demands for inclusion of "their" diseases in their state's screening panel. Instead, they often argue for the most inclusive possible screening programs, and for both policy shifts and normative shifts that would allow mandatory screening for conditions that have no proven treatment.
>
> (Grob 2011b: 232)

For instance, one non-profit foundation, concerned with a condition which is effectively treatable, argued that "all children should be screened for all diseases that technology can provide for at this time" (ibid.: 242). Obviously, such demands support, advertently or not, the dominant technoscientific culture of biomedicine which favors high-tech diagnostic tools and treatments along with creating more or less subtle and tacit moral obligations to actually use these tools, even in those cases where this, unlike the use of NBS in the USA (Timmermans and Buchbinder 2013: 7) and many other countries, is not in fact mandatory.

At first sight, it is quite understandable that parents should react to a terrible personal experience (the loss of a child due to the fact that a treatable disorder has not been included in NBS programs) by making a general, political claim (maximum expansion of NBS): this is prompted above all by the moral impulse to spare others suffering by avoiding such a mismatch (Grob 2011b: 231). However, NBS for conditions that are hitherto untreatable, where diagnosis is fundamentally uncertain or which are late-onset diseases, may have undesirable and unwanted impacts on the affected families (see Timmermans and Buchbinder 2013). As Grob points out, the voices of these parents and families have scarcely been heard in what she terms the "discourse of urgency" in favor of the expansion of NBS programs. She argues that "the dynamics of parental advocacy around NBS have made it very difficult to achieve polyvocal, broadly participatory advocacy" (Grob 2011b: 248ff.). The problem of representation mentioned by Epstein thus resurfaces in a broader perspective: which patients' voices are heard in public and political debates or in the media, and why are other, quieter voices not heard? For Grob, arriving at more comprehensive and just participation of parents and patients "requires more … than willingness to grant entree to those who speak loudest. What is needed is a serious commitment of time, attention, and resources so that we are able to hear the quiet as well as the forceful voices of personal experience" (ibid.: 251).

Our second example relates to the development of a DNA chip for what is termed "preconception" carrier testing for a large number of recessively inherited rare genetic diseases, which has been co-funded by the self-help organization Beyond Batten Disease Foundation (BBDF).[9] BBDF was founded by a couple in the United States after their five-year-old daughter had been diagnosed with Batten disease, a degenerative and fatal neurological disorder. Since Batten disease is a rare and recessively inherited condition, parents in most cases do not have any family history of the disease, which is why the diagnosis of a child usually comes as a complete and painful surprise. In order to protect other parents from experiencing such a devastating situation, BBDF initiated and supported the development of a comprehensive DNA chip designed to test for up to almost 600 recessively inherited conditions (Kingsmore 2012). However, these conditions include not only incurable, fatal and early-onset diseases such as Batten disease and Tay-Sachs disease but also a considerable number of treatable, less severe, highly variable or late-onset disorders such as phenylketonuria (PKU), Wilson's disease, hemochromatosis, and cystic fibrosis (CF), for which a remarkable increase in life expectancy has been achieved in recent decades. Quite a few of these treatable diseases are now included in NBS programs. One can easily imagine that not all patients suffering from diseases of this latter type would agree to integrate their conditions into a technology for preconception testing that ultimately focuses on the possibility of prevention, which means preventing the birth of affected individuals.

Both examples point to a problem which might to some extent be symptomatic of activist, interest- and experience-based engagement with (not only) science and technology. We would like to describe this as a tendency or shift towards overhasty and unjustified generalization of personal or group-specific experiences and interests. Grob and Mark Schlesinger (2011: 285) have argued on similar lines, warning against a tendency among advocacy groups to simplify the existing diversity of interests and experiences "to a singular perspective in order to enhance the coherence of their message". Such tendencies lead to a problematic situation in which one group of patients or advocates de facto speaks for others whose position appears to be similar but actually is different in important respects. At first sight, this phenomenon seems to correspond to Prior's preoccupation with the "idiosyncratic" or outright mistaken nature of laypeople's and patients' experiential knowledge, as quoted at the start of this chapter. However, we would like to suggest that this issue should be understood somewhat differently, namely as a problem of balanced representation and participation in public discourse and decision-making rather than merely a cognitive problem. What is problematic is not patients' experiential knowledge in itself, but rather the uncoordinated generalization of the conclusions some advocacy groups draw from their individual and particular experiences. Consequently, the way to counter this threat to the legitimacy of activist engagement is not so much to provide better medical knowledge but rather, as Grob indicates, to improve the opportunities to participate for all affected groups and to institutionally support and intensify the exchange of communication between them.

Outlook

In conclusion, we would like to outline two suggestions for dealing with the problem of legitimate representation among different patient associations (as well as within them). We see one possibility of doing this in giving a stronger, more active role to intermediary and umbrella organizations regarding the discussion of these far-reaching questions, as addressed in both of the previously mentioned examples. For the field of rare diseases, umbrella organizations exist on a national level (e.g. NORD in the USA, AMR in France, ACHSE in Germany) as well as on a supranational level (such as EURORDIS in Europe).[10] In our view these organizations have, to date, been understandably reluctant to concern themselves with topics such as prevention, prenatal diagnosis, or preimplantation genetic diagnosis because it is to be expected that individual member groups will have very different opinions regarding these practices, making consensus almost impossible.[11] However, arguing for a stronger commitment by umbrella organizations concerning these issues is not necessarily intended to achieve consensus by all means, or to suggest that all groups should adopt and support the majority's view. Rather, the goal is to create interactive and democratic forums in which all of the various views can be openly expressed and it is possible to discuss how individual advocacy groups can and should legitimately act and react in the face of apparently unresolvable disagreement. This could prevent individual groups from speaking for others or de facto acting on their behalf with regard to these controversial topics, for example by supporting the maximum expansion of NBS or preconception carrier screening without actually being legitimized to do so.

Our second suggestion pertains to finding new ways and formats for civil society to participate in the decision-making processes in science or research policy. As already mentioned, there has been considerable dissatisfaction with established procedures of "invited participation" in the last few years; here, forms of uninvited and spontaneous engagement have been shown to exhibit a number of advantages (see Wehling 2012; Wehling and Viehöver 2013). However, this should not be interpreted as an essentialist contrast between "good" uninvited and "bad" invited participation. Instead, it might be fruitful to develop and test new procedures for participation that are able to combine the benefits of both invited and uninvited participation. Invited participation, at least in principle, offers greater transparency and inclusiveness compared to market-style structured public discourse where those groups "who speak loudest" have the advantage, that is to say those groups that are able to mobilize more resources in order to gain public, political, or scientific attention. Contrary to this "market of attention", political institutions could place an emphasis on deliberately involving quieter voices in public debates and political decision-making, and in particular those voices whose demands are not fully compatible with the dynamics of biomedicine. Uninvited participation, on the other hand, has highlighted the importance of independent expertise, strong self-interest, and long-term commitment as crucial preconditions for meaningful and effective participation in matters of medical knowledge production and technology development.

Two partly overlapping, concrete examples of procedures that seek to combine and mutually reinforce the respective virtues of invited and uninvited participation are, first, processes of participatory research agenda setting as developed and proven effective in practice, particularly in the Netherlands, and second, the new format of a "dissensus conference" as suggested by David J. Hess (2011).

Where participatory research agenda setting is concerned, social scientists in several pilot projects relating to various diseases have "developed and tested a methodology for patient participation that is radically dialogical in its orientation and offers clear prescriptive guidelines on how to consult and integrate the issues of various stakeholders, including patients, in research agenda setting" (Abma and Broerse 2010: 161). Even if these approaches will never be able to fully overcome existing power imbalances or prevent patients from being marginalized (see Elberse et al. 2011), they show us that it is potentially feasible to include the interests and points of view of (almost) all affected parties when formulating research objectives and priorities. As the social scientists who are involved in such procedures emphasize, this often means giving special attention to the interests and views of the least influential group of participants, which is usually the patients (Abma and Broerse 2010: 168). This may often require empowering patients prior to a dialogue meeting with scientists: "Often, the problems and needs of patients are quite similar. Awareness of this fact creates empowerment among patients and refutes the accusation of subjectivity that is used to exclude them" (Elberse et al. 2011: 236). This may also help to overcome merely "idiosyncratic" views and to develop common positions as well as to find out on which aspects there is disagreement among patients or patient associations themselves.

The second example, the "dissensus conference", offers an alternative to public deliberation procedures oriented towards arriving at a consensus on the relevant facts and certainties. David J. Hess argues that, especially in highly contested and politicized medical fields, instead of holding a consensus conference one might initiate a dissensus conference

> to draw attention to and analyze the perspectives of a scientific counterpublic. The object of the conference would not be to produce a report that provides input from a random selection of laypeople into a technical decision but instead to produce a publicized controversy that draws attention to the power–knowledge issues in a given scientific field.
>
> (Hess 2011: 639)

Participants in the dissensus conference would be stakeholders such as leaders of dominant and subordinate networks in the relevant scientific fields, potential sponsors, patient and social movement representatives, industry representatives, journalists, and regulators. The goal here would be to make the diversity of perspectives and perceptions visible and to explore them in a process that is as open and inclusive as possible in order to, among other things, prevent a premature closure of the research agenda or the establishment of a "dominant epidemiological paradigm". Instead, a dissensus conference could result in the development of complementary and contrasting research programs which would then be supported politically as well as financially.

Although there are a number of open questions that need to be further investigated experimentally, we believe that both of these approaches are, in principle, suited to the task of bringing about a higher degree of transparency, inclusiveness, and representativeness of patient participation without jeopardizing the strengths of "uninvited", interest- and experience-based engagement – and without any intention to undermine or replace this engagement. In this way, the effectiveness and impact of patient participation can not only be increased, but simultaneously its democratic and epistemic legitimacy can be reinforced and defended – not least against the danger that diversity and disagreement will be marginalized by patient associations and advocacy organizations themselves.

Notes

1 For instance, we do not agree with the statement that patients' experiential knowledge is necessarily idiosyncratic. It regularly develops within a larger social group as well as in interaction with scientific knowledge so that idiosyncratic traits can be corrected (although, in some cases, they will of course be reinforced through interaction within a group of like-minded people). In addition, the statement that knowledge is "invariably limited" applies both to lay knowledge and to scientific knowledge. There can be little doubt that scientists too "can be wrong", and the field of medicine, in particular, offers numerous examples of this.

2 By using the term "activist", we mainly refer to Iris Marion Young's insightful paper "Activist Challenges to Deliberative Democracy" (2001). While Young conceives of "the activist" primarily in terms of spectacular political protest and opposition, many of the traits she ascribes to this ideal type also apply to activism in science and technology, for instance the belief that the normal workings of existing (scientific) institutions produce inadequate results and have unjust effects for certain groups of people and patients (ibid.: 673).

3 Especially since the 1990s, many rare disease patient associations have intensified their involvement in biomedical research and research policies, for instance by funding research projects or offering research awards in order to draw the attention of biomedicine to this class of previously underinvestigated diseases. To date, however, there exists no comprehensive account of rare disease patients' or advocates' engagement with medical research, but instead a number of case studies and "middle-range" comparative analyses (see for instance Rabeharisoa and Callon 1999; Callon and Rabeharisoa 2004, 2008; Stockdale and Terry 2002; Wailoo and Pemberton 2006; Terry et al. 2007; Huyard 2009a, 2009b, 2012; Panofsky 2011; Wehling 2011). Although there is a feeling of togetherness among these groups based on the shared state of "being rare", one must bear in mind that "rare disease" is ultimately merely a statistical category referring to the prevalence of a disease (in Europe, for instance, a disease is termed rare when no more than 5 in 10,000 people are affected), thus lumping together an estimated number of 5,000 to 7,000 diseases which may differ considerably in many other respects such as severity, age of onset and availability of treatment.

4 However, such interactions and discussions do not necessarily lead to consensus about collective interests. They can also result in dissent and the acknowledgement that the formation of a common interest is impossible, either in principle or temporarily. Even such dissent, though, does not simply follow from a pre-existing incompatibility of individual preferences but rather is the outcome of a process of collective reflection within the social group.

5 More precisely, it is usually the interplay of external influences and internal priorities that shapes the agenda of science; see also Proctor 1995; Frickel and Moore 2006; Frickel et al. 2010.

6 This applies, for instance, to the case of the residents of Woburn in Massachusetts, USA, who in the 1980s detected a cluster of leukemia among their children and correctly connected it to the contamination of their drinking water (Brown and Mikkelsen 1997).

7 According to Moore et al. (2011: 520) the concept of epistemic modernization "is intended to capture the shifts in the governance of science that have involved escalating levels of scrutiny by civil society actors toward scientific research and technology regulation, the growing permeability of the scientific and industrial fields to both partnerships with and opposition from various civil society actors, and the increasing legitimacy and institutionalization of such relationships through innovative collaborative arrangements and new forms of governance".

8 In the United States, NBS currently tests for about 50, but in some cases even up to 80 mostly genetic disorders (Grob 2011a: 1f.; Timmermans and Buchbinder 2013: 1f.).

9 Preconception carrier testing means that future parents are tested before pregnancy (or conception) in order to determine whether both of them are genetic carriers of the same genetic variation related to one of the up-to-600 recessively inherited rare conditions that are expected to be testable in the near future by a single DNA chip. In case of a positive result, each child of the couple has a 25 percent chance of having this condition. In this situation, apart from ignoring the test result, the couple has a number of reproductive options, ranging from not having children to the use of medical technologies such as prenatal diagnosis with possible termination of pregnancy, preimplantation genetic diagnosis (PGD), and sperm or egg donation.

10 NORD stands for *National Organization for Rare Disorders*, AMR for *Alliance Maladies Rares*, ACHSE for *Allianz Chronischer Seltener Erkrankungen*, and EURORDIS is Rare Diseases Europe.

11 One such disagreement emerged during a conference of the German rare disease umbrella organization ACHSE on PGD in 2011. Although a majority of the participating member groups argued in favor of PGD, ACHSE itself did not

take a position on this technology because it wanted to respect the diversity of voices within the organization.

References

Abma, Tineke A. and Broerse, Jacqueline (2010) Patient participation as dialogue: setting research agendas, *Health Expectations*, 13(2), 160–173.

Bogner, Alexander (2012) The paradox of participation experiments, *Science, Technology & Human Values*, 37(5), 506–527.

Braun, Katrin and Schultz, Susanne (2010) "… A certain amount of engineering involved": constructing the public in participatory governance arrangements, *Public Understanding of Science*, 19(4), 403–419.

Brown, Phil (1992) Popular epidemiology and toxic waste contamination: lay and professional ways of knowing, *Journal of Health and Social Behavior*, 33(3), 267–281.

Brown, Phil (2007) *Toxic Exposures: Contested illnesses and the Environmental Health Movement*, New York and Chichester: Columbia University Press.

Brown, Phil and Mikkelsen, Edwin J. (1997) *No Safe Place: Toxic Waste, Leukemia, and Community Action*, 2nd edition, Berkeley, CA: University of California Press.

Brown, Phil; McCormick, Sabrina; Mayer, Brian; Zavestoski, Stephen; Morello-Frosch, Rachel; Gasior Altman, Rebecca and Senier, Laura (2006) "A lab of our own": environmental causation of breast cancer and challenges to the dominant epidemiological paradigm, *Science, Technology & Human Values*, 31(5), 499–536.

Brown, Phil; Morello-Frosch, Rachel; Zavestoski, Stephen and the Contested Illnesses Research Group (2012) *Contested Illnesses: Citizens, Science, and Health Social Movements*, Berkeley, CA: University of California Press.

Bucchi, Massimiano and Neresini, Federico (2008) Science and public participation, in E. Hackett; O. Amsterdamska; M. Lynch and J. Wajcman (eds) *Handbook of Science and Technology Studies*, 3rd edition, Cambridge, MA: MIT Press, 449–473.

Callon, Michel and Rabeharisoa, Vololona (2003) Research "in the wild" and the shaping of new social identities, *Technology in Society*, 25(2), 193–204.

Callon, Michel and Rabeharisoa, Vololona (2004) Patients and scientists in French muscular dystrophy research, in S. Jasanoff (ed.) *States of Knowledge: The Co-production of Science and the Social Order*, London and New York: Routledge, 142–160.

Callon, Michel and Rabeharisoa, Vololona (2008) The growing engagement of emergent concerned groups in political and economic life: lessons from the French Association of Neuromuscular Disease Patients, *Science, Technology & Human Values*, 33(2), 230–261.

Callon, Michel; Lascoumes, Pierre and Barthe, Yannick (2009) *Acting in an Uncertain World: An Essay on Technical Democracy*, Cambridge, MA, and London: MIT Press.

Caron-Flinterman, Francisca; Broerse, Jacqueline and Bunders, Joske (2005) The experiential knowledge of patients: a new resource for biomedical research? *Social Science and Medicine*, 60(11), 2575–2584.

Elberse, Janneke; Caron-Flinterman, Francisca and Broerse, Jacqueline (2011) Patient-expert partnerships in research: how to stimulate inclusion of patient perspectives, *Health Expect*ations, 14(3), 225–329.

Epstein, Steven (2011) Measuring success: scientific, institutional, and cultural effects of patient advocacy, in B. Hoffman; R. Grob; M. Schlesinger and N. Tomes (eds) *Patients as Policy Actors*, New Brunswick, NJ, and London: Rutgers University Press, 257–277.

Frickel, Scott and Moore, Kelly (eds) (2006) *The New Political Sociology of Science: Institutions, Networks, and Power*, Madison, WI: University of Wisconsin Press.

Frickel, Scott; Gibbon, Sahra; Howard, Jeff; Kempner, Joanna; Ottinger, Gwen and Hess, David J. (2010) Undone science: charting social movement and civil society challenges to research agenda setting, *Science, Technology & Human Values*, 35(4), 444–473.

Fung, Archon (2003) Associations and democracy: between theories, hopes, and realities, *Annual Review of Sociology*, 29, 515–539.

Grob, Rachel (2011a) Testing Baby: The Transformation of Newborn Screening, Parenting, and Policy Making, Camden: Rutgers University Press.

Grob, Rachel (2011b) A house on fire: newborn screening, parents' advocacy, and the discourse of urgency, in B. Hoffman; N. Tomes; M. Schlesinger and R. Grob (eds) *Patients as Policy Actors*, New Brunswick, NJ, and London: Rutgers University Press, 231–256.

Grob, Rachel and Schlesinger, Mark (2011) Epilogue: principles for engaging patients in U.S. health care and policy, in B. Hoffman; N. Tomes; M. Schlesinger and R. Grob (eds) *Patients as Policy Actors*, New Brunswick, NJ, and London: Rutgers University Press, 278–291.

Hess, David J. (2009) The potentials and limitations of civil society research: getting undone science done, *Sociological Inquiry*, 79(3), 306–327.

Hess, David J. (2010) Environmental reform organizations and undone science in the united states: exploring the environmental, health, and safety implications of nanotechnology, *Science as Culture*, 19(2), 181–214.

Hess, David J. (2011) To tell the truth: on scientific counterpublics, *Public Understanding of Science*, 20(5), 627–641.

Huyard, Caroline (2009a) How did uncommon disorders become "rare diseases?" History of a boundary object, *Sociology of Health & Illness*, 31(4), 463–477.

Huyard, Caroline (2009b) Who rules rare disease associations? A framework to understand their action, *Sociology of Health & Illness*, 31(7), 979–993.

Huyard, Caroline (2012) *Rare: sur la cause politique des maladies peu fréquentes*, Paris: Editions de l'Ecole des Hautes Etudes en Sciences Sociales.

Kingsmore, Stephen (2012) Comprehensive carrier screening and molecular diagnostic testing for recessive childhood diseases, *PLOS Currents, Evidence on Genomic Tests.* Available online at: <http://currents.plos.org/genomictests/article/comprehensive-carrier-screening-and-molecular-diagnostic-testing-for-recessive-childhood-diseases> (accessed 23 May 2014).

Kitcher, Philip (2011) *Science in a Democratic Society*, New York: Prometheus Books.

Ley, Barbara (2009) *From Pink to Green. Disease Prevention and the Environmental Breast Cancer Movement*, New Brunswick, NJ: Rutgers University Press.

McCormick, Sabrina (2009a) *No Family History: The Environmental Links to Breast Cancer*, New York: Rowman and Littlefield.

McCormick, Sabrina (2009b) *Mobilizing Science: Movements, Participation, and the Remaking of Knowledge*, Philadelphia, PA: Temple University Press.

Mansbridge, Jane; Bohman, James; Chambers, Simone; Estlund, David; Føllesdal, Andreas; Fung, Archon; Lafont, Cristina; Manin, Bernard and Martí, José Luis (2010) The place of self-interest and the role of power in deliberative democracy, *Journal of Political Philosophy*, 18(1), 64–100.

Martin, Graham (2008) "Ordinary people only": knowledge, representativeness, and the publics of public participation in healthcare, *Sociology of Health and Illness*, 30(1), 35–54.

Moore, Kelly; Frickel, Scott; Hess, David and Kleinman, Daniel (2011) Science and neoliberal globalization: a political sociological approach, *Theory and Society*, 40(5), 505–532.

Moss, Pamela and Teghtsoonian, Katherine (eds) (2008) *Contesting Illness: Process and Practices*, Toronto and London: University of Toronto Press.

Müller-Wille, Staffan and Rheinberger, Hans-Jörg (2012) *A Cultural History of Heredity*, Chicago: University of Chicago Press.

Panofsky, Aron (2011) Generating sociability to drive science: patient advocacy organizations and genetics research, *Social Studies of Science*, 41(1), 31–57.

Powell, Maria C. and Colin, Mathilde (2009) Participatory paradoxes: facilitating citizen engagement in science and technology from the top-down? *Bulletin of Science, Technology & Society*, 29(4), 325–342.

Prior, Lindsay (2003) Belief, knowledge and expertise: the emergence of the lay expert in medical sociology, *Sociology of Health and Illness*, 25(3), Silver Anniversary Issue, 41–57.

Prior, Lindsay; Evans, Meirion R. and Prout, Hayley (2011) Talking about colds and flu: the lay diagnosis of two common illnesses among older British people, *Social Science & Medicine*, 73(6), 922–928.

Proctor, Robert N. (1995) *Cancer Wars: How Politics Shapes What We Know and Don't Know about Cancer*, New York: Basic Books.

Rabeharisoa, Vololona and Callon, Michel (1999) *Le Pouvoir des malades: l'Association française contre les myopathies et la recherche*, Paris: Presses de l'Ecole des Mines.

Stockdale, Alan and Terry, Sharon (2002) Advocacy groups and the new genetics, in J. Alper; C. Ard; A. Asch, J. Beckwith; P. Conrad and L. N. Geller (eds) *The Double-Edged Helix: Social Implications of Genetics in a Diverse Society*, Baltimore, MD and London: Johns Hopkins University Press, 80–101.

Terry, Sharon F.; Terry, Patrick F.; Rauen, Katherine A.; Uitto, Jouni and Bercovitch, Lionel G. (2007) Advocacy groups as research organizations: the PXE International example, *Nature Reviews Genetics*, 8(2), 157–164.

Timmermans, Stefan and Buchbinder Mara (2013) *Saving Babies? The Consequences of Newborn Genetic Screening*, Chicago: University of Chicago Press.

Tomes, Nancy and Hoffman, Beatrix (2011) Introduction: patients as policy actors, in B. Hoffman; N. Tomes; R. Grob and M. Schlesinger (eds) *Patients as Policy Actors*, New Brunswick, NJ, and London: Rutgers University Press, 1–16.

Viehöver, Willy and Wehling, Peter (eds) (2011) *Entgrenzung der Medizin: Von der Heilkunst zur Verbesserung des Menschen?* Bielefeld: Transcript Verlag.

Wailoo, Keith and Pemberton, Stephen (2006) *The troubled dream of genetic medicine*, Baltimore, MD: Johns Hopkins University Press.

Wehling, Peter (2011) The "technoscientization" of medicine and its limits: technoscientific identities, biosocialities, and rare disease patient organizations, *Poiesis & Praxis: International Journal of Technology Assessment and Ethics of Science*, 8(2–3), 67–82.

Wehling, Peter (2012) From invited to uninvited participation (and back?): rethinking civil society engagement in technology assessment and development, *Poiesis & Praxis: International Journal of Technology Assessment and Ethics of Science*, 9(1–2), 43–60.

Wehling, Peter and Viehöver, Willy (2013) "Uneingeladene" Partizipation der Zivilgesellschaft: ein kreatives Element der Governance von Wissenschaft, in E. Grande; E. Jansen; O. Jarren; A. Rip; U. Schimank and P. Weingart (eds) *Neue Governance der Wissenschaft: Reorganisation – externe Anforderungen – Medialisierung*, Bielefeld: Transcript Verlag, 213–234.

Wynne, Brian (2007) Public participation in science and technology: performing and obscuring a political–conceptual category mistake, *East Asian Science, Technology and Society: An International Journal*, 1(1), 99–110.
Wynne, Brian (2014): Further disorientation in the hall of mirrors, *Public Understanding of Science*, 23(1), 60–70.
Young, Iris Marion (1996) Communication and the other: beyond deliberative democracy, in S. Benhabib (ed.) *Democracy and Difference: Contesting the Boundaries of the Political*, Princeton, NJ: Princeton University Press, 120–135.
Young, Iris Marion (2001) Activist challenges to deliberative democracy, *Political Theory*, 29(5), 670–690.

13 The ethical legitimacy of patient organizations' involvement in politics and knowledge production

Epistemic justice as a conceptual basis[1]

Silke Schicktanz

Introduction

In 2011, the leading US American Alzheimer's advocacy group, the Alzheimer's Association, launched a campaign for 'A world free of Alzheimer's'.[2] The Alzheimer's Association supports academic research with grants of up to ten million US dollars per year for research, particularly in the fields of biomedicine and the neurosciences. On its website it offers a 'find-a-clinical-trial' database to encourage its members and visitors – mostly family members and sometimes patients themselves – to become engaged with biomedicine. In contrast, the leading German Alzheimer's advocacy group Deutsche Alzheimer Gesellschaft e.V.[3] provides grants mainly for integrative care or psycho-social research. On its website, it provides position papers and statements[4] problematizing the involvement of Alzheimer's patients in research and clinical trials – especially if it is third-party research, which means there is no individual benefit to a research participant or this is very unlikely.

The shaping of dementia research by these two patient organizations thus differs with regard to both the epistemic and ethical dimension of research. On the one hand, they differ in their prioritization of the kind of research needed to 'solve' the serious problems dementia causes for patients, their families and societies, while on the other hand, they have different opinions about whether involving severely cognitively impaired patients such as Alzheimer's patients in clinical, pharmaceutical, psychological or even sociological research is ethically acceptable, as can be seen from the different ways they balance risks against benefits and agency against self-determination.

These differences in grant policy, priority setting for research topics and bioethical positions between two advocacy groups working in the same field are remarkable. Advocacy groups not only strive for a particular kind of research allocation or challenge epistemic premises about illness or its etiology (see Brown et al. 2012) but also play an important role in bioethical and biopolitical discourses. This biopolitical engagement is certainly embedded in a broader politico-legal and cultural framework, as a comparison would reveal. While in the USA, third-interest research with patients who are cognitively impaired is allowed under restrictions for proxy consent (see National Bioethics Advisory Commission 1998), the German expert discourse on ethics and law is less permissive. Concerns, also raised by patient associations, about misuse and imbalanced risk-benefit assessment have led to Germany's rejection of the Oviedo Convention of Human rights and Bioethics by the Council of Europe (1997), as the convention does allow third-interest research with cognitively impaired patients. In this case, advocacy groups are not per se 'research friendly'.

This example shows the possible variations of positions towards ethical, scientific and political issues that can be held by 'similar' advocacy groups. This diversity is thus a strong motive to reflect upon the role and impact patient organizations and health advocacy groups can and should have in the public-political sphere. From a sociological or political perspective, there are immense cultural differences in how advocacy groups engage with the public, scientific and political spheres (Wood 2000; Raz et al. 2012). Skeptical voices might immediately ask: why should we include advocacy perspectives at all if they differ so much? The inclusion or exclusion of such positions therefore needs a particular normative justification.

In the following, I will not seek to answer the question of the dynamics or factors explaining such cultural differences, but will examine the ethical question of what, given this heterogeneity, justifies the inclusion of patients' perspectives. Such ethical-normative considerations of inclusion rely on sociological research on patient organizations with respect to their empirical relevance and their understanding of dynamics and conflicts. In this regard, ethical-normative considerations are located between the empirical analysis of the impact of patient advocacy and the critical assessment of that impact. Is there too much or too little impact? Are the positions one-sided, balanced, arbitrary, or justified?

In the following chapter, I will refer to a more general level of argumentation as to why the involvement of patient advocacy is ethically needed and justified. I will do so by showing, first, that this is still a marginalized perspective in the political and ethical expert discourse, and will then criticize the often implicit and sometimes explicit expertocratism that exists in mainstream medical research. The main argument here for the political involvement of patient organizations – or, more generally, the inclusion of patients' and advocates' perspectives – is 'epistemic justice'. Epistemic *in*justice, as the philosopher Miranda Fricker has argued, pre-structures many public, political and scientific discourses, especially where knowledge and experience constitute the factual basis within ethical or legal frameworks (Fricker 2009). By applying Fricker's reasoning to the particular situation of being 'a patient' or an 'affected person' in a context where expert opinions still dominate the discourse, we find a strong argument for the inclusion of patients. Subsequently, this general point of view is confronted with the social fact mentioned above: that advocacy groups can differ strongly in their political power, ways of lobbying, and positions adopted. This will be discussed with regard to some more practical implications.

Some background assumptions: why applied ethics needs epistemics

Ethics is often understood as ethical reasoning and reflection upon the normative meaning of statements and moral assessments, but without empirical considerations because of the need to avoid the 'is-ought gap'. I want to critically revise this assumption by introducing the concept of *applied ethics.* In applied ethics, we attempt to make an ethical judgment in the form of an imperative: 'X should do Y in the context of Z'. This judgment is a *mixed* judgment which relies on premises that are prescriptive (normative, e.g. 'it is good to save a human life') *and* descriptive (empirical, e.g. 'by this pharmaceutical treatment, individual life can be prolonged for 10 years').[5] These premises are concerned with different kinds of criticism: the former raises the question of (basic) justification (e.g. what is the final source of our moral assumption), while the latter has to grapple with epistemological doubts (e.g. how valid and robust is the empirical evidence for the descriptive statements). The relationship between the premises is difficult in two respects. First, it is important to avoid the is-ought fallacy. One can do this by explicating the underlying moral assumption. Second, it is important to reflect how far the descriptive premise is really 'ethically neutral', e.g. how our assumption of what counts as valid epistemics depends on normative assumptions of what is good science, or how trustworthy such a descriptive statement can be. In this sense, the two forms of modern skepticism do not appear as independent, but co-exist in a reflexive relationship.

In the following, my focus will lie on the interface of epistemic and ethical fundamental conditions, which are also labeled 'epistemic duties' (Lübbe 2002) or, to be more specific, epistemic justice (Fricker 2009). A number of feminist epistemologists have argued that it is important to reflect upon this relation in order to gain a better understanding of how to deal with science in the public sphere (for an overview, see Intemann 2010). What I am arguing here is congruent with feminist epistemological stances that argue for an understanding of knowledge production that is context-sensitive, social, and normatively loaded. However, my argumentation goes beyond this stance in two ways. I argue from a normative perspective of ethical reasoning (and not in an epistemological way of understanding knowledge production), and I suggest that we need to interpret the idea of 'situated knowledge' (Haraway 1988) as a morally relevant form of 'being affected'. The focus will be on the inclusion of certain *perspectives*, namely those of affected persons.[6]

The inclusion of those perspectives can happen by different means. Whether for such an inclusion direct political forms such as social protests, public hearings and consultations, participatory and deliberative elements or indirect ways such as empirical research in social sciences are more appropriate is the subject of debate from theoretical and pragmatic points of view. I will set aside these debates, and here focus on the basic assumptions that justify the inclusion of such perspectives.[7]

The spectrum of 'lay' perspectives in health and science discourse

According to the classical sociological lay-expert division, there seems to be no particular difference between lay people, citizens and people affected directly, indirectly or potentially. However, the rise of new concepts such as 'lay expert' or 'scientifi c citizen' means that we need to differentiate the spectrum of knowledge and experience non-professionals can have. While the scientifi c citizen has been virtually made into the ideal of European science policy, its basic assumption is that there should be something called a knowledge economy in which citizens informed on scientifi c topics are willing and able to take part in debates and discourses (Felt 2003: 18):

> The concept of the scientifi c citizen is a much more active concept which contains the idea of rights and duties: that is, the right to be informed on science and technology, to take part in debates and decisions, but to some extent also the duty to be informed, to reflect on subjects, to take responsibility, to position oneself as part of a collective and according to its interests.
>
> (author's translation)

In contrast, lay experts, as Epstein (1995, 1996) labeled HIV activists, constitute a new phenomenon of public actors, namely patients who engage actively in knowledge construction and even reform clinical research and health care.

From a political-ethical point of view it is debatable whether these new types of lay actors already constitute a democratization of knowledge production or even of science policy. But what can be said is that they characterize attempts to classify and analyze new emerging relationships between epistemic (knowledge, expertise) and political-normative categorizations (citizenship). While the debate on the scientifi c citizen means significantly turning away from the *passive* consumer, user or patient, the concept is highly controversial with regard to its idealization and to normative claims about how citizens have to be. The discussion about lay expertise, instead, illuminates the existing power relations related to expertise. When only used in an affi rmative way, it runs the risk of underestimating the still-existing power asymmetry between lay persons and professionals. Moreover, it also can lead to reducing the interests and opinions of these patients to epistemic claims, while neglecting the important moral dimensions linked to patients' perspectives. These moral dimensions include, for example in the cases of HIV activists and Alzheimer's advocacy groups, protection against discrimination or social exclusion and the right to be medically treated and socially respected.

A theoretical category that encompasses both the epistemic and the normative dimension of a lay person's relevance in a better way is the term 'affected person'. While the term 'lay person' emphasizes the epistemic aspect of not possessing any prior scientifi c education, the complex term 'being affected' implies the claim to an epistemically and normatively exclusive position, based on the two factors of having experience *and* bearing the consequences (see also Schicktanz et al. 2008).[8] According to the sociologist Otthein Rammstedt (1981), the term has two basic but only partly related meanings. On the one hand, 'being affected' establishes a causal relationship, the (positive or, more often than not, negative) impact of an event on a person or a group of people. In this respect, the relationship may even be independent of the awareness of the person(s) involved. For example, patients suffering from chronic renal disease are 'affected' with regard to the political debate on organ transplantation. This is the case even if the patients do not feel directly addressed, but experts and politicians justify legal reforms aiming at fostering organ donation argumentatively using those patients as a statistical factor in order to emphasize the moral problems resulting from organ shortage.

On the other hand, 'being affected' denotes an emotional reaction to an event. This will usually include emotions such as compassion, care and empathy. Thus someone can be affected by the pain or discrimination which ill or disabled persons experience without ever having undergone these him or herself. This kind of being affected becomes explicitly normatively relevant when we argue for solidarity and social responsibility.

Even if the two meanings of being affected are structurally different, they are nevertheless connected in some cases. We can observe, for example, that feelings of being affected emotionally by others will be stronger and more enduring if this person is also affected objectively. Thus, in the field of social movements, 'being affected' can be seen as another major factor in changing social awareness and politics on behalf of social solidarity with and the attaining of social power by affected persons. Overall, epistemically, being affected is characterized with reference to experiences, personal insights and actual knowledge of circumstances, but also involves bearing the material or psychological consequences of an event or condition.

These two meanings become related by the way in which the emotional component supports and encourages the principle of adopting others' perspectives and standpoints, in other words, putting oneself in someone else's position.[9] This change of perspective implies, on the one hand, anticipating and empathizing with strong and basic convictions, with physical and psychic suffering or actual experiences of discrimination. But it may also lead to the insight that some experiences cannot be easily understood or anticipated. This 'asymmetrical reciprocity', as Iris Marion Young (1997: 41ff.) calls it, accepts insurmountable differences, ruptures and the specific localization of the other in a relationship of mutual recognition.

Health advocacy groups encompass a broad spectrum of affected persons. Here, the term 'advocacy group' is used as an umbrella term for different kinds of patient organizations and associations that tend to include family members or semi-professionals who speak on behalf of patients. As 'advocacy' groups they can be distinguished by their political engagement from non-political, mainly local, short-term self-help groups. However, we need a critical perspective on what constitutes the social and political background of the majority in advocacy groups. As Susan Chandler (1990) has convincingly shown in relation to the controversy about advocates for persons with mental illness, 'advocates' can claim to speak on behalf of the patients but sometimes rather advocate their own interests. The development of self-advocacy by persons with autism (e.g. as promoted by the Autistic Self Advocacy Network (ASAN) – http://autisticadvocacy.org), who have publicly criticized the power and particular positions taken towards research and care by established 'advocates' (mainly parents of autistic children), illustrates the importance of such differences (Wehmeyer et al. 2000).

The concept of 'being affected' therefore needs to be distinguished in terms of different stages or passages in the field of health care. We can speak of 'directly affected persons' when we mean patients suffering from a particular illness, and can distinguish 'indirectly affected persons' such as close family members or care givers who care emotionally about the patients and whose social life is also seriously affected by the illness. Moreover, a third category is useful in the context of predicting genetic diseases, risks for age-related impairments, or end of life planning. It is necessary to distinguish 'anticipated affected persons' who are not yet ill but on whom the anticipation of future prospects has already had a psychological or social impact.

The need for a plurality of perspectives and the inclusion of situated knowledge

The professional expertise of health professionals, ethicists, and social scientists is broadly applied in health policy advice. This practice is, however, a source of criticism and skepticism based on different premises, which may be related to democratic theory or political theory (Gutmann and Thompson 1997; Dodds and Thomson 2006), epistemology (Feyerabend 1989), or metaethical questions (Steinkamp et al. 2008; Archard 2011). The last two kinds of considerations are often put forward as a way of challenging the ideal of truth or the objectivity of science as such, and particularly as challenges to *normative* expertise (Schicktanz et al. 2012). Whether skepticism about any kind of professional expertise must result in denial of any knowledge-informed political decision is, however, questionable. Rather, it is important to note that professional knowledge cannot serve alone as a legitimating basis for external, social decisions (Lübbe 2002: 153). This argument includes any kind of expertise, whether it is of natural scientific, social scientific or philosophical nature.

From a theoretical point of view, the solution to this problem of legitimacy lies not in simple, practical forms of lay participation in research and policy making[10] but in a conceptual analysis of the kind of perspectives needed. In practice, we do not yet have such perspectives. We are assuming here that there is no single, ultimate perspective; only a combination of different perspectives can offer us an approximation of the 'whole picture'. But how does this joint pluralism of perspectivism come into play? It requires a systematic adoption of others' perspectives – the whole gaze has to switch to another person.

Being sensitive to the problem of adopting others' perspectives is a central element in feminist epistemology. Here, Donna Haraway's work in science and technology studies from the 1980s occupies a prominent place. Critically referring to the postmodern sense of superficiality and relativism on the one hand and the rather materialist-reductionist, formal analytical tradition of rationality on the other, she develops the concept of the social situatedness of knowledge (Haraway 1988). Her concept of 'situated knowledge' stands in the tradition of feminist criticism of science, which is especially interesting from an ethical perspective. Science is critically challenged in relation to power structures and the problematic separation of knowledge production and application (Harding 1987) by using historical, Marxist and social constructivist approaches. However, Haraway goes a step further as she also includes the morally motivated engagement *with* science. What is at stake is not purely deconstruction and criticism, but a

> successor science project that offers a more adequate, richer, better account of the world, in order to live in it well and in a critical, reflexive relation to our own as well as others' practices of domination and the unequal parts of privilege and oppression that make up all positions.
> (Haraway 1988: 579)

As Haraway points out, what is called epistemology in feminist criticism is understood as 'ethics and politics' in philosophy (ibid.: 579). This point must be emphasized, as it signals a joint interest but a different disciplinary practice of labeling. Haraway's method of choice is a critical-empirical one which does not reduce differences; it acknowledges and creates the radical multiplicity of local knowledge and values it as a source of comprehensive knowledge. In contrast to the classic assumption of distant, abstract knowledge, she proposes particular, embodied knowledge. But this knowledge is not 'innocent' (ibid.: 582), meaning morally neutral. Rather, the aim is to challenge *every* form of positioning and representation, to deconstruct and to analyze it.

Consequently, an acceptable discourse when deciding about aims and means of Alzheimer's disease research requires much more than various experts' reflections (e.g. ethicists or lawyers saying what kind of research is ethically acceptable) combined with objective facts about the disease, compiled by medical, neuroscience and public health experts. The underlying 'morally thick concepts' and their everyday life experience such as 'health', 'illness', 'normality' or 'quality of life' must be collected, scrutinized and compared in their theoretical richness *and* lived diversity (on diversity in Alzheimer's experience, see Innes et al. 2004). In a second step, the ideal of a 'point of view' as a 'view from nowhere' (which Haraway ironically terms the 'God's eye position'), a stance which many modern, cognitivistic approaches share, whether in ethics (Baier 1958) or science (Popper 2005), must be questioned. Under the premise of power relations and hegemonic structures of public and professional debates, particularly marginalized positions must be sufficiently recognized.

Understanding epistemic injustice in existing discourses

While the ideal of freedom from power sometimes seduces normative ethics into negating or ignoring the problem of existing power relations, the critique of power is almost ubiquitous in the social sciences. This minefield is entered by the philosopher Miranda Fricker (2009) in a promising way. In Fricker's view, questions of epistemology are closely linked to questions of justice. Referring to the above-mentioned concept of situated knowledge, she is concerned with tracing problems of the social distribution of power in ethically relevant discourses right in the construction of knowledge. In doing so, she argues from the assumption of the existence of concrete subjects, communicative interactions and social interdependencies between the parties concerned instead of abstract frameworks. The actors and parties involved do not have to have an explicit, rational or direct understanding of these interdependencies but they can still turn them into a source of epistemic injustice. Fricker summarizes this central assumption of her approach by saying that 'a socially situated account of human practice is an account such that participants are conceived not in abstraction from relations of social power (as they are in traditional epistemology, including most social epistemology) but as operating as social types who stand in relation of power to one another' (ibid.: 3).[11]

The concept of the social situatedness of knowledge allows for a closer scrutiny of power relations and epistemic authority, and a critical evaluation of their influence on the ethical framework of our epistemic practice. Only by doing this, Fricker argues, can we achieve an epistemic procedure that is in fact more rational and fair. This approach helps us to understand and justify the need for fair mechanisms and participatory procedures in shaping science and health policies. For this, one has to identify the two major different types of epistemic injustice Fricker has classified: testimonial and hermeneutic injustice.

When would our epistemic procedure be ethically problematic? According to Fricker, this would be the case if it were 'unjust'. Assuming that the *epistemological* conditions of the descriptive elements of judgment and subsequent decisions are important, this poses a serious problem. These epistemological conditions refer to descriptions of, for example, risks, expected benefit, social impact, questions of practicability, desirability, the existence of opposition or opinions etc. in relation to a particular practice (e.g. in health care: organ transplantation, predictive genetic testing, or a particular pharmaceutical therapy). Statements made about this by those taking part in the discourse, e.g. experts, are not detached from but dependent on the social reality; and this reality is not free of power constellations. Power should not be conceived as abstract or structural,[12] but as the capacity of concrete agents. Fricker defines it as 'a practically socially situated capacity to control others' actions, where this capacity may be exercised (actively or passively) by particular agents, or alternatively it may operate purely structurally' (2009: 13).

Testimonial injustice: undermining or underrepresenting social group members' credibility by means of stereotypes

As already mentioned, one very relevant form is 'testimonial injustice', which might be paraphrased as an unjust evaluation of credibility. This includes all situations in which someone is not trusted, for example when he or she is not taken seriously as a witness because of the unjustified prejudice that the person concerned is incompetent, irrational, partial, dishonest, etc. Testimonial injustice arises when the listener *underestimates* or *overestimates* the speaker regarding his or her credibility. The importance of a speaker's credibility to the recognition of his or her statements can be exemplified with reference to the role of an expert or witness in court. Fricker argues that injustices occur when the listener systematically misinterprets the speaker because of prejudices and stereotypes (2009: 17ff.). According to Fricker, injustice only exists in the case of an unjustified lack of credibility, but not in the reverse case of overestimating credibility: 'The primary characterization of testimonial injustice … remains such that it is a matter of credibility deficit and not credibility excess' (ibid.: 21). Overestimation would in fact *benefit* the other person and would thus be something like undeserved luck. However, Fricker's limitation of injustice to underestimation is not convincing. Many prejudices are based on socially contained, antagonistic assumptions of traits. The overestimation of one group often goes along with the systematic underestimation of another group. This is particularly the case in conflicts between lay and professional or advocacy and 'neutral' experts. Giving greater credibility to experts because they are 'expert' is an overestimation of their credibility, and it is systematically associated with an underestimation of the credibility of lay persons. Especially in medical and health care issues, this is problematic as the situated knowledge lay persons and patients have about illness or care for ill family members is not systematically less credible. It simply differs from the expert explanation of a disease and its social implications.

Such systematic misjudgments are based on mistaken assumptions about others' capacity to know (ibid.: 20). These assumptions feed on prejudices regarding social identity, that is to say the speaker's social involvement in class, gender, and ethnicity but also in education, religion, politics, or (sub) culture and so on. In our case, it also includes prejudices regarding illness or disability. Prejudices concerning social identities are based on *stereotypes*. In terms of social psychology, stereotypes are an elementary concept of cognitive heuristics used to deal with social complexity (Tversky and Kahneman 1974; Greenwald and Banaji 1995). Therefore it is sometimes hard to identify stereotypes or to eliminate the reference to stereotypes from the range of human behaviors. In an epistemic sense, stereotypes turn into a problem when they lead to wrong or unreliable statements about the seriousness or competence of individual members of a social group (Fricker 2009: 23ff.). Typically, negative social stereotypes attribute excessive emotionality, low intelligence, evolutionary inferiority, lack of logic, ignorance, being uninformed, or moral dubiousness. Historical stereotypes relating to socially marginalized groups such as women, senior citizens or certain ethnic communities often use one or more of these attributes. Stereotypes about chronically ill patients or their advocates work in the same way, suggesting that they are too emotional, too partial, too egoistic, uninformed, cognitively impaired, etc.

In the field of dementia, this becomes even more relevant. The social representation of dementia is dominated by ageism, negative stereotypes, moral panic and a biomedical model of disease. Being elderly or demented is hence associated with being totally socially dependent, cognitively totally incompetent, and behaving in a totally 'unusual' way (McColgan 2004: 171ff.). Such imputations have been predominant in the USA for many years and are increasingly becoming relevant in Germany as well. The negative stereotype also impacts on caregivers for people with dementia; they are conceptualized as socially dependent, overwhelmed, emotional, suffering and socially isolated.

Depending on the context, stereotypes can have positive as well as negative connotations. The crucial problem which numerous social psychological studies have shown lies in the fact that stereotypes influence not only formal ascriptions but also the listener's (and to a certain degree also the speaker's) entire cognitive disposition. This makes it especially hard to identify them. In their review, the social psychologists Anthony Greenwald and Mahzarin Banaji (1995) refer to a number of studies which show how test persons are implicitly (in the sense of unconsciously) influenced by positive and negative stereotypes of race and gender. The effects of social stereotypes, especially historically evolved ones, may even be seen in persons who explicitly distance themselves from such stereotypes. Social stereotypes also affect self-images and active performance (e.g. in cognitive tests). This supports Fricker's statement that we must assume that injustices in the ascription of credibility are widespread in the discourses of our everyday life (Fricker 2009: 39).

To what extent, then, are these considerations helpful in analyzing the relevance of expertise and of 'being affected' in debates related to science? Assumptions about who is an expert, a lay person or an affected person can be crucial to the practical discourse and the inclusion of different voices. Lay persons, affected persons and professionals constitute social groups which categorize one another by using stereotypes. These social categories and their attendant attributes are constantly being performed and confirmed in public discourse. Thus experts tend to describe lay persons as ignorant, uninformed and rather emotional (see, for example, Rippe 2000). Affected persons such as the representatives of patient associations are usually considered to be informed, but there is a fear that they will be partial, susceptible and even corruptible (e.g. by the pharmaceutical industry) (cf. Paul 2008), whereas experts are described as intelligent, rational, logical, analytical, etc. – whether by themselves or by others.

These attributes can be crucial for the way certain statements on risks, the needs, the means or objectives of patients and the underlying values are assessed. Epistemic injustice often occurs when experts (but also other listeners such as lay persons and politicians) discredit statements by lay or affected persons as less credible *because* they were voiced by lay or affected persons. A first step to counter epistemic injustices therefore consists of uncovering these stereotypes and raising consciousness about them.[13]

Hermeneutic injustice: the impossibility of naming a problem

A second form of epistemic injustice can be understood as hermeneutic injustice (Fricker 2009: 248ff.). Compared to testimonial injustice, the first form of epistemic injustice, it represents a more complex case because injustice here arises from the fact that a whole society is *unable* to call a serious problem by its name. Thus, it implies situations in which a certain problem is not yet culturally conceptualized or linguistically defined. Accordingly, Fricker defines hermeneutic injustice as 'the injustice of having some significant area of one's social experience obscured from collective understanding owing to a structural identity prejudice in the collective hermeneutical resource' (ibid.: 155). Thus, affected persons have difficulties recognizing their fears and the injustice they suffer as well as communicating these or demanding changes. The concept of physical disability, which has dominated the debate for a long time, can be an example of hermeneutic injustice. Only the disability rights movement of the late 1970s brought about a change of perspective by arguing that external and social factors are the things that actually disable people (cf. Charlton 2000). Since then the social model of disability has suggested that for wheelchair users, for example, it is urban planning and social and architectural ignorance that are disabling – while they themselves are not per se disabled.

Hermeneutic injustice as structural discrimination means that certain social groups are prima facie marginalized. The articulation of problems they are striving for is systematically ignored or pushed aside because the problem they are trying to articulate touches a culturally blank space with no generally recognized concepts. Their suffering already exists as an experience, but neither the affected persons nor their environment can accurately name it. Thus it is hard for the affected persons to clearly articulate their concern among themselves, and even more difficult to communicate it to other social groups.

Using the concept of hermeneutic limitations in the wide field of medicine and technology development might cover several dimensions. First, it might be related to yet unknown risks related to the introduction of modern technologies and their impact on bodies, life and social interaction. Unknown risks can also be understood as a problem of a certain inability to describe something in words, and as long as they are not adequately labeled they do not count.[14] Second, it might help in understanding the problem of contested illness (Brown et al. 2012). Here, affected persons want to strive for labels and etiology of a particular illness experience and therefore start talking about their experiences. This can result in heated debates with scientists if they are seen to neglect the shared experience. The affected persons' claiming for such a label, however, can be understood as a claim to hermeneutic justice. Nevertheless, there are also examples where the opposite happens, and an existing biomedical description of a disease is criticized or even radically rejected by a community of affected people. They resist the way a labeling normally causes a socially negative 'career' (Thoits 2011) because it does not address their experience adequately, e.g. deaf communities rejecting any attempts to be classified as deviant (Blume 2010). Other reasons for resistance are high levels of coping strategies, effective treatment, or multiple role-identities (Thoits 2011).

Practical implications of epistemic justice: including marginalized perspectives of health advocacy groups

According to Fricker, by using a procedural approach epistemological injustices can be revealed and avoided. This means that *just epistemological* conditions must be created. The ethically problematic epistemological limitations also imply a need for action in scientific practice itself. We must counterbalance these limitations or altogether avoid them.

In social practice, three strategies have been established to avoid such forms of discrimination: identity blindness, raising consciousness and affirmative action (Greenwald and Banaji 1995: 19). Identity blindness can be practiced in assessments or experiments which actually make it possible to eliminate all social information on the 'speaker'. In a public discourse, however, this is hardly possible. Consciousness raising is very successful in a number of respects, especially to reduce hermeneutic injustices. This has been shown in successful campaigns on consciousness raising and education in the women's, civil rights and disability movements which have repeatedly pointed out grievances and offered successful alternatives. This, however, needs socially mobilized groups who fight for the implementation of strategies of consciousness. This shows the limits for contained or small groups whose perspective is marginalized. Affirmative action is defended as a strategy for use when the first two strategies fail. Moreover, it can be regarded as compensating for past, present and future implicit forms of injustice (ibid.: 19).

It should be noted, however, that including particular perspectives goes well beyond the idea of what Steven Epstein (2007) has described as the new inclusion paradigm in recent medical research. Here, inclusion is reduced to the systematic recruitment of diverse populations in research settings. Examples of such new research participants are women, elderly patients, children, or patients with different ethnic backgrounds, and the goal is to overcome the physiological bias in pharmaceutical research if only white, young men are included as research participants. However, this form of bodily inclusion does not necessarily address the particular interests, experiences or opinions those groups have. According to Caroline Cantley and Alison Bowes (2004), any adequate social inclusion requires value commitments, including the recognition of personhood, valuing relationships and citizenship, service development and specialization to address individual needs.

In this sense, the inclusion of perspectives can only be achieved by including representatives of those perspectives. Advocacy groups in dementia (and mental illness) have been criticized for paying too much attention to the carer's perspective (for the UK: Cantley and Bowes 2004: 268f.; for the USA: Beard 2004). But this is beginning to change, with people with dementia in different stages being enabled to play an active role in such advocacy groups. Although carers are not the natural representatives of people with dementia, their experiences and interests are of importance and are often overlooked by experts. They unanimously demand better and sufficient resources for care, more individualized service, and local support. There is a major difference between these demands and recent political and professional activities, which have mainly focused on the neuroscience basis of dementia and neglected the social dimensions of this illness. In this case, overcoming epistemic injustice would mean including the voices and perspectives of people with dementia by respecting their wishes and needs for individualized care, and challenging the medical model of dementia which only focuses on loss, risk, and dependency.[15]

All three strategies for avoiding discrimination can be transferred to the problem outlined at the beginning. In public and policy debates about health care, scientific experts' perspectives receive more attention while the perspectives of affected persons, both carers and people with dementia, are marginalized. Therefore the contrasting of the views of the US and German Alzheimer's advocacy groups is closely related to questions of epistemic (in) justice, both in its testimonial and hermeneutic form. To whom should be given more credibility and authority when it comes to defining research priorities, the scientists, the carers or the patients? How (and by whom) can the hitherto hardly communicable needs and experiences of both dementia patients and carers be publicly and politically articulated? Thus, reflecting on epistemic justice can sensitize us for the possibly unjust and unjustified marginalization and exclusion of certain perspectives from 'rational' political and scientific communication.

In contrast to social movement theory, which mainly reflects on the social fact of whether or not activists are putting forward their own positions, the object of this ethical-normative approach is to illuminate more generally the need for different perspectives. This is particularly true in contexts where social groups are weakly represented in debates on health care and sciences. This approach therefore goes beyond historically and culturally contingent events such as bottom-up social movements. It seeks instead to problematize the absence of such movements, and looks for alternatives, such as top-down perspectives, e.g. within a deliberative model of a democratic shaping of science.

Future directions

Patient organizations and advocacy groups, particularly in their diversity, are an important mediator between individual patients' interests and public stakeholder activism. However, a critical perspective on their particular perspective is needed. The argument developed above can serve as a general framework for the analysis of existing power relations and discursive strategies for combating epistemic injustice. However, it also provides a basis for more scrutiny regarding the question of who should be involved. Given the diversity and plurality of patient associations and advocacy groups, including their sometimes contradictory positions on serious medical or ethical problems, a fair and balanced politics of inclusion would be required. For example, in the case of Alzheimer's disease and the increasing public efforts to 'deal' with this disease, there is a whole complex spectrum of crucial, unsolved ethical and practical problems. This includes the important question in many countries of providing sufficient and human medical care facilities. Moreover, it also means reflecting on the emerging technologies being used to look for a pre-symptomatic prediction of Alzheimer's disease, e.g. by genetic tests (which is rather unlikely because the APOE susceptibility tests used are very vague predictors) or (more likely) by new neuroimaging biomarkers. Nevertheless, the need to develop effi cient and affordable treatments should not be underestimated. Hence, it is important to critically assess existing positions and to identify what they may leave out. Any politics of inclusion must be justified against existing epistemic injustices, not only between affected lay persons and experts but even within the often broad spectrum of advocacy groups.

Recent legal developments, e.g. in Germany and the UK, to include representatives of patient associations in health policy committees on the regional and even national level, raise the serious question of whether only a few perspectives will be represented. Once again, there is a risk that some groups will be more strongly 'marginalized' than others. A balanced and transparent selection process therefore is an ethical necessity. How such a process can be guided and organized will be a delicate question of participatory governance structures (see Wehling and Viehöver in Chapter 12 of this volume), but is not an unsolvable problem as such.

Acknowledgement

I would like to thank Wendy Sarvasay, Berkeley, and Mark Brown, Sacramento, for instructive discussions on an earlier version of this chapter, and the editors of this volume for helpful comments.

Notes

1 Some parts of this contribution draw on my considerations in Schicktanz 2012 (in German).

2 See <www.alz.org> (accessed 14 June 2013).

3 German Association for Alzheimer's, author's translation, see <www.deutsche-alzheimer.de> (accessed 14 June 2013), only available in German.

4 See <www.deutsche-alzheimer.de/unser-service/archiv-alzheimer-info/ethik-und-alzheimer.html> (accessed 14 June 2013).

5 This form of argumentation goes back to Aristotle's concept of the practical syllogism in ethics, which is a three-point argument. It is based first on a general, major theory (here: normative premise such as a moral maxim) and is combined with a particular instance (here: descriptive premise such as a description of particular facts). For example, a practical ethical judgment saying 'there should be socially funded health care providing basic health care to all citizens' brings together normative assumptions such as 'citizens have a right to health care' or 'ensuring a health status in citizens is morally good', and particular empirical assumptions such as 'there are financial capacities to provide health care' or 'socially funded health care will improve health status (not make it worse)' and so on. Of course, the more complex and concrete a judgment is, the more different layers of assumptions can be identified. But this is not the major point here: what counts here is the fact that only the combination of the (sometimes hidden) moral and empirical joint assumptions together form a practical ethical judgment, and this is what distinguishes applied ethics from ethical theory.

6 The term 'affected person' – as I will argue – must be distinguished from the rather narrow meaning of the 'affective turn' in sociology, which mainly addresses emotions in social relations (Clough and Halley 2007) but shares the basic idea of the importance of personal experience and how this state is based on a mixture of cognitive, emotional, and moral aspects.

7 I have argued in detail elsewhere for a particular integration of social sciences and bioethics as a way of overcoming the expertocratism and 'arm-chair' philosophy that characterizes academic discussions. Our proposal includes participatory elements in public debates on bioethics (Schicktanz 2009; Schicktanz et al. 2012).

8 The concept of 'being affected' shares with feminist standpoint theory the idea of a potential for epistemic advantage; it is not per se advantageous, as Intemann rightly says, but it 'can be … understood as the claim that epistemic communities that include members of marginalized groups will have epistemic advantages, or more rigorous critical consciousness, than communities that do not (at least in some contexts)' (Intemann 2010: 787). However, this must be distinguished from the feminist epistemic idea of giving just voice to those oppressed (see ibid.: 788), because the concept of 'being affected' is less dependent on the social assessment of who now counts as a marginalized group but of course also needs a particular contextual justification relating to who is 'affected' under which conditions.

9 This principle corresponds to Hannah Arendt's 'enlarged thought' and Seyla Benhabib's interpretation of the liberal, deliberative principle of impartiality toward all experiences. Benhabib, convincingly, criticizes the idea of an objective, 'universal' position of impartiality and replaces it by a reflection based on more contextualized narratives (cited in Young 1997; see for further discussion ibid.: 38ff.).

10 The participatory alternative, namely to increasingly include lay people and patients directly in ethical-political debates (among others: Joss 1999), has however been received skeptically by many experts. Approaches arguing for a structural heterogeneity with regard to science and politics try to mediate between the two antagonistic positions, the expertocracy on the one hand and direct democracy on the other (Brown 2009; Schicktanz 2011). These models advocate an 'opening up' instead of a 'closing down' of deliberation and public debate (Stirling 2008). However, they do not claim the exclusivity of particular approaches.

11 This concept, as Fricker argues, can be reconciled with moral-cognitivist approaches in ethics if one recognizes that, in the perception of a moral problem, emotions (often termed moral intuitions) and cognition do not exclude but supplement each other. It presupposes that we are able to communicate them in language and interactions. In the case of those who cannot speak on behalf of themselves, e.g. young children or severely cognitively impaired patients, the construction of advocacy can bridge this condition, but it is of course a challenge with regard to authenticity and representativity.

12 This requires the pre-assumption of the existence of embodied agents, not only of non-individual, structural power.

13 Whether it is possible, practically and theoretically, to eliminate all social categories of identity as a consequence can be doubted. However, this reservation does not contradict attempts to overcome existing limitations.

14 Overseeing such unknown risks can be ethically problematic and has therefore led to the introduction of the 'precautionary principle'. However, this principle is criticized for its hyper-alarming and reactionary tendency in ethical judgment.

15 Social science studies are an important way of including these voices, but they cannot replace political inclusion. Such studies can, however, contribute greatly to the way we identify bias, stereotypes, and social and epistemic injustice in public and private life.

References

Archard, David (2011) Why moral philosophers are not and should not be moral experts, *Bioethics*, 25(3), 119–127.

Baier, Kurt (1958) *The Moral Point of View*, Ithaca, NY: Cornell University Press.

Beard, Renée L. (2004) Advocating voice: organisational, historical and social milieux of the Alzheimer's disease movement, *Sociology of Health & Illness*, 26(6), 797–819.

Blume, Stuart (2010) *The Artificial Ear: Cochlear Implants and the Culture of Deafness*, New Brunswick, NJ: Rutgers University Press.

Brown, Mark (2009). *Science in Democracy: Expertise, Institutions, and Representation*, Cambridge, MA: MIT Press.

Brown, Phil; Morello-Frosch, Rachel and Zavestoski, Stephen (2012) *Contested Illnesses: Citizens, Science, and Health Social Movements*, Berkeley, CA: University of California Press.

Cantley, Caroline and Bowes, Alison (2004) Dementia and social inclusion: the way forward, in A. Innes, C. Archibald and C. Murphy (eds) *Dementia and Social Inclusion: Marginalised Groups and Marginalised Areas of Dementia Research, Care and Practice*, London and Philadelphia: Jessica Kingsley, 255–271.

Chandler, Susan Meyers (1990) *Competing Realities: The Contested Terrain of Mental Health Advocacy*, New York: Praeger.

Charlton, James (2000) *Nothing About Us Without Us: Disability Oppression and Empowerment*, Berkeley, CA, Los Angeles, CA, and London: University of California Press.

Clough, Patricia Ticineto and Halley, Jean (eds) (2007) *The Affective Turn: Theorizing the Social*, Durham, NC: Duke University Press.

Council of Europe (1997) *Convention on Human Rights and Biomedicine*, Oviedo, Spain: European Union.

Dodds, Susan and Thomson, Colin (2006) Bioethics and democracy: competing roles of national bioethics organisations, *Bioethics*, 20(6), 326–338.

Epstein, Steven (1995) The construction of lay expertise: AIDS activism and the forging of credibility in the reform of clinical trials, *Science, Technology, & Human Values*, 20(4), 408–437.

Epstein, Steven (1996) *Impure Science: AIDS, Activism, and the Politics of Knowledge*, Berkeley, CA: University of California Press.

Epstein, Steven (2007) *Inclusion: The Politics of Difference in Medical Research*, Chicago, IL: Chicago University Press.

Felt, Ulrike (2003) Scientific Citizenship: Schlaglichter einer Diskussion, *Gegenworte*, 11, 16–20.

Feyerabend, Paul (1989) *Irrwege der Vernunft*, Frankfurt a.M.: Suhrkamp.

Fricker, Miranda (2009) *Epistemic Injustice: Power and the Ethics of Knowing*, Oxford: Oxford University Press.

Greenwald, Anthony and Banaji, Mahzarin (1995) Implicit social cognition: attitudes, self-esteem, and stereotypes, *Psychological Review*, 102(1), 4–27.

Gutmann, Amy and Thompson, Dennis (1997) Deliberating about bioethics, *Hastings Center Report*, 27(3), 38–41.

Habermas, Jürgen (1996) *Die Einbeziehung des Anderen*, Frankfurt a.M.: Suhrkamp.

Haraway, Donna (1988) Situated knowledge: the science question in feminism and the privilege of partial perspective, *Feminist Studies*, 14(3), 575–599.

Harding, Sandra (1987) *The Science Question in Feminism*, Ithaca, NY: Cornell University Press.

Innes, Anthea; Archibald, Carole and Murphy, Charlie (eds) (2004) *Dementia and Social Inclusion: Marginalised Groups and Marginalised Areas of Dementia Research, Care and Practice*, London and Philadelphia: Jessica Kingsley.

Intemann, Kristin (2010) 25 years of feminist empiricism and standpoint theory: where are we now? *Hypatia*, 25(4), 778–796.

Joss, Simon (1999) Public participation in science and technology policy- and decision-making: ephemeral phenomenon or lasting change? *Science and Public Policy*, 26(5), 290–293.

Leidinger, Friedrich (1999) 'Überzeugende Alternative beflügeln den Widerstand' Forschung für Menschen, an Menschen und mit Menschen mit Demenzerkrankungen, in U. Bach and A. de Kleine (eds) *Auf dem Weg in die totale Medizin? Eine Handreichung zur 'Bioethik'*, Debatte, Neukirchen-Vluyn: Neukirchner Verlag, 70–75.

Lübbe, Weyma (2002) Epistemische Pflichten in der 'Wissensgesellschaft', in C. Engel, J. Halfmann and M. Schulte (eds) *Wissen – Nichtwissen – Unsicheres Wissen*, Baden-Baden: Nomos Verlag, 146–160.

McColgan, Gillian (2004) Images, constructs, theory and method: including the narrative of dementia, in A. Innes, C. Archibald and C. Murphy (eds) *Dementia and Social Inclusion. Marginalised Groups and Marginalised Areas of Dementia Research, Care and Practice*, London and Philadelphia, PA: Jessica Kingsley, 169–183.

National Bioethics Advisory Commission (1998) *Research Involving Persons with Mental Disorders that may Affect Decisionmaking Capacity*, Washington, DC: National Bioethics Advisory Commission.

Nowotny, Helga; Scott, Peter and Gibbons, Michael (2001) *Re-Thinking Science: Knowledge and the Public in an Age of Uncertainty*, Cambridge: Polity Press.

Paul, Diane (2008) Patient advocacy in newborn screening: continuities and discontinuities, *American Journal of Medical Genetics*, 148C(1), 8–14.

Popper, Karl (2005) *Logik der Forschung*, 11th edition, Tübingen: Mohr Siebeck.

Rammstedt, Otthein (1981) Betroffenheit – was heißt das?, *Politische Vierteljahreszeitschrift*, 22 (Special Issue 12), 452–463.

Raz, Aviad; Jordan, Isabella and Schicktanz, Silke (2012) Exploring the positions of German and Israeli patient organizations in the bioethical context of end-of-life policies, *Health Care Analysis*, 22(2), 143–159.

Rippe, Klaus-Peter (2000) Ethikkommissionen in der deliberativen Demokratie, in M. Kettner (ed.) *Angewandte Ethik als Politikum*, Frankfurt a.M.: Suhrkamp, 140–164.

Schicktanz, Silke (2009) Zum Stellenwert von Betroffenheit, Öffentlichkeit und Deliberation im *empirical turn* der Medizinethik, *Ethik in der Medizin*, 21(3), 223–234.

—— (2012) Epistemische Gerechtigkeit: Sozialempirie und Perspektivenpluralismus in der Angewandten Ethik, *Deutsche Zeitschrift f. Philosophie*, 60(2), 269–284.

Schicktanz, Silke; Schweda, Mark and Wynne, Brian (2012) The ethics of 'public understanding of ethics': why and how bioethics expertise should include public and patients' voices, *Medicine, Health Care and Philosophy*, 15(2), 129–139.

Schicktanz, Silke; Schweda, Mark and Franzen, Martina (2008) 'In a completely different light'? The role of being affected for epistemic perspectives and moral attitudes of patients, relatives and lay people, *Medicine, Health Care and Philosophy*, 11(1), 57–72.

Steinkamp, Norbert L.; Gordijn, Bert and ten Have, Henk A. J. M. (2008) Debating ethical expertise, *Kennedy Institute of Ethics Journal*, 18(2), 173–192.

Stirling, Andrew (2008) 'Opening up' and 'closing down': power, participation, and pluralism in the social appraisal of technology, *Science, Technology, & Human Values*, 33(2), 262–294.

Thoits, Peggy (2011) Resisting the stigma of mental illness, *Social Psychology Quarterly*, 74(1), 6–28.

Tversky, Amos and Kahneman, Daniel (1974) Judgment under uncertainty: heuristics and biases, *Science*, 185, 1124–1131.

Wehmeyer, Michael; Bersani, Hank and Gagne, Ray (2000) Riding the third wave: self-determination and self-advocacy in the 21st Century, *Focus on Autism and Other Developmental Disabilities*, 15(2), 106–115.

Wood, Bruce (2000) *Patient Power? The Politics of Patients' Associations in Britain and America*, Buckingham and Philadelphia, PA: Open University Press.

Young, Iris Marion (1997) *Intersecting Voices: Dilemmas of Gender, Political Philosophy, and Policy*, Princeton, NJ: Princeton University Press.

Conclusion

Effects of and challenges to the public shaping of medical research

Willy Viehöver, Peter Wehling, and Matthias Roche

As the contributions to this volume have illustrated, the ways in which patient associations, local communities, advocacy groups, and health social movements shape medical science differ greatly and therefore can be accounted for with a variety of theoretical concepts and models. In addition, the authors of the chapters have emphasized different facets and aspects of the complex phenomenon of the public shaping of medical research. While some have focused on the many opportunities and successes of science-related patient activism, others have drawn our attention to problems, perils, and potential backlashes and still others have pointed to emerging challenges and possible future directions of patient and social movement activism. In quite few chapters, all of these aspects are addressed and their interconnections examined. It is therefore not an easy task to summarize (some of) the findings presented and to address the question of what lessons we can learn from the wide range and different types of patient participation in biomedical knowledge production.

In the following, we would like to address some focal points of the ongoing debates which are mirrored in the chapters of this volume. Perhaps a good way to start is by taking a look at Steven Epstein's (2011) criteria for the "success" – taken in its broadest sense – of patient activism and health social movements. As Epstein points out, the activities of patient organizations and health social movements cannot be reduced solely to aspects of *resource mobilization* and *identity politics*. He argues that the spectrum of assessment criteria should be expanded to take into account intended and non-intended effects and subsequent socio-cultural impacts, without limiting the analysis to determining whether or not activists "succeeded" in achieving or "failed" to achieve the goals they set for themselves (Epstein 2011: 258–263). At the same time, the requirements and opportunities for effective collective action within the field of biomedical research and corresponding science and research policies remain an important area of study. The *capacities* of patients and activists to actually break the "barriers of expertise" cannot be taken as a given (see for example Parthasarathy 2010). In addition, it is important to note that health activism, as practiced by patient organizations and health social movements, cannot be reduced to their relationships to the scientific or the political field (in the stricter sense). Rather, health activism takes place in a multi-institutional field (Armstrong and Bernstein 2008) or, as we prefer to say, in a *polycentric arena of discourse* and *decision making* (Wehling and Viehöver 2012, 2013), within which a variety of – often conflicting – actors raise their voices or mobilize their (embodied) knowledge resources and expertise, as a number of our contributors have highlighted.

Shifting opportunities for mobilizing science

A first observation concerning the "success" of patient activism (which we regard, however, as requiring more research and systematic exploration) relates to the *requirements for mobilization* that must be met by patient-based activism, as well as the meaning of the *opportunity structures* (Tarrow 2011: 157–180) which promote or prevent socio-cultural and institutional impact on science and science policy. Among the most important factors are problems related to mobilizing and utilizing resources, establishing (inter-)organizational structures (such as umbrella organizations) (see Nourissier et al. in Chapter 3), conceiving of framing strategies, and the perceived and actual resonance of these strategies in institutions and the media. Beyond that, however, experiences in the field of rare diseases show that although fundraising is indeed important, this also applies to building organizational capacities and mobilizing knowledge resources. Lori Baralt reminds us in Chapter 1 that the constitution of environmental breast cancer movements was ultimately made possible by networking different social movements and organizations (e.g., the women's rights movement, health movement activists, and environmentalists), that is, by connecting different cultures of knowledge (see also Hess' study on complementary and alternative medicine (CAM) approaches to cancer treatment). However, Mercedes C. Lyson and Stephen Zavestoski have shown in Chapter 5 that problematic, paternalistic effects can also emerge when existing social movements adopt (putative) health issues such as obesity and use them in order to put forward their own, particular agendas. In addition, in Chapter 6, Peter Conrad and Catherine Tan point to the fact that the new (social) media have completely changed opportunities for mobilization. In showing how the internet has become a factor with a persistent capacity to structure and restructure patient activism, they demonstrate that this has been a decisive development in opening up possibilities for mobilizing patient activists and constructing collective illness identities (Barker 2002). The new media not only offer new opportunities on local or national levels but also enable the constitution and mobilization of patient activism across national boundaries, which is particularly important in those cases where only a small number of affected people live in a given country. A possible flipside might be that transnational communication via the internet also seems to foster the exchange and reinforcement of idiosyncratic and esoteric views on the etiology or therapy of illnesses.

Furthermore, the case of environmental breast cancer activism (Baralt in Chapter 1 and Batt in Chapter 7) shows that the effects and effectiveness of patient engagement is highly dependent on local conditions, media resonance, cultural contexts and, not least, adequate political preconditions of patient activism. However, considering Epstein's warning, one should also note that a (partial) failure can also provide useful suggestions for other health movement activists (in the sense of "anti-models"). For example, Sharon Batt uses the case of Canadian breast cancer movements to show that changes in government subsidization structures and strategies not only have economic ramifi cations but also, and more importantly, lead to a sustained influence of the pharmaceutical industry on the framing of breast cancer activism. She outlines some of the pitfalls and difficulties activists may encounter, and thus shows how they may be able to avoid such problems in future.

The diversity of patient activism

What the different contributions to this volume clearly show is that current patient activism has actually crossed the boundaries of science and science policy, sometimes leading to conflicts, and in other instances has forged new citizen science alliances or patient-based epistemic communities (see Akrich et al., Baralt, Batt, Hess and Reimann in this volume). Health activists substantially challenge science/society boundaries by changing traditional self-conceptions and self-descriptions of patient organizations, becoming *experts of experience* or *evidence-based activists* (Akrich et al. in Chapter 4). These patient activists are no longer viewed as passive objects of research, or viewed as patients at all. Rather, they become (self-)empowering active *subjects* and co-producers of health (care)-related (bio-)medical knowledge. Moreover, patient activism has fundamentally changed the interrelations of society with science and technology; it has become an important counterbalancing power to economic stakeholders and political decision makers. Health movements and patient associations mobilizing science (McCormick 2007, 2009a) and questioning established institutional routines and often *dominant epidemiological paradigms* (Brown 2007) are a rather new type of patient activism, one that is widening the scope of more traditional constituency-based self-help activism campaigning for better health access or public recognition. If the social contours of the public shaping and participatory governance of biomedical research are currently changing, this immediately affects the roles, quality, effi cacy, and legitimacy of patient activism (see Bucchi in Chapter 11, Wehling and Viehöver in Chapter 12, and Schicktanz in Chapter 13).

What we can conclude from these contributions is that the activities involved in mobilizing science are limited neither to agenda building and agenda setting processes nor to the formation of new biosocial identities (see Lemke, Lyson and Zavestoski, and Conrad and Tan in this volume).

Patient activism in biomedical research has itself become diversified. Patient activists and health social movements are not only active in research politics and related policy making processes, but also establish important organizational resources as well as different forms of knowledge resources (see Nourissier et al. and Reimann in this volume). Beyond the aspect of collecting and distributing knowledge, they are also actively involved in processes of knowledge production, e.g., pointing out areas of undone science (see Hess, Chapter 8, and Hess 2009, 2011). Furthermore, they are key providers of neglected forms of experiential knowledge (Akrich et al. in Chapter 4; see also Callon and Rabeharisoa 2003), forging *citizen-science alliances* (Brown 2007), reframing disease-related causal stories (Conrad and Tan in Chapter 6), carrying out independent research and taking on urgent ethical, moral and legal questions (see Baralt, Batt, Conrad and Tan; Lyson and Zavestoski and Schicktanz in this volume). Others in turn are initiating research (e.g., by fundraising), but are rarely themselves doing or interpreting science, as was the case with early breast cancer activism in the US, for instance.

This shows that there are different forms and degrees to which civil society actors contribute to producing, shaping, contesting and using (bio-)medical knowledge; this brings us to another important point in health activism: the varieties of (patient) knowledge, which we will examine in the next section. Given the diversity of patients' engagement in biomedical research and research policy, it is important to keep in mind that there is some danger that public involvement in science will tend to become a latent (or even manifest) normative model for what it means to be an "active patient". Therefore, one lesson that could be extrapolated from the findings presented in this volume is that there are different kinds of active patients, as Janine Barbot's (2006) case study on AIDS activism has pointed out, and not all activists address science in the first place. Barbot distinguishes four types of active patients: the patient as *manager of their illness*, the *empowered patient*, the *science-wise activist*, and the *experimenter*. The last two groups appear to be well attuned to scientific knowledge and practices or are even involved in the processes of doing science and interpreting scientific data – and in doing so they may sometimes run the risk of adopting a "technoscientific illness identity" (Sulik 2009). The first two types, by contrast, focus on the experience of illness, on health care and self-help, and/or construct new and independent collective illness identities. In this sense they may create new forms of solidarity among and between patients and their carers, but they also represent a counterbalance to medical, economic, and political institutions that exclude certain types of sufferers, neglect their interests, or prevent equal access to the health care system. Although our focus in this volume has been on the public shaping of science, we think patient activists, as well as those in social science who observe them, should not consider public involvement in science as a "magic bullet" which leads to automatic success for patient advocacy or even as a superior form of patient activism (see also Stockdale and Terry 2002).

Varieties of knowledge and knowledge-based patient activism

Since patient activism has crossed the boundaries of science, as the different pieces presented in this volume underscore, patient advocacy and health social movements' engagement provide established biomedical research with a variety of knowledge forms. Thus, the involvement of patients and concerned groups has not only accentuated and increased the moral authority of patients (e.g., in terms of self-help and advocacy groups) in recent decades but also transformed and diversified the role of patients' knowledge. The distinction between *lay experts* and *experiential experts* – as discussed in the introduction as well as in many individual chapters – is an initial point of reference, but is still too imprecise in that it, first, suggests a clear boundary between patients' experience and scientific knowledge and, second, does not suffi ciently account for the variations and different roles of patient knowledge. To understand "patient knowledge" as a hybrid and "messy" form of knowledge, as recently suggested by Jeannette Pols (2014), is a step in the right direction but still remains too general and does not embrace the varying constellations and entanglements of patient and scientific knowledge. In the following we would therefore like to propose a more detailed, yet still tentative typology of patients' knowledge and expertise.

Embodied experiential knowledge

A first form of patient knowledge can be categorized as *embodied experiential knowledge* with regard to the specific bodily illness experience patients feel, express, and possibly share with other sufferers. For example, the activism of the Canadian women's health movement and breast cancer activism, as Batt shows in her paper, was able to contest and demystify much of the existing medical and societal canon about women's bodies. On the one hand, by expressing and mobilizing embodied experiential knowledge, "lay" women were able to regain the right to possess valuable self-knowledge about their own bodily condition. One the other hand, as a result of this new-found ability to mobilize embodied experiential knowledge, breast cancer activists have been able to challenge dominant knowledge frames, thereby urging the research community to re-examine basic assumptions about women's biology, e.g., by reclaiming the power of definition on normal states like pregnancy and menopause. Likewise, some groups of autism and obesity "patients" refer to their bodily experience when they claim that their conditions fall into the normal range of human diversity and should not be addressed as diseases or disorders. In any event, as these and other examples highlight, even this form of patient knowledge, although ultimately based on "first-hand" individual bodily experience, is far from being purely self-sufficient and idiosyncratic but instead is articulated and expressed in more or less conscious interaction (and sometimes confrontation) with existing medical knowledge.

Patient driven epistemic communities, citizen science alliances and the co-production of knowledge

There is, however, another type of patient knowledge which is of major importance to the current forms of public shaping of science. This kind of knowledge has to be seen as a body of collective knowledge which cannot be taken for granted or simply be run through processes of awareness or recognition, as in the case of embodied knowledge. Nor is it a strategic knowledge which is appropriated by patient activists in order to mobilize organizational or individual capacities. What is particular to this kind of knowledge, as Madeleine Akrich and her colleagues (see also Rabeharisoa and O'Donovan 2013; Rabeharisoa et al. 2014) underline, is that rather than taking knowledge as a mere resource which patient advocates and organizations rely on for advocating or defending their causes, it needs to be viewed as "something" to be (co-)produced and discussed within processes of "mobilizing science" (McCormick 2009a, 2009b) and building "citizen-science alliances" (Brown 2007). This very process of knowledge production has various characteristics and effects. It (a) reconfigures the epistemic networks patient activists are a part of, (b) combines patient experience with scientific (or "proto-scientific") methods of inquiry (lay mapping, research in the wild) and transforms the modalities of research (research designs or paradigm shifts), sometimes leading to an institutionalization of these forms of co-production, and (c) results in a new politics of knowledge, based on new evidence for grounding health policies in the different condition areas in which patient associations and organizations are active. Leaving aside all conceptual differences, we think that we can find similar evidence for co-produced and reflexive knowledge in the cases examined by Akrich et al., as well as the cases of the environmental breast cancer movement and the CAM approaches to cancer therapy (see Baralt and Hess in this volume). This kind of knowledge must be gathered, compiled, produced or co-produced by patient activists. Frequently, this works by self-organized research (such as lay mapping), self-projected research designs, or forging partnerships. The formation and mobilization of the processes of knowledge co-production are often, though not always, the result of a conflicted process, which might encompass different levels and degrees. Patient activism efforts first uncover what David J. Hess has termed "undone science". According to Hess, one of the focal points of health social movements is to identify neglected fields of knowledge production, propose funding for those areas of undone science, or even contribute to the formulation of related research designs. A second central factor in processes of knowledge co-production is the linking of different strands of knowledge. Baralt (in Chapter 1) points to the fact that by networking activities between women's health movements and environmental organizations, the environmental breast cancer movement has been able to merge different knowledge resources and thereby formulate new causal stories as well as a *popular epidemiology*. Lyson and Zavestoski (in Chapter 5) point to a third important step, namely how co-produced knowledge is translated into actions as in the complete streets movement. Whereas Baralt, Hess, Lyson and Zavestoski as well as Conrad and Tan point to partially conflicted processes of knowledge co-production, Akrich and coauthors, like Christel Nourissier and her colleagues and Andreas Reimann, show that the production of patient-centered knowledge can just as easily result from more collaborative partnership models. In these models, groups are able to problematize their divergent illness conditions and have formed affiliated networks of expertise. As Akrich et al. have shown in their research on evidence-based activism, the continuous efforts of experts of experience in discussion with given biomedical knowledge formulates new research issues and might even lead to a radical redefinition of diseases or the emergence of new nosographic categories.

Organizational knowledge

In recent decades, health activism and patient advocacy have generated, mobilized, and disseminated a third type of knowledge. This has to do with the fact that in order to become effective, patient activism and health social movements undergo processes of institutionalization and even professionalization, as is best demonstrated in Reimann's contribution on how to initiate and fund medical research on Cystic Fibrosis. The studies in this volume by Reimann and Nourissier et al., but also Baralt's case study of environmental breast cancer activism, all show that patient organizations are capable of shaping and institutionalizing a type of knowledge that is difficult to fit into the categories of *lay* and *experiential knowledge*. It is instead a form of organizational and strategic knowledge that does not necessarily compete with scientific knowledge, but primarily serves the purpose of mobilizing and stabilizing the resources and capacities of patient activism. Accordingly, building affiliation capacities becomes an important factor of empowerment. In this sense, it is a valuable form of organizational, technical, and strategic knowledge which is intended to enable patient activists to become lay experts or experts of experience, but also to be able to interact with researchers on an equal footing as well as to translate patients' experiences into research questions and priorities. One way this may be achieved is by using new communication technologies (e.g., Nourissier et al. in Chapter 3). Moreover, this type of knowledge relates to organizational fundraising and networking strategies, but also to problems of (cognitive and institutional) capacity building. In this sense national or transnational umbrella organizations have been helpful in organizing, institutionalizing and supplying (e.g., in terms of workshops and seminars) knowledge in order to deal with urgent problems of patient activism.

Patient knowledge as a countervailing power in public discourse

There is a fairly obvious but nonetheless important point that should not be overlooked: knowledge is always inevitably linked to power.

For good reasons, Phil Brown (2007) places a major focus of his studies on whether and under what circumstances patient organizations and health advocates are able to challenge and question the respective dominant epidemiological paradigm. In these cases, patient knowledge directly opposes biomedical knowledge claims and aims to subvert established definitions of disease or disorder. Historically, this has happened, more or less successfully, with (male) homosexuality (Conrad 2007). This is also true for many mental disorders, as well as disabilities whose established medical definitions have been challenged by the emerging disability movement. In these cases, patient knowledge and activism do not primarily aim at initiating or contributing to alternative or more comprehensive medical research. Instead, activists may claim that their condition or identity should be demedicalized, that is to say it must not be understood as an object of medical research (or scientific research at all).[1] Or instead, they may advocate for quite different types of research; for example, this can include social science research intended to protect affected people against discrimination (as is demanded by the "neurodiversity" wing of the autism advocacy groups), or research on urban planning and transport aimed at removing barriers which prevent disabled people from fully participating in public life. Thus, attempts at demedicalization need not necessarily be linked with a radically anti-scientific attitude but can also result in alliances with non-mainstream medical researchers or scientists from fields other than medicine.

In these instances, patients' knowledge or knowledge claims do not form part of a process of scientific knowledge production but rather are statements or interventions in public and political debates in society at large about how to frame and understand health and illness, normality and aberrance. Unsurprisingly, these interventions made by patients often encounter attempts at re-establishing biomedical illness narratives and re-integrating alternative views into technoscientific or industry-driven research programs (see Chapters 7, 9 and 10 by Batt, Langstrup and Lemke, respectively). In this respect, Silke Schicktanz rightly warns against reducing patient knowledge in a cognitivist manner to factual knowledge about illness and disease; as she emphasizes, we should instead acknowledge that patients, activists and advocates also command normative knowledge and that their state of "being affected" (by an illness as well as by social discrimination and marginalization) is not only epistemically but also morally and ethically relevant. This holds true, for instance, when it comes to debates or decision making on issues such as pre-implantation or prenatal genetic testing or the inclusion of impaired patients into medical research. However, as Peter Wehling and Willy Viehöver emphasize in Chapter 12, patient and advocacy activists must be particularly careful to reflect on and become aware of the "situatedness" of their knowledge (Haraway 1988), both factual and normative, in order to avoid imprudently and illegitimately speaking or acting on behalf of other patients.

Changing cultures of patient activism

Obviously the contributions to this volume also offer important pointers toward the wider social and cultural effects of health activism, a topic recently raised by Epstein (2011: 263). Without pretending to give anything close to a full account here, we can at least distinguish four socio-cultural impacts resulting from patient activism. The first effect could be understood as a reconfiguration of the "passive" biomedical research "object" to an actively participating subject; a second meso-level vein of cultural effects results in a transformation of biomedical knowledge cultures. Third, biomedical knowledge and related patient activism flow into new illness identities and biosocialities. Last but not least, the emergence of a new culture of participation must be acknowledged as a kind of macro-effect of the public shaping of science. We will briefly discuss these points in the following.

A new image of the patient

First and foremost, the various chapters show how patient activism successfully challenges a scientific and medical culture that views patients predominantly as passive objects of research, treatment and education, as has been the background assumption of the so-called "deficit model" of science-society relations (see Bucchi in Chapter 11). Most scholars clearly indicate that, contrary to such paternalistic models, patient activists restore, empower, and publicly reshape the idea of *active* patients as knowledgeable subjects or even powerful partners and they examine different movement cultures of participating in knowledge production.

Transformations of biomedical knowledge cultures and research practices

Patient activism has had even more far-reaching meso-level effects on standard scientific cultures of knowledge production and related policies. Processes of transformation take place in different arenas, however, and at different social as well as institutional levels. Also, they vary in societal range and impact. This is illustrated by (partly) successful attempts of local environmental breast cancer movements to introduce alternatives to dominant scientific approaches, methods, and standards of proof, thereby challenging and possibly even transforming the seemingly well-founded background assumptions and unquestioned epistemic routines of scientific cultures of knowledge production, as discussed by Baralt and Batt respectively.

Beyond that, as shown by most of the case studies, patient organizations contribute as experts of experience in terms of their specific illness experience (see for example Reimann, and Akrich et al. in Chapters 2 and 4, and also Epstein 1995, 2008), in order to provide patients, doctors, health professionals, and research networks with new, competing or additional information. Similarly, the suggestions put forward by Reimann and Nourissier et al., as well as Akrich et al., regarding the field of rare disease research can be understood as strategies for transforming established research cultures and their realignment with the needs and desires of those affected and their advocates.

David J. Hess' study in Chapter 8 on the case of advocacy for complementary and alternative medicine (CAM) approaches to cancer is a good example not only of how counterpublics mobilize in opposition to pharmaceutical industries, but also of how these can effect changes in prevailing approaches to cancer research, even though the articulation of an alternative public interest is hardly innocent of sectional interests. In addition, patient organizations become actively involved as interest-based and politicized stakeholders in health care and research policy and also play a role in governing biomedical research itself (e.g., through data collection and interpretation) (see Baralt in Chapter 1). Furthermore, when supported on a clearly defined and sufficiently extensive knowledge base, patient advocacy, patient organizations, and health social movements are able to directly shape cultures of funding and financing strategies, as well as research programs and design, sometimes by way of forging multiple alliances and even new "communities of practice" between researchers, pharmacological industry, health professionals and policy makers (see for example Reimann, and Nourissier et al. in Chapters 2 and 3; Callon et al. 2009; Akrich 2010; Akrich et al. 2008; Rabeharisoa et al. 2014), or even challenge dominant epidemiological paradigms and related knowledge cultures (Zavestoski et al. 2004; Brown 2007; Brown et al. 2012). Both cooperative interactions (partnership model) and competitive or even conflicted interrelations (contested illness model; Brown et al. 2012) with science and technology may transform the pre-existing institutionalized health regimes, knowledge cultures and related practices (Klawiter 2008).

Emerging biosocialities and illness identities

Social and cultural effects also encompass the creation of new illness identities (Barker 2002; Callon and Rabeharisoa 2003; Rabeharisoa 2003) and biosocialities (Rabinow 1996, 2008; Gibbon and Novas 2008). In this regard, ongoing processes of biomedicalization and "technoscientization" (Clarke et al. 2010) such as the expansion of genetic testing appear to have a substantial influence on how social groups or networks form and reform within society. While these new identities and socialities do of course bring about new opportunities and directions for collective action (see Callon and Rabeharisoa 2008), they may also have some questionable aspects, as Henriette Langstrup and Thomas Lemke illustrate in Chapters 9 and 10, such as the engagement of patient associations with long-term technoscientific projects (or "hypes") whose success is anything but guaranteed, or the assumption of a stable and unequivocal biology (see also Wehling 2011a, 2011b). However, as both these authors as well as other contributors to this volume underline, patients' identities are not determined by biomedicine but develop in complex interactions with medical knowledge and sometimes even in outright opposition to it. Examples of this include the "social model" of disability and the self-understanding of the deaf community as a specific culture of its own which is based on the use of sign language (Blume 2010).

Changing cultures of participation

The socio-cultural effects of the public shaping of science can also be understood in a much more extensive sense by conceiving of them as part of a constantly changing, differentiating, and dynamic culture of civil society participation in science and politics. One might even understand this as a macro- or meta-change in regard to concepts, forms and procedures of public involvement in biomedical science. The chapters presenting case studies offer implicit evidence of this, whereas the contributions by Massimiano Bucchi, Wehling and Viehöver, and by Schicktanz in the third section of this volume give an explicit analysis of participation cultures and problems involved in legitimizing them.

One can trace the ongoing trends and transformations of science/society interactions back to long-standing controversies about *participatory democracy* (Pateman 1970) that have touched science and technology issues since the 1970s. These debates have now developed into a rethinking of the very meaning of public/science interaction, as the institutionalization of new participatory exercises or dialogue formats in different arenas on behalf of governments or (national) parliaments shows (e.g., roundtables, consensus conferences, stakeholder-dialogues). Since at least the 1990s there has been criticism of the core assumptions of the so-called deficit model of science-public interactions, which is that expert knowledge is superior to the knowledge of patients and the latter are ignorant of and therefore inimical to science. As patient activists became experts on their own (Epstein 1995), the seemingly clear-cut division between lay and expert knowledge has increasingly been called into question. In this respect one could speak of a new culture of participation emerging since the 1990s. Yet, as Bucchi and other contributors remind the reader, one ought also to consider that the emerging culture of participation is not necessarily to be grasped as a harmonious or consensual culture. Moreover, one should be equally careful not to read the emergence of new participatory models in biomedical research in a strict evolutionary perspective leading from paternalistic deficit models (science as a mode of educating the public) to sponsored dialogue or invited forms of participation (round tables etc.) and subsequently to spontaneous or uninvited modes of participation (e.g., citizen-science alliances, partnership models).

With regard to this question, Bucchi proposes an interpretative framework for science and public participation which discerns *intensity of cooperation* among different actors in knowledge production processes on the one hand, and *spontaneous (uninvited)* and *invited forms* of participation on the other (see also Wehling 2012). But whether and when (spontaneous or invited) forms of participation emerge and succeed or whether traditional deficit models appear to picture specific science/society interrelations more appropriately depends heavily on the respective contexts. These include, for example, the structure of (social, cultural, economic, as well as political) opportunities, degrees of scientific controversy, the public salience of biomedical issues and related media coverage, the "access points" (Callon et al. 2009) provided within research and research policy processes, existing mobilization cultures and their definitions of the situation, and also the (mobilization) capacities of patient activists, their allies and supporters.

Problems, perils, and emerging challenges

In the previous sections of this conclusion, we have focused primarily on successes and positive effects of public involvement in knowledge production in biomedical research. Although the productive contributions towards the democratization of science that have been made by patient organizations, advocacy groups, and health social movements are certainly to be held in high regard, there are also a number of problems or obstacles which, we believe, should not be tacitly ignored or casually overlooked. While examining the contributions to this volume, we encountered three central patterns of problems regarding the current landscape of how civil society actors are engaged in the process of shaping biomedical research.

Institutional persistence

In some cases, scientific institutions and their well-rehearsed research practices and routines appear to be much more stable than the civil society protagonists of participatory governance of science (and, also, some social science analysts) had initially hoped. As Baralt points out, although environmental breast cancer activists were successful in mobilizing science and setting the agenda for possible environmental links to breast cancer, and were also effective in urging governmental offi cids to support targeted research, they have been less successful in reversing the burden of proof in regulatory science. Their calls for regulation of putatively carcinogenic chemicals based on the existing, inconclusive evidence have been widely disregarded, and the process of establishing a link between environmental factors and breast cancer still follows conventional research concepts and models. Thus, as Robert Proctor noted almost 20 years ago, we can observe that the process of regulating carcinogens still favors "scientific conservatism", which demands definite proof of harm, over "public health conservatism", which urges for precautionary regulation even in the absence of definite proof (Proctor 1995: 264). Hess, in his contribution, also identifies obstacles to patients' and advocates' engagement by showing that out of 147 studies that were sponsored by the National Center for Complementary and Alternative Medicine between 2001 and 2011, only two were actually clinical studies on CAM cancer therapy. Hess goes on to show that certain findings produced by alternative cancer research were not accepted by mainstream medicine, which led to a substantial loss of trust between CAM research teams and conventional research teams. A certain degree of skepticism is also warranted regarding the presumed change in societal or institutional cultures of participation, as noted by Bucchi as well as Wehling and Viehöver. The general trend towards a pronounced participatory rhetoric described by Bucchi and others is often revealed, under closer inspection, to be mere lip service (see also Wynne 2014). This suggests that the change in keywords in European policy documents, e.g., from "public awareness of science" to "citizen engagement", from "communication" to "dialogue", and from "science and society" to "science in society", as observed by Bucchi, can at best be seen as leading only partway to an effective and sustainable policy change or to real institutional transformations.

Hopes and hypes: ambiguities of biomedical research

It also seems prudent to adopt a careful approach when discussing the hopes invested in the success of biomedical research by patients and by representatives of patient organizations. As much as these hopes may be justified when faced with the severity of many illnesses (Novas 2006): whether rare diseases, Alzheimer's, AIDS, or cancer, the positions held by patient organizations themselves show that after a decade of exaggerated biomedical promises, enthusiasm has been replaced with a more skeptical stance on short-term therapeutic breakthroughs. As Reimann's Chapter 2 illustrates, a substantial percentage of research sponsored by the German Mucoviszidosis Institute never leads to any gain in knowledge about the illness or even to negative findings. As Hess shows in Chapter 8, this case is reminiscent of the expectations that were placed on CAM. Langstrup, in her contribution on the relationships between stem cell research and Danish patient organizations (Chapter 9), shows that at least two important organizations (the Danish Alzheimer's Association and the Multiple Sclerosis Association) have resisted interpellation by biomedicine, not least because they did not want their members to invest their hopes in exorbitant and unrealistic claims. Thus, we are able to observe – across a number of contributions, and covering a variety of illnesses – just how much the rhetoric of future development and institutionally launched promises of breakthroughs in research had become a driving force of current patient activism, without, however, being sufficiently supported by evidence. Reimann's contribution (Chapter 2) shows that patients react to this dilemma by carefully evaluating research proposals and ventures according to how plausible and credible these high expectations of success actually are.

As Batt's Chapter 7 indicates, it was also the promise of fast and direct access to new treatments (and not only financial support) that led several patient groups to seek a problematic proximity to the pharmaceutical industry. However, the understandably high hopes placed in new medications are frequently disappointed, as Batt shows using the example of "high-dose chemo" treatments. Furthermore, the fact that the development of medicines is increasingly embedded in asymmetrical transnational power structures must also be considered, as Lemke notes in his Chapter 10. This is the case, for example, when the testing of medical compounds is outsourced to poorer countries, relatively speaking, such as India and Russia – resulting in the questionable situation which has test participants in these countries carrying the risk of suffering from unforeseen side effects, but usually not profiting from successfully tested drugs because their national health systems are unable to finance these often prohibitively expensive treatments.

Tensions within and among patient associations

Conrad and Tan show in their chapter that new media of communication have allowed actors with very different (scientific and normative) positions to become publicly visible and network with each other across regional boundaries. On the other hand, they also demonstrate that these forms of media and public spaces allow some patient or advocacy groups to gain a kind of public resonance regarding perspectives on illnesses which must appear questionable due to a shortage of evidence or, at the very least, very controversial findings (as noted also by Hess in his contribution on CAM). Conrad and Tan themselves refer, in Chapter 6, to the lack of evidence for alternative causal stories surrounding autism, such as a connection with Mumps, Measles, and Rubella (MMR) vaccines, which is championed by some patient advocates on internet platforms. Additionally, the developments they described are indicative of an erosion of the hitherto valid and established organizational model of patient activism and advocacy, i.e., a single national association for a certain condition. Instead, patients now are able to connect transnationally across borders, especially thanks to the internet, and in the future it is conceivable that different groups and virtual networks with competing interests and goals will arise in this way, as we have seen with autism spectrum disorder. It is plain to see that such developments harbor new opportunities for representing patient interests, especially concerning very rare or highly contested conditions. From another perspective, however, this tendency to virtuality, plurality and competition could also contain risks for patient associations, e.g., by leading to new doubts as to their legitimacy and representativeness or endangering their recognition by national political or scientific actors.

Furthermore, the factor of access or non-access to new media appears to point towards another problem related to the phenomenon of epistemic injustice described by Schicktanz in Chapter 13. On the one hand, access to media and public arenas can offer an alternative forum to actors in civil society whose voices would otherwise be ignored by science and scientific policy. On the other hand, due to differences in available financial resources, organizational capacities, rhetorical skills, political positions, etc., not all civil society actors are afforded the same degree or quality of access to media, politics, and scientifi c forums. This applies, for instance, to the case of missionary medicalization of obesity as discussed by Lyson and Zavestoski in Chapter 5. It appears that the alternative food and complete streets movements have been much more visible and able to make their respective claims than those advocating against the medicalization of obesity such as the Fat Acceptance Movement. An emerging problem, therefore, seems to be whether and how patient advocates legitimize their public and political claims-making activities. Against this background, it is not a coincidence that a number of chapters ask critical questions about the related problems of representation. Schicktanz is fully justified in Chapter 13 in pointing out the ethical implications of epistemic injustices, not only regarding the relationship between "lay people" and scientific "experts" but also between different groups of affected individuals or advocates.

A brief look ahead

Taking into account all the findings presented in this volume, we must acknowledge that a process of participatory governance of medical research – described by Vololona Rabeharisoa and Michel Callon (2002) as a "third way" which might be able to compensate for the one-sidedness and limitations of state- and market-driven research funding – has spread in a variety of ways and has, in some cases, become an indispensable perspective for understanding how patients, advocates, and health movement activists engage with biomedicine. Nevertheless, it is important that, especially in medical contexts, public engagement in science should not tacitly become a normative ideal that supplants or diminishes other forms of commitment, such as self-help groups, which primarily concentrate on care and emotional support for those affected by illness.

Further studies are required in order to clarify whether this third way of research governance "can be transposed to other fields than health, such as the environment, energy, or food security" (ibid.: 64). Furthermore, urgently needed are additional comparative international studies (see Akrich et al. in Chapter 4 and Akrich et al. 2008) focusing on diverging contexts and conditions for mobilization and success in Europe and North America, and also on new patient-based movements and research initiatives in Asia, Africa, and South America. The same applies to the efforts to institutionally transnationalize or even globalize patient-based activism, for which Christel Nourissier, Monica Ensini and Maria Mavris offer some initial suggestions in Chapter 3, referring to the example of EURORDIS, the European umbrella organization of rare disease patient associations. Thus, in our view, there is little doubt that the public shaping of research will continue to be a powerful social phenomenon as well as an important object of social science studies, although its aims, organizational infrastructures, and conditions of (and obstacles to) success are likely to change considerably in the future.

Note

1 It is important to note, however, that biomedicine does not always aim at medicalizing certain conditions in order to expand its definitional domain. Sometimes biomedical explanations argue for demedicalization while sufferers demand medicalization, as for instance in the cases of so-called "electrosensitivity" or multiple chemical sensitivity (MCS).

References

Akrich, Madeleine (2010) From communities of Practice to Epistemic Communities: Health Mobilizations on the Internet, *Sociological Research Online*, 15(2). Available online at: <www.socresonline.org.uk/15/2/10.html> (accessed 8 June 2013).

Akrich, Madeleine; Nunes, João; Paterson, Florence and Rabeharisoa, Vololona (2008) *The Dynamics of Patient Organizations in Europe*, Paris: Presses de l'Ecole des Mines.

Armstrong, Elizabeth and Bernstein, Mary (2008) Culture, Power, and Institutions: A Multi-Institutional Politics Approach to Social Movements, *Sociological Theory*, 26(1), 74–99.

Barbot, Janine (2006) How to Build an "Active" Patient? The Work of AIDS Associations in France, *Social Science & Medicine*, 62(3), 538–551.

Barker, Kristin (2002) Self-Help Literature and the Making of an Illness Identity: The Case of Fibromyalgia Syndrome (FMS), *Social Problems*, 49(3), 279–300.

Blume, Stuart (2010) *The Artificial Ear: Cochlear Implants and the Culture of Deafness*, New Brunswick, NJ: Rutgers University Press.

Brown, Phil (2007) *Toxic Exposures: Contested Illnesses and the Environmental Health Movement*, New York: Columbia University Press.

Brown, Phil; Morello-Frosch, Rachel; Zavestoski, Stephen and the Contested Illnesses Research Group (2012) *Contested Illnesses: Citizens, Science, and Health Social Movements*, Berkeley, CA: University of California Press.

Callon, Michel; Lascoumes, Pierre and Barthe, Yannick (2009) *Acting in an Uncertain World: An Essay on Technical Democracy*, Cambridge, MA and London: MIT Press.

Callon, Michel and Rabeharisoa, Vololona (2003) Research "in the Wild" and the Shaping of New Social Identities, *Technology in Society*, 25(2), 193–204.

—— (2008) The Growing Engagement of Emergent Concerned Groups in Political and Economic Life: Lessons from the French Association of Neuromuscular Disease Patients, *Science, Technology & Human Values*, 33(2), 230–261.

Clarke, Adele; Mamo, Laura; Fosket, Jennifer Ruth; Fishman, Jennifer R. and Shim, Janet K. (eds) (2010) *Biomedicalization: Technoscience, Health, and Illness in the U.S.*, Durham, NC: Duke University Press.

Conrad, Peter (2007) *The Medicalization of Society: On the Transformation of Human Conditions into Treatable Disorders*, Baltimore: Johns Hopkins University Press.

Epstein, Steven (1995) The Construction of Lay Expertise: AIDS Activism and the Forging of Credibility in the Reform of Clinical Trials, *Science, Technology & Human Values*, 20(4), 408–437.

___ (2008) Patient Groups and Health Movements, in E. J. Hackett, O. Amsterdamska, M. Lynch and J. Wajcman (eds): *The Handbook of Science and Technology Studies*, 3rd edition, Cambridge, MA and London: MIT Press, 499–539.

___ (2011) Measuring Success: Scientific, Institutional, and Cultural Effects of Patient Advocacy, in B. Hoffman, N. Tomes, R. Grob and M. Schlesinger (eds) *Patients as Policy Actors*, New Brunswick, NJ, and London: Rutgers University Press, 257–277.

Gibbon, Sahra and Novas, Carlos (eds) (2008) *Biosocialities, Genetics and the Social Sciences: Making Biologies and Identities*, London and New York: Routledge.

Haraway, Donna (1988) Situated Knowledges: The Science Question in Feminism and the Privilege of Partial Perspective, *Feminist Studies*, 14(3), 575–599.

Hess, David J. (2009) The Potentials and Limitations of Civil Society Research: Getting Undone Science Done, *Sociological Inquiry*, 79(3), 306–327.

___ (2011) To Tell The Truth: On Scientific Counterpublics, *Public Understanding of Science*, 20(5), 627–641.

Klawiter, Maren (2008) *The Biopolitics of Breast Cancer: Changing Cultures of Disease and Activism*, Minneapolis, MN: University of Minnesota Press.

McCormick, Sabrina (2007) Democratizing Science Movements: A New Framework for Mobilization and Contestation, *Social Studies of Science*, 37(4), 609–623.

___ (2009a) *Mobilizing Science: Movements, Participation, and the Remaking of Knowledge*, Philadelphia, PA: Temple University Press.

___ (2009b) *No Family History: The Environmental Links to Breast Cancer*, Lanham, MD: Rowman & Littlefield.

Novas, Carlos (2006) The Political Economy of Hope: Patients' Organizations, Science and Biovalue, *Biosocieties*, 1(3), 289–305.

Parthasarathy, Shobita (2010) Breaking the Expertise Barrier: Understanding Activist Strategies in Science and Technology Policy Domains, *Science and Public Policy*, 37(5), 355–367.

Pateman, Carol (1970) *Participation and Democratic Theory*, Cambridge: Cambridge University Press.

Pols, Jeannette (2014) Knowing Patients: Turning Patient Knowledge into Science, *Science, Technology & Human Values*, 39(1), 73–97.

Proctor, Robert N. (1995) *Cancer Wars: How Politics Shapes What We Know and Don't Know About Cancer*, New York: Basic Books.

Rabeharisoa, Vololona (2003) The Struggle Against Neuromuscular Diseases in France and the Emergence of the "Partnership Model" of Patient Organization, *Social Science and Medicine*, 57(11), 2127–2136.

Rabeharisoa, Vololona and Callon, Michel (2002) The Involvement of Patients' Associations in Research, *International Social Science Journal*, 54(3), 57–65.

Rabeharisoa, Vololona and O'Donovan, Órla (2013) *Europe of Patients, Europe for Patients: The Europeanization of Healthcare Policies by European Patients' Organizations*, CSI Working Paper Series, 030, 1–33.

Rabeharisoa, Vololona; Moreira, Tiago and Akrich, Madeleine (2013) Evidence-Based Activism: Patients' users' and activists' groups in knowledge society, *BioSocieties*, 9(2), 111–128.

Rabinow, Paul (1996) Artificiality and Enlightenment: From Sociobiology to Biosociality, in P. Rabinow, *Essays in the Anthropology of Reason*, Princeton, NJ: Princeton University Press, 91–111.

___ (2008) Afterword: Concept Work, in S. Gibbon and C. Novas (eds) *Biosocialities, Genetics and the Social Sciences: Making Biologies and Identities*, London and New York: Routledge, 188–192.

Stockdale, Alan and Terry, Sharon (2002) Advocacy Groups and the New Genetics, in J. S. Alper, C. Ard, A. Asch, J. Beckwith, P. Conrad and L. N. Geller (eds) *The Double-Edged Helix: Social Implications of Genetics in a Diverse Society*, Baltimore, MD: Johns Hopkins University Press, 80–101.

Sulik, Gayle (2009) Managing Biomedical Uncertainty: The Technoscientific Illness Identity, *Sociology of Health and Illness*, 31(7), 1059–1076.

Tarrow, Sidney G. (2011) *Power in Movement: Social Movements and Contentious Politics*, Cambridge: Cambridge University Press.

Wehling, Peter (2011a) Biology, Citizenship and The Government of Biomedicine: Exploring the concept of Biological Citizenship, in U. Bröckling, S. Krasmann and T. Lemke (eds) *Governmentality: Current Issues and Future Challenges*, London: Routledge, 225–246.

___ (2011b) The "Technoscientization" of Medicine and its Limits: Technoscientific Identities, Biosocialities, and Rare Disease Patient Organizations, *Poiesis & Praxis: International Journal of Technology Assessment and Ethics of Science*, 8(2–3), 67–82. Available online at: <http://link.springer.com/content/pdf/10.1007%2Fs10202-011-0100-3.pdf.> (accessed 11 February 2014).

___ (2012) From Invited to Uninvited Participation (and Back?): Rethinking Civil Society Engagement in Technology Assessment and Development, *Poiesis & Praxis: International Journal of Technology Assessment and Ethics of Science*, 9(1–2), 43–60.

Wehling, Peter and Viehöver, Willy (2012) Zivilgesellschaft und Wissenschaft: Ein Spannungsfeld zwischen Konflikt und Kooperation, *Sozialwissenschaften und Berufspraxis (SuB)*, 35(2), 216–232.

___ (2013) "Uneingeladene" Partizipation der Zivilgesellschaft – ein kreatives Element der Governance von Wissenschaft, in E. Grande, D. Jansen, O. Jarren, A. Rip, U. Schimank and P. Weingart (eds) *Neue Governance der Wissenschaft: Reorganisation – externe Anforderungen – Medialisierung*, Bielefeld: Transcript Verlag, 213–234.

Wynne, Brian (2014) Further Disorientation in the Hall of Mirrors, *Public Understanding of Science*, 23(1), 60–70.

Zavestoski, Stephen; Morello-Frosch, Rachel; Brown, Phil; Mayer, Brian; McCormick, Sabrina and Gasior-Altman, Rebecca (2004) Health Social Movements and the Challenge to the Dominant Epidemiological Paradigm, in D. Myers and D. Cress (eds) *Authority in Contention: Research in Social Movements, Conflict and Change*, Oxford: Elsevier JAI, 253–278.

Index

Note: page numbers in italics refer to figures; page numbers in bold refer to tables

For Product Safety Concerns and Information please contact our EU representative GPSR@taylorandfrancis.com
Taylor & Francis Verlag GmbH, Kaufingerstraße 24, 80331 München, Germany

www.ingramcontent.com/pod-product-compliance
Ingram Content Group UK Ltd
Pitfield, Milton Keynes, MK11 3LW, UK
UKHW022022180926
475701UK00005B/991

* 9 7 8 0 3 6 7 3 4 1 4 1 1 *